AF703387

Aging and Aging-Related Diseases: Mechanisms and Interventions

Aging and Aging-Related Diseases: Mechanisms and Interventions

Editor: Oliver Fincher

AMERICAN
MEDICAL PUBLISHERS
www.americanmedicalpublishers.com

AMERICAN
MEDICAL PUBLISHERS
www.americanmedicalpublishers.com

Cataloging-in-Publication Data

Aging and aging-related diseases : mechanisms and interventions / edited by Oliver Fincher.
p. cm.
Includes bibliographical references and index.
ISBN 978-1-63927-579-3
1. Geriatrics. 2. Older people--Diseases. 3. Older people--Health and hygiene.
4. Aging. 5. Gerontology. I. Fincher, Oliver.
RC952 .A35 2023
618.97--dc23

© American Medical Publishers, 2023

American Medical Publishers,
41 Flatbush Avenue,
1st Floor, New York,
NY 11217, USA

ISBN 978-1-63927-579-3 (Hardback)

This book contains information obtained from authentic and highly regarded sources. Copyright for all individual chapters remain with the respective authors as indicated. All chapters are published with permission under the Creative Commons Attribution License or equivalent. A wide variety of references are listed. Permission and sources are indicated; for detailed attributions, please refer to the permissions page and list of contributors. Reasonable efforts have been made to publish reliable data and information, but the authors, editors and publisher cannot assume any responsibility for the validity of all materials or the consequences of their use.

Trademark Notice: Registered trademark of products or corporate names are used only for explanation and identification without intent to infringe.

Contents

Preface

Aging refers to the physiological changes that are endured by an organism, which results in the deterioration of biological functions and the capability to adjust with the metabolic stress. It is a progression, which takes place during the life span of a living organism. Cells and organs, or the whole organism undergoes aging with the passage of time. Diseases related with age are basically difficulties that arise with senescence and they differ from the process of aging. Age related diseases include cancer, cardiovascular disease, cataracts, hypertension, atherosclerosis, osteoporosis, Alzheimer's disease, and type-2 diabetes. The frequency of such diseases tends to increase with age. This book aims to understand the clinical perspectives of aging. Also included herein is a detailed explanation of the various mechanisms and interventions of aging and aging-related diseases. This book will prove to be immensely beneficial to students and researchers in the field of aging and geriatric medicine.

This book is a result of research of several months to collate the most relevant data in the field.

When I was approached with the idea of this book and the proposal to edit it, I was overwhelmed. It gave me an opportunity to reach out to all those who share a common interest with me in this field. I had 3 main parameters for editing this text:

1. Accuracy - The data and information provided in this book should be up-to-date and valuable to the readers.

2. Structure - The data must be presented in a structured format for easy understanding and better grasping of the readers

3. Universal Approach - This book not only targets students but also experts and innovators in the field, thus my aim was to present topics which are of use to all

Thus, it took me a couple of months to finish the editing of this book.

I would like to make a special mention of my publisher who considered me worthy of this opportunity and also supported me throughout the editing process. I would also like to thank the editing team at the back-end who extended their help whenever required.

Editor

1

The Association between Home Healthcare and Burdensome Transitions at the End-of-Life in People with Dementia: A 12-Year Nationwide Population-Based Cohort Study

Ping-Jen Chen [1,2,3,*], Chung-Han Ho [4,5], Jung-Yu Liao [6], Lisanne Smits [1,7], Chao A. Hsiung [6], Sang-Ju Yu [8], Kai-Ping Zhang [9], Irene Petersen [10] and Elizabeth L. Sampson [1,11]

1 Centre for Dementia Palliative Care Research, Marie Curie Palliative Care Research Department, Division of Psychiatry, University College London, London W1T 7NF, UK; lisannesmits94@gmail.com (L.S.); e.sampson@ucl.ac.uk (E.L.S.)
2 Department of Family Medicine and Division of Geriatrics and Gerontology, Kaohsiung Medical University Hospital, Kaohsiung Medical University, Kaohsiung 807, Taiwan
3 School of Medicine, Kaohsiung Medical University, Kaohsiung 807, Taiwan
4 Department of Medical Research, Chi-Mei Medical Center, Tainan 710, Taiwan; ho.c.hank@gmail.com
5 Department of Hospital and Health Care Administration, Chia Nan University of Pharmacy and Science, Tainan 717, Taiwan
6 Institute of Population Health Sciences, National Health Research Institutes, Miaoli 350, Taiwan; jyliao@nhri.edu.tw (J.-Y.L.); hsiung@nhri.edu.tw (C.A.H.)
7 Faculty of Medicine, University of Amsterdam, 1105 AZ Amsterdam, The Netherlands
8 Home Clinic Dulan, Taitung 959, Taiwan; bebe.yu@gmail.com
9 Home Clinic Dulan, Taipei 106, Taiwan; falcony910425@gmail.com
10 UCL Department of Primary Care and Population Sciences, University College London, London NW3 2PF, UK; i.petersen@ucl.ac.uk
11 Barnet Enfield and Haringey Mental Health Trust Liaison Psychiatry Team, North Middlesex University Hospital, London N18 1QX, UK
* Correspondence: ping-jen.chen.18@ucl.ac.uk

Abstract: Background: For people with dementia, burdensome transitions may indicate poorer-quality end-of-life care. Little is known regarding the association between home healthcare (HHC) and these burdensome transitions. We aimed to investigate the impact of HHC on transitions and hospital/intensive care unit (ICU) utilisation nearing the end-of-life for people with dementia at a national level. Methods: A nested case-control analysis was applied in a retrospective cohort study using a nationwide electronic records database. We included people with new dementia diagnoses who died during 2002–2013 in whole population data from the universal healthcare system in Taiwan. Burdensome transitions were defined as multiple hospitalisations in the last 90 days (early transitions, ET) or any hospitalisation or emergency room visit in the last three days of life (late transitions, LT). People with (cases) and without (controls) burdensome transitions were matched on a ratio of 1:2. We performed conditional logistic regression with stratified analyses to estimate the adjusted odds ratio (OR) and 95% confidence interval (CI) of the risks of transitions. Results: Among 150,125 people with new dementia diagnoses, 61,399 died during follow-up, and 31.1% had burdensome transitions (50% were early and 50% late). People with ET had the highest frequency of admissions and longer stays in hospital/ICU during their last year of life, while people with LT had fewer hospital/ICU utilisation than people without end-of-life transitions. Receiving HHC was associated with an increased risk of ET (OR = 1.14, 95 % CI: 1.08–1.21) but a decreased risk of LT (OR = 0.89, 95 % CI 0.83–0.94). In the people receiving HHC, however, those who received longer duration (e.g., OR = 0.50, 95 % CI: 0.42–0.60,

>365 versus ≤30 days) or more frequent HHC or HHC delivered closer to the time of death were associated with a remarkably lower risk of ET. Conclusions: HHC has differential effects on early and late transitions. Characteristics of HHC such as better continuity or interdisciplinary coordination may reduce the risk of transitions at the end-of-life. We need further studies to understand the longitudinal effects of HHC and its synergy with palliative care, as well as the key components of HHC that achieve better end-of-life outcomes.

Keywords: dementia; end-of-life; home healthcare; hospitalisation; national health program; palliative care; patient transfer

---

1. Introduction

1.1. Background/Rationale

Dementia is currently one of the commonest causes of death in Western countries and will be one of the major and increasing global causes of serious health-related suffering [1–3]. People with dementia are at a high risk of experiencing hospitalisation or other care transitions [4], particularly towards the end-of-life [5–7]. Transitions and life-prolonging treatments near the end-of-life may be caused by the fragmentation of care, are burdensome for people with dementia, and may indicate poor-quality end-of-life care [8,9].

Burdensome end-of-life transitions for people with dementia, mainly investigated in the US and Europe [8–10], are defined as "early transitions (ET)" when there are multiple hospitalisations during the last 90 days of life or "late transitions (LT)" when occurring in the last three days of life. Gozalo et al. reported that burdensome transitions for Medicare nursing home residents with cognitive issues were associated with poorer-quality end-of-life care, including stays in intensive care units (ICU) in the last 30 days of life or late referrals to hospice care [9]. Using a linked administrative and clinical database in London, Leniz et al. found people with ET had a higher level of hospital use throughout the last year of life than people with LT [10]. However, there is a lack of population-based data of burdensome end-of-life transitions for people with dementia in Asia.

Previous observational studies have shown that palliative care was associated with fewer referrals to the emergency room (ER) and reduced use of life-sustaining treatments at the end-of-life for people with dementia [11–13]. However, access to palliative care for people with dementia in different countries is still very limited and is often implemented close to the time of death, because the end-of-life trajectory is difficult to predict [11,14,15]. Besides, evidence of the effectiveness of palliative care for people with dementia living outside nursing homes is still poor [16]. Strategies and interventions to reduce avoidable transition and acute healthcare utilisation at the end-of-life for people with dementia living in the community are therefore vital.

Home healthcare (HHC) is increasingly recognised as important in supporting people with dementia living in the community [17]. HHC mostly comprises services that rehabilitate after an illness or injury or help to manage chronic diseases and their complications [18]. The services may include some aspects of social care but primarily focus on medical services provided by healthcare professionals or staff, such as physicians, registered nurses, pharmacists, or qualified therapists. Various programs are included in the category of HHC, such as Medicare skilled home healthcare, home-based primary care, physician house calls, or hospital at home. These vary in terms of acuity, type of care provided, and the degree of physician involvement [18–20].

Previous studies that investigated HHC interventions for similar end-of-life outcomes in people with dementia were mostly in small samples or followed a short period before death [21,22]. Jennings et al. reported a longitudinal nurse practitioner dementia care programme in the Los Angeles community that enrolled 322 people and achieved a more than 90% rate of advance care planning (ACP) in decedents. Programme recipients experienced fewer ICU stays and recurrent hospitalisations, consistent with their preferences for less aggressive care [21]. Mitchell et al. found that people aged 65 years or older with advanced dementia who died within one year of receiving HHC (n = 290) had fewer end-of-life hospitalisations than those that died within one year of admission to nursing homes (n = 2730) [22]. HHC service models in Taiwan are similar to the mix of home-based primary care and skilled home healthcare in the US Medicare system and have been reimbursed by the Taiwan National Health Insurance (NHI) scheme since 1995. The impact of "routine" HHC on end-of-life transitions in people with dementia in a larger-scale study for a longer follow-up has not been well-investigated.

1.2. Objectives

Our population-based cohort study aimed to investigate the patterns and characteristics of HHC utilisation, burdensome transitions, and hospital/ICU use at the end-of-life for people with dementia following from the point of their dementia diagnosis. We examined the association between HHC and burdensome end-of-life transitions and the impact of characteristics of HHC on these transitions at a national level in Taiwan.

Our hypothesis was that more continuous or more interdisciplinary collaboration in HHC may be associated with a lower risk of burdensome transitions in people with dementia at the end-of-life.

2. Materials and Methods

2.1. Setting

The NHI in Taiwan, initiated in 1995, provides single-payer healthcare services and covers 99.9% of Taiwan's legal residents [23]. Almost all healthcare providers have contracts with the NHI, and all kinds of healthcare services are unified, with corresponding fees and reimbursements by the NHI mainly based on a fee-for-service model. By law, every beneficiary pays the NHI premium according to their income. The premiums of those who have no salary (so-called "dependent" group), such as spouses or elderly people, are paid by a family member who has a salary. The contents of healthcare services are the same regardless of the premium paid, and 10 percent of the cost of each healthcare service is co-payed by the beneficiaries unless the beneficiary has a "catastrophic illness certificate" where co-payment is waived.

HHC in Taiwan covers nurses' and physicians' visits, drug injections, respiratory therapy, and laboratory tests (before 2015), with extended services provided by more disciplines added after 2015 [24]. HHC is provided by HHC teams affiliated to hospitals, by independent HHC organisations, or by community health centres from the public sector [25]. The eligibility criteria for HHC in Taiwan cover those people who have (1) a limited ability to self-care, e.g., needing help with more than half of their daily activities; (2) definite medical or nursing care needs assessed by both physicians and nurses at outpatients clinics, on hospital admission, or at home; and (3) chronic conditions requiring long-term nursing care or continual post-discharge healthcare needs [25,26]. HHC in this study did not include the home-based palliative care (HBPLC) program in Taiwan.

2.2. Data Source and Ethics

This is a nationwide cohort study using Taiwan's National Health Insurance Research Database (NHIRD), which is a routinely collected, claim-based, and anonymised electronic record database, including the entire inpatient and ambulatory healthcare services between 2000 and 2013. In the NHIRD, information about any utilisation of NHI-reimbursed healthcare services or drug prescriptions for an individual is obtained by tracing specific administrative codes and is linked by an encrypted identification code. Disease diagnoses are based on the International Classification of Diseases, Ninth Revision, Clinical Modification (ICD-9-CM) codes before 2016. The study protocol was approved by the institutional review board of Chi-Mei Medical Center in Taiwan (Approval No. 10410-E01) and informed consent waived due to the anonymous nature of NHIRD analysis.

2.3. Cohort Definition

The study cohort included people aged 40 years and older who had a new dementia diagnosis from the whole country from 2002 to 2013. Individuals with dementia were identified by the ICD-9-CM codes for dementia (Table A1 in the Appendix A), followed by at least one inpatient record of an ICD-9-CM dementia code or at least three outpatient records within 1 year. Cohort entry date was defined as the date on which the first diagnosis code of dementia appeared. We excluded people aged older than 105 years, individuals who had a previous history of dementia or stroke, had a stroke diagnosed on the same day of the dementia diagnosis, received HHC or palliative care before the cohort entry date, or received the last HHC in the follow-up more than 2 years before death. Those who had errors in the data registration, such as stroke, HHC, or palliative care recorded after death, were also excluded (Figure 1).

Next, people with dementia who died by the end of 2013 were selected as the study focus. Death was determined when a patient was coded as "in-hospital death" or "sudden death" at the ER or withdrew from the NHI programme without any other healthcare visits in the following 6 months, as is a common working criteria for the NHIRD [11].

2.4. Case Identification

A nested case-control analysis in cohort decedents was applied to minimise the bias of identifying end-of-life outcomes. We identified people with dementia who experienced end-of-life burdensome transitions before death, including ET or LT. ET was defined as three or more hospitalisations in the last 90 days of life, while LT was defined as any ER visit or hospitalisation in the last three days of life [9]. This pattern of transition was used as a binary variable in the analysis.

2.5. Exposure Measurements and Covariates

We examined all records of HHC received by people with dementia during the follow-up period before death (for the claim codes for HHC, see Table A2 in the Appendix A). Characteristics of HHC, including resource utilisation groups (RUG); total counts of services or services provided by different professionals; and time-related factors for services, such as the period from cohort entry, duration of HHC, and the period from last HHC to death, were presented and used in the subgroup analyses. HHC services by nurses can be classified into four levels according to RUG [26]. The first level RUG is intended for those who only require ordinary healthcare visits to the home, and levels 2–4 of RUG are aimed at people who require one, two, three, or more specialised care services, respectively. The predefined specialised care services include tracheostomy care; urinal indwelling catheterisation and/or catheter change; insertion and/or change of a nasogastric tube; bladder irrigation; wound care or debridement for stage 3 or 4 pressure injuries; intravenous fluid supply; colostomy, ileostomy, or urostomy care (e.g., an ileal conduit); or post-colon resection care. The reimbursement for physician visits is a fixed payment regardless of the RUG of HHC that patients receive [26].

Covariates included age, sex, socioeconomic status (personal income and urbanisation level of residence), comorbidities, and age-adjusted Charlson Comorbidity Index (aCCI) at baseline [27]. The aCCI scores were calculated with different comorbid conditions that were weighted and additional points added for age. Each decade over the age of 40 years was assigned a comorbidity score of 1 to risk and so on. Comorbidities and aCCI were defined based on information from at least one inpatient record or three outpatient records within 1 year before the cohort entry date and classified by ICD-9-CM codes (Table A1 in the Appendix A). Income was classified by insurance premiums, and urbanisation level was considered according to population density and medical resource [28].

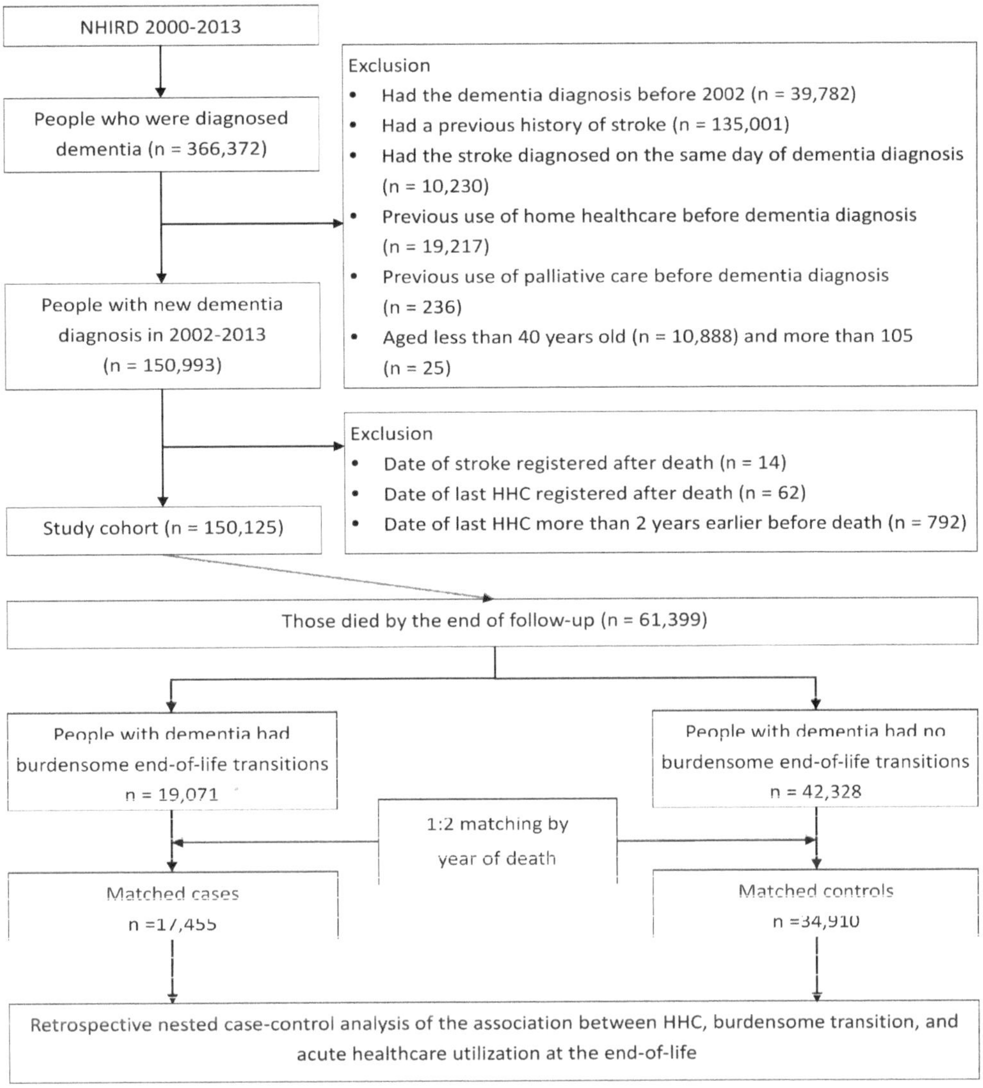

Figure 1. Schematic illustration of the study cohort and patient selection criteria. HHC = home healthcare and NHIRD = National Health Insurance Research Database.

2.6. *Statistical Analysis*

The mean and standard deviation (SD) or median and interquartile range was estimated for continuous variables. Discrete variables were described as the frequency with percentage. People with (cases) and without (controls) burdensome end-of-life transitions were matched on a ratio of 1:2 by year of death to diminish the influence of changes to policy or end-of-life care practice over time. Conditional logistic regression was then used to estimate the adjusted odds ratio (OR) and 95% confidence interval (CI) of risks of transitions between cases and controls. Stratified analyses for potential factors of interest were estimated and presented as forest plots. In addition, characteristics of HHC among people who received HHC were estimated using unconditional logistic regression analysis. All regression analyses were adjusted for age, gender, socioeconomic status, aCCI, and listed comorbidities. SAS 9.4 (SAS Institute, Cary, NC, USA) was used for all statistical analyses.

3. Results

3.1. *Participants*

Among 150,125 people with a new dementia diagnosis, a total of 61,399 decedents were identified. The mean age of decedents was 83.2 years at death, and the mean survival period was 1030.7 days after the diagnosis of dementia, 48.2% of whom were female (Table 1). The percentage of burdensome end-of-life transitions in the decedents was 31.1% (19,071), including 9533 with ET (15.5%) and 9538 with LT (15.5%). We further included 17,455 cases with burdensome end-of-life transitions, who were divided into different groups according to ET, LT, or both (Figure A1 in the Appendix A), and 34,910 controls for the nested case-control analysis.

3.2. Descriptive Data

Most characteristics at the time of dementia diagnosis were significantly different in proportions between cases and controls, and the group with ET had a much higher proportion of males (Table 1). For the characteristics at follow-up, the groups with ET had a shorter time from dementia diagnosis to death or to receiving the first HHC, shorter duration of HHC, and lower frequency of HHC compared to the group with LT only or controls.

Figure 2 presents the utilisation pattern of ER visits and hospital and ICU admissions in the last year of life for each group of cases and controls. The group with ET had more hospital/ICU admissions and longer hospital/ICU stays. The group with LT only had fewer hospital/ICU admissions than the control group during their last year.

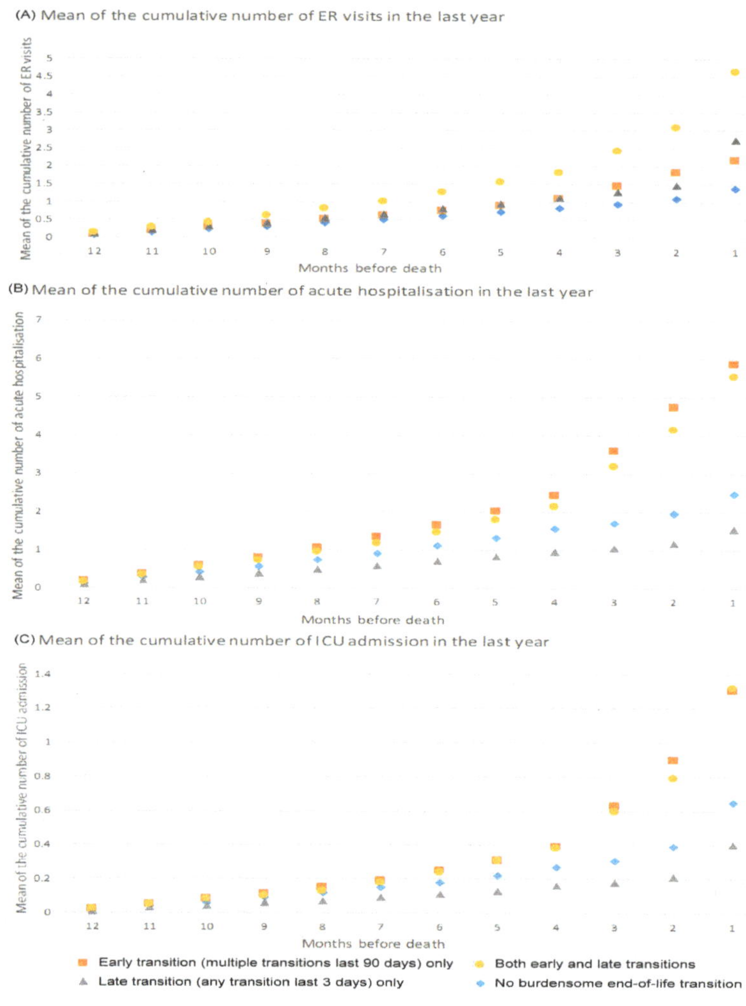

Figure 2. The utilisation of acute healthcare in the last year for people with dementia by type of burdensome end-of-life transition. ER = emergency room and ICU = intensive care unit.

Table 1. Characteristics of people with dementia and matched groups with or without burdensome end-of-life transition.

	All Decedents N = 61,399	Decedents Included in the Nested Case-Control Analysis			
		No Burdensome End-of-Life Transitions (Matched Controls) N = 34,910	Burdensome End-of-Life Transitions (Matched Cases) N = 17,455		
			Early Transition Only (Multiple Transitions Last 90 Days) N = 7891	Late Transition Only (Any Transition Last 3 Days) N = 8752	Both Early and Late Transitions N = 812
Age when death, mean (SD)	83.2 (9.7)	83.5 (9.6)	82.3 (9.6)	82.7 (10.1)	82.2 (10.2)
Gender (female), *n* (%)	29,595 (48.2)	17,099 (49.0)	3266 (41.4)	4486 (51.2)	339 (41.8)
Characteristics at time of dementia diagnosis					
SES—Income #, *n* (%)					
Dependent	11,934 (19.4)	6968 (20.0)	1307 (16.6)	1776 (20.3)	143 (17.6)
Fair	32,609 (53.1)	18,575 (53.2)	4660 (59.1)	4212 (48.1)	426 (52.5)
High	16,076 (26.2)	8955 (25.7)	1828 (23.2)	2621 (30.0)	239 (29.4)
Very high	780 (1.3)	412 (1.2)	96 (1.2)	143 (1.6)	4 (0.5)
SES—Urbanisation, *n* (%)	(Missing, *n* = 25,381; 41.3%)	(Missing, *n* = 14,722; 42.2%)	(Missing, *n* = 3153; 40.0%)	(Missing, *n* = 3580; 40.9%)	(Missing, *n* = 316; 38.9%)
1 most urbanised	15,745 (43.7)	8806 (43.6)	2005 (42.3)	2356 (45.6)	211 (42.5)
2	15,494 (43.0)	8733 (43.3)	2060 (43.5)	2170 (42.0)	218 (44.0)
3	4097 (11.4)	2281 (11.3)	580 (12.2)	538 (10.4)	55 (11.1)
4 most ruralised	682 (1.9)	368 (1.8)	93 (2.0)	108 (2.1)	12 (2.4)
Age-adjusted CCI, mean (SD)	7.4 (2.8)	7.3 (2.8)	7.7 (2.9)	7.3 (2.8)	7.9 (3.0)
Comorbidities					
Cancer, *n* (%)	8520 (13.9)	4699 (13.5)	1323 (16.8)	1101 (12.6)	158 (19.5)
Heart failure, *n* (%)	10,806 (17.6)	5998 (17.2)	1484 (18.8)	1573 (18.0)	174 (21.4)
COPD, *n* (%)	21,466 (35.0)	12,033 (34.5)	3066 (38.9)	2875 (32.9)	339 (41.8)
Liver cirrhosis/ chronic liver Disease, *n* (%)	11,946 (19.5)	6552 (18.8)	1768 (22.4)	1634 (18.7)	177 (21.8)
Renal failure, *n* (%)	1565 (2.6)	886 (2.5)	230 (2.9)	203 (2.3)	23 (2.8)
Hypertension, *n* (%)	40,441 (65.9)	22,805 (65.3)	5266 (66.7)	5720 (65.4)	555 (68.4)
Diabetes, *n* (%)	18,953 (30.9)	10,413 (29.8)	2664 (33.8)	2775 (31.7)	259 (31.9)
Coronary artery disease, *n* (%)	22,871 (37.3)	12,755 (36.5)	3082 (39.1)	3265 (37.3)	330 (40.6)

Table 1. *Cont.*

	All Decedents N = 61,399	Decedents Included in the Nested Case-Control Analysis			
		No Burdensome End-of-Life Transitions (Matched Controls) N = 34,910	Burdensome End-of-Life Transitions (Matched Cases) N = 17,455		
			Early Transition Only (Multiple Transitions Last 90 Days) N = 7891	Late Transition Only (Any Transition Last 3 Days) N = 8752	Both Early and Late Transitions N = 812
Hyperlipidaemia, *n* (%)	13,578 (22.1)	7408 (21.2)	1647 (20.9)	2181 (24.9)	174 (21.4)
Atrial fibrillation, *n* (%)	3954 (6.4)	2192 (6.3)	559 (7.1)	581 (6.6)	56 (6.9)
Depression, *n* (%)	8015 (13.1)	4321 (12.4)	1019 (12.9)	1313 (15.0)	121 (14.9)
Characteristics in the follow-up					
Time from cohort entry to death (days), mean (SD)	1030.7 (872.8)	1038.7 (859.4)	841.0 (770.4)	1093.5 (898.8)	887.2 (816.6)
HHC related factors					
HHC, *n* (%)	17,046 (27.8)	9670 (27.7)	2197 (27.8)	2277 (26.0)	251 (30.9)
HHC (total counts/person), mean (SD)	22.2 (27.4)	22.8 (27.3)	16.8 (21.8)	23.8 (28.8)	17.0 (24.1)
Duration of HHC (days), median (Q1–Q3)	234 (57–648)	245 (61–654)	151 (28–496)	256 (59–728)	127 (15–499)
Frequency of HHC (counts /year/person), mean (SD)	9.8 (6.7)	10.1 (6.7)	8.4 (6.4)	10.0 (6.8)	8.3 (6.5)
Resource utilisation group of first HHC, *n* (%)	(missing n = 20; 0.1%)	(missing *n* = 10; 0.1%)	(missing *n* = 4; 0.2%)	(missing *n* = 5; 0.2%)	
1	895 (5.3)	487 (5.0)	118 (5.4)	147 (6.5)	11 (4.4)
2	11,958 (70.2)	6766 (70.0)	1458 (66.5)	1663 (73.2)	168 (66.9)
3	3888 (22.8)	2242 (23.2)	567 (25.9)	437 (19.2)	68 (27.1)
4	285 (1.7)	165 (1.7)	50 (2.3)	25 (1.1)	4 (1.6)
Time from cohort entry to first HHC (days), median (Q1–Q3)	520 (145–1179)	520 (147–1165)	455 (133–1020)	578 (151–1255)	488 (115–1068)
Time from last HHC to death, (days), median (Q1–Q3)	29 (15–67)	30 (17–69)	46 (22–89)	18 (9–32)	22 (9–52)

COPD = chronic obstructive pulmonary disease, HHC = home healthcare, SD = standard deviation, SES = socioeconomic status, Q1 = first quartile, Q3 = third quartile, and CCI = Charlson Comorbidity Index. # Insurance premium-related income.

3.3. Main Results

The risk of burdensome end-of-life transitions between those with and without HHC and the stratified group analysis are shown in Figure 3 (for the number of cases and controls, see Table A3 in the Appendix A). People who received HHC had a higher risk of ET than those without HHC (OR = 1.14, 95 % CI 1.08–1.21), whereas people with HHC had a lower risk of LT (OR = 0.89, 95 % CI 0.83–0.94). In the stratified group analysis, considering the age groups, survival period, or stroke event after dementia diagnosis and year of death, the risk of transitions between those with and without HHC is in keeping with the risk in the primary analysis. The only exception was in people whose survival period was less than one year after dementia diagnosis; those with HHC had a higher risk of LT than those without HHC (OR = 1.13, 95 % CI 0.98–1.31). A sensitivity analysis suggested similar results with the primary analysis after excluding people with missing values on urbanisation (Table A4 in the Appendix A).

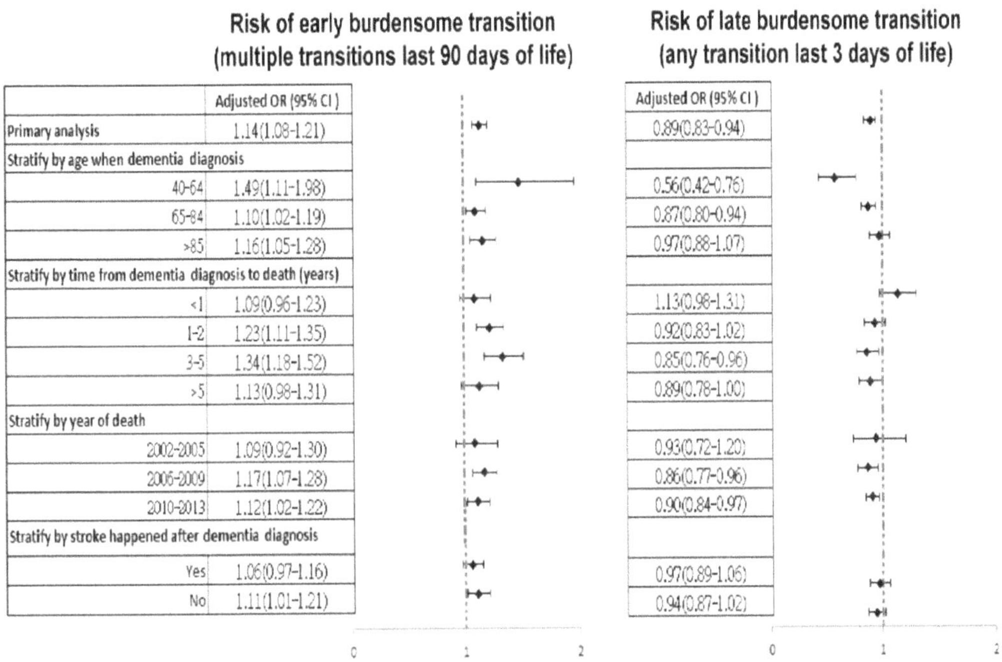

Figure 3. Risk of burdensome end-of-life transition in people with dementia who received home healthcare compared with those who had no home healthcare services (reference group). CI = confidence interval, HHC = home healthcare, ICU = intensive care unit, and OR = odds ratio. In the regression model, the early burdensome transition represents those with early transition only and those with both early and late transition; the late burdensome transition represents those with late transition only. All the analyses were adjusted for age, gender, socioeconomic status, age-adjusted Charlson Comorbidity Index, and comorbidities.

Table 2 shows the influence by characteristics of HHC on the risk of burdensome end-of-life transitions in people who received HHC. The risk of transitions did not significantly differ between RUG levels or the period from dementia diagnosis to the first HHC. HHC that was more frequent (e.g., OR = 0.52, 95 % CI 0.45–0.61, >16 versus ≤4 times per year), of longer duration (e.g., OR = 0.50, 95 % CI 0.42–0.60, >365 versus ≤30 days), or delivered closer to the time of death (e.g., OR = 0.73, 95 % CI 0.62–0.84, >90 versus 0–15 days) was associated with a remarkably lower risk of ET. HHC that was of longer duration or provided by both physicians and nurses was associated with a lower risk of LT.

Table 2. Subgroup analysis of burdensome end-of-life transition in people with dementia who received home healthcare stratified by the characteristics of home healthcare.

	Early Burdensome Transition (Multiple Transitions Last 90 Days of Life)				Late Burdensome Transition (Any Transition Last 3 Days of Life)			
	Cases (n)	Controls (n)	Adjusted OR	95 % CI	Cases (n)	Controls (n)	Adjusted OR	95 % CI
RUG								
1	105	229	(Reference)		147	258	(Reference)	
2	1278	3223	0.85	0.67–1.08	1663	3543	0.94	0.81–1.10
3	486	1106	0.96	0.74–1.24	437	1136	0.91	0.80–1.03
4	29	88	0.71	0.44–1.15	25	77	0.91	0.79–1.06
HHC by professionals								
HHC by nurse only	410	783	(Reference)		410	748	(Reference)	
HHC by physician and nurse	2034	3863	1.01	0.88–1.15	1862	4266	0.80	0.70–0.91
Duration of HHC (days)								
≤30	670	861	(Reference)		413	894	(Reference)	
>30 and ≤120	471	821	0.80	0.66–0.98	404	840	0.69	0.56–0.85
>120 and ≤365	528	1157	0.58	0.48–0.71	504	1208	0.56	0.46–0.69
>365	779	1812	0.50	0.42–0.60	956	2077	0.60	0.50–0.73
Frequency of HHC (counts/year)								
≤4	933	1263	(Reference)		636	1318	(Reference)	
5–8	435	899	0.66	0.57–0.76	407	899	0.94	0.81–1.10
9–16	744	1598	0.64	0.56–0.72	789	1801	0.91	0.80–1.03
>16	336	891	0.52	0.45–0.61	445	1001	0.91	0.79–1.06
Time between the dementia diagnosis and receiving the first HHC (years)								
<1	1084	2079	(Reference)		895	1943	(Reference)	
1–2	804	1478	1.03	0.92–1.15	697	1526	0.99	0.87–1.11
3–4	210	434	0.91	0.76–1.10	230	566	0.87	0.73–1.03
>4	350	660	1.00	0.86–1.17	455	984	0.99	0.86–1.14
Time between receiving the last HHC and death (days)								
>90	569	999	(Reference)		265	994	(Reference)	
31–90	944	1303	1.28	1.12–1.46	334	1534	0.82	0.68–0.98
16–30	484	1245	0.69	0.59–0.80	692	1384	1.88	1.59–2.21
0–15	451	1104	0.73	0.62–0.84	986	1107	3.35	2.85–3.93

CI = confidence interval, HHC = home healthcare, RUG = resource utilisation groups, and OR = odds ratio. In the regression model, the early burdensome transition represents those with early transition only and those with both early and late transition; the late burdensome transition represents those with late transition only. All the analyses were adjusted for age, gender, socioeconomic status, age-adjusted Charlson Comorbidity Index, and comorbidities.

4. Discussion

We used a large database to conduct the first national-level cohort study on the impact of HHC on burdensome end-of-life transitions in people with dementia, following from dementia diagnosis to death. HHC, in general, is not specifically targeted at end-of-life care needs and, thus, is seldom investigated for its effect on end-of-life outcomes. Our findings have important implications for focusing interventions on those who experience ET and have the highest acute healthcare needs at the end of life. We need to understand further the differential effects of routine HHC on ET and LT and the specific components of HHC that reduced the risk of end-of-life transitions.

4.1. End-of-Life Transitions and Hospital/ICU Utilisations

Overall, in Taiwan, 31.1% of decedents with dementia experienced end-of-life transitions, a much higher proportion than the counterparts reported in US Medicare (19%) or Finish nursing home residents (9.9%), as well as in the UK (16%) [8–10]. The proportions of ET and LT among people with dementia were equal in our cohort, which is different to the LT-predominant pattern in the US and UK [9,10]. Previous studies found that younger age and male sex increase the risk of burdensome transitions, especially ET, in people with dementia [8–10]. Our findings on age and sex are in keeping with the existing literature. In addition, Leniz et al. reported that ET was associated with the presence of physical illness and depressed mood [10], which may explain the higher proportion of physical and mental comorbidities and higher aCCI score in cases with ET in our study.

A tendency towards aggressive healthcare at the end of life for people with dementia in Taiwan is associated with cultural norms of avoiding the discussion on end-of-life issues in advance, lack of recognition of dementia as a terminal illness, and the fee-for-service predominant design of the healthcare system, which we illustrated in our previous publications [5,11]. The remarkably higher utilisation and longer length of stay of hospital/ICU admissions in the ET group echoed findings from the UK [10] and highlighted the urgent need to identify and develop preventive interventions such as HHC for those at high risk of ET. Further details on the pattern of avoidable aggressive interventions or life-sustaining treatments associated with the increased use of ICU services should be explored in the Asian context.

4.2. Impact of HHC on Burdensome End-of-Life Transitions

Much research on burdensome transitions or acute healthcare utilisation at the end of life has focused on residents living in long-term care facilities [8,9,29]. Sleeman and Leniz et al. analysed an electronic health records database in a mental health trust in London and, further, found that people with dementia at home are at a higher risk of burdensome end-of-life transitions than those in care homes [7,10]. To our knowledge, our study is the first one that targets the unmet need of these high-risk people with dementia by investigating the impact of HHC intervention on both ET and LT defined by Gozalo et al. [9].

The percentage of ET and LT in the group who received HHC in our study were 34.5% and 31.2%, respectively. In comparison with previous studies, Mitchell et al. included only those people with advanced dementia who died within 12 months after admissions to either the HHC programme or nursing home care and found that the ratio of hospitalisation within the 90 days prior to their last minimum dataset assessment was 31.5% in the HHC group, which was lower than the ratio of 43.7% in the nursing home group [22]. Jennings et al. followed a longitudinal cohort with dementia receiving a nurse practitioner-led comprehensive community care programme and showed 38% of the decedents were hospitalised in the last six months of life, whereas 69% died with hospice care, and 66% died at home [21]. The aforementioned two studies did not specifically report data on LT.

In our study, the HHC intervention had an opposite effect on ET and LT in people with dementia. The slightly higher risk of ET in the HHC group compared to those who did not have HHC may have occurred because people who received HHC may have had more multi-morbidities, more complex care needs, or have been at increased risk of using acute healthcare services before the HHC service [30,31]. For example, disabled people who received HHC in Taiwan had a higher risk of hospitalisation or ER transition after HHC (OR = 1.6, 95 % CI 1.41–1.83 and OR = 1.16, 95 % CI: 1.04–1.30, respectively) compared to the non-HHC group, even though HHC reduced hospital admissions by 80% and ER visits by 65% for people in the HHC group within the year after HHC service [30]. Another explanation is that better care coordination in home-based services compared with the usual care may identify more cases with unmet needs, leading to an increase in admissions for elderly people [32,33].

This interesting phenomenon of divergence between HHC and end-of-life transitions in different periods prior to death (early or late) may reflect the results of Jennings' research [21]. This study showed that people with dementia who received the HHC programme and engaged in completion of the Physician Orders for Life-Sustaining Treatment (POLST) were more likely to be hospitalised in the last six months of life (43% versus 31%; $p = 0.04$) than those who received HHC but did not complete the POLST; however, the former group were also more likely to have had a discussion about hospice care (78% versus 64%; $p = 0.01$), die with hospice care (74% versus 62%; $p = 0.03$), and die at home (70% versus 59%; $p = 0.04$).

Our key finding is that the characteristics of HHC impacts on burdensome end-of-life transitions for people with dementia. HHC with longer duration, higher frequency, or that was provided continuously closer to the time of death may be factors indicating a better continuity of care (CoC) [34], and CoC is related to fewer hospitalisations and ER visits for people with dementia in the US Medicare system and a non-HHC population in Taiwan [35,36]. Continuous HHC may enhance the communication and relationship between patients, family members, and medical professionals and facilitate the ACP of substitute decision-makers and decision-making regarding do-not-resuscitation and do-not-hospitalise [21,37,38]. The obligated 24-h telephone support for clients in the Taiwanese HHC programme, which offers basic triage and care advice, may also contribute to the reduction of transitions [39].

4.3. Integration of Various Home-Based Services for Better End-of-Life Care

Although HBPLC showed increased odds of home death and had a heterogeneous effect on reduced hospitalisations at the end of life for people with different diseases [40,41], the evidence among people with dementia is unclear [16]. A recent Japanese cross-sectional nationwide death certificate study found that the density of primary care physicians in a region had a much stronger association with increased odds of home/nursing home death than the density of HBPLC did for people in chronic conditions, including dementia [42]. In our study, we found that HHC provided by both physicians and nurses was associated with a decreased risk of LT in contrast with nurse-only HHC. This implies that interdisciplinary coordination, which is also a core feature in HBPLC, leads to better outcomes and may reduce hospitalisation when death is approaching [43].

Considering the low coverage and late referral to specialist palliative care in people with dementia [11,14,42], especially for those living at home or in a care home, HHC should be embedded within a needs-orientated palliative care framework. HHC complements earlier delivery, broader interdisciplinary practice, better referral, or coordination with specialist palliative care to build up a seamless, integrated care model for supporting people in the long disease trajectory of dementia [44]. It is also important for health policymakers to design a value-based payment scheme to make this home-based integrated and continuous care model possible. To better understand this, the authors initiated the "Home-based Longitudinal Investigation of the Multidisciplinary Team Integrated Care (HOLISTIC)" in Taiwan [45], collecting data on a cohort served by an innovative "Integrated HHC programme" launched in 2016, which may provide more solid evidence in the future.

Our study has several limitations. With the fundamental weaknesses of an administrative database, we were unable to obtain information about the severity of cognitive impairment or comorbidities, lifestyle and social support factors, or functional status, which may lead to confounding. We were unable to define the place of residence of participants, which means an analysis of transitions between home and care home and the influence of place of care is not possible. A lack of detailed clinical information on the reasons for acute healthcare utilisation made the judgment of avoidable admissions or transitions difficult. There were no records of patients' preferences and advance directives, nor the process of surrogate decision-making. It may be difficult to compare the results to other countries due to differences in healthcare delivery, reimbursement, or resources allocation. Finally, using old claims data for this study could lead to an incomplete depiction of the current situation. Future research will include more updated datasets. Despite these limitations, the association between routine HHC and the risk of end-of-life transition from a 12-year nationwide population-based cohort in Taiwan is novel and provides a key step for further investigation.

5. Conclusions

For people with dementia, HHC has contrasting effects on early and late burdensome end-of-life transitions prior to death. Characteristics of HHC such as intensity, continuity, or interdisciplinary coordination may reduce the risk of transitions at the end of life. We suggest that researchers and policymakers explore the synergy between routine HHC and specialist palliative care, and how they interact, to impact on acute healthcare utilisation in longitudinal studies through the trajectory from dementia diagnosis to death.

Author Contributions: Study concept and design: P.-J.C., C.-H.H., L.S., C.A.H., S.-J.Y., K.-P.Z., I.P. and E.L.S. Acquisition of data: P.-J.C., C.-H.H., C.A.H. and J.-Y.L. Analysis and interpretation of data: All authors. Drafting of the manuscript: P.-J.C., C.-H.H. and L.S. Critical revision of the manuscript for important intellectual content: All authors. All authors have read and agreed to the published version of the manuscript.

Acknowledgments: This study was based on data from the Taiwan NHIRD, which has been transferred to the HWDC, Department of Statistics, Ministry of Health and Welfare, Taiwan. We thank Katherine Sleeman at King's College London for her advice about the study approach and Victoria Vickerstaff at University College London for her statistical consultation at an earlier stage of the analysis.

Appendix A

Table A1. List of International Classification of Diseases, Ninth Revision, Clinical Modification (ICD-9-CM) code of the diseases.

Disease	ICD-9-CM code
Dementia	290.1x–209.4x, 291.2, 292.82, 294.1x, 294.8, 331.0, 331.1x, 331.2, 331.82
Stroke	430–438
Cancer	140–208
Heart Failure	428
Chronic obstructive pulmonary disease	491, 492, 494, 496
Liver cirrhosis/ chronic liver disease	571
Renal failure	585.4, 585.5, 585.6, 586
Hypertension	401, 402, 403, 404, 405
Diabetes	250, 251
Coronary artery disease	410–414
Hyperlipidaemia	272
Atrial fibrillation	427.31
Depression	296.2–296.36, 300.4, 311

Table A2. List of administrative claim codes for home healthcare in the National Health Insurance Research Database (NHIRD).

Code in NHIRD	Definition
	A. In common area
05307C	Fee for physician visit (per time)—for the first to fourth patient visited by one physician on the same day
05309C	Fee for physician visit (per time)—for the fifth to eighth patient visited by one physician on the same day
05301C	Fee for nurse visit (per time)—RUG 1, within reasonable caseload
05328C	Fee for nurse visit (per time)—RUG 1, beyond reasonable caseload
05303C	Fee for nurse visit (per time)—RUG 2, within reasonable caseload
05330C	Fee for nurse visit (per time)—RUG 2, beyond reasonable caseload
05305C	Fee for nurse visit (per time)—RUG 3, within reasonable caseload
05332C	Fee for nurse visit (per time)—RUG 3, beyond reasonable caseload
05321C	Fee for nurse visit (per time)—RUG 4, within reasonable caseload
05334C	Fee for nurse visit (per time)—RUG 4, beyond reasonable caseload
	B. In specific rural area

Table A2. *Cont.*

Code in NHIRD	Definition
05308C	Fee for physician visit (per time)—for the first to fourth patient visited by one physician on the same day
05310C	Fee for physician visit (per time)—for the fifth to eighth patient visited by one physician on the same day
05302C	Fee for nurse visit (per time)—RUG 1, within reasonable caseload
05329C	Fee for nurse visit (per time)—RUG 1, beyond reasonable caseload
05304C	Fee for nurse visit (per time)—RUG 2, within reasonable caseload
05331C	Fee for nurse visit (per time)—RUG 2, beyond reasonable caseload
05306C	Fee for nurse visit (per time)—RUG 3, within reasonable caseload
05333C	Fee for nurse visit (per time)—RUG 3, beyond reasonable caseload
05322C	Fee for nurse visit (per time)—RUG 4, within reasonable caseload
05335C	Fee for nurse visit (per time)—RUG 4, beyond reasonable caseload

RUG = Classification of resource utilization groups.

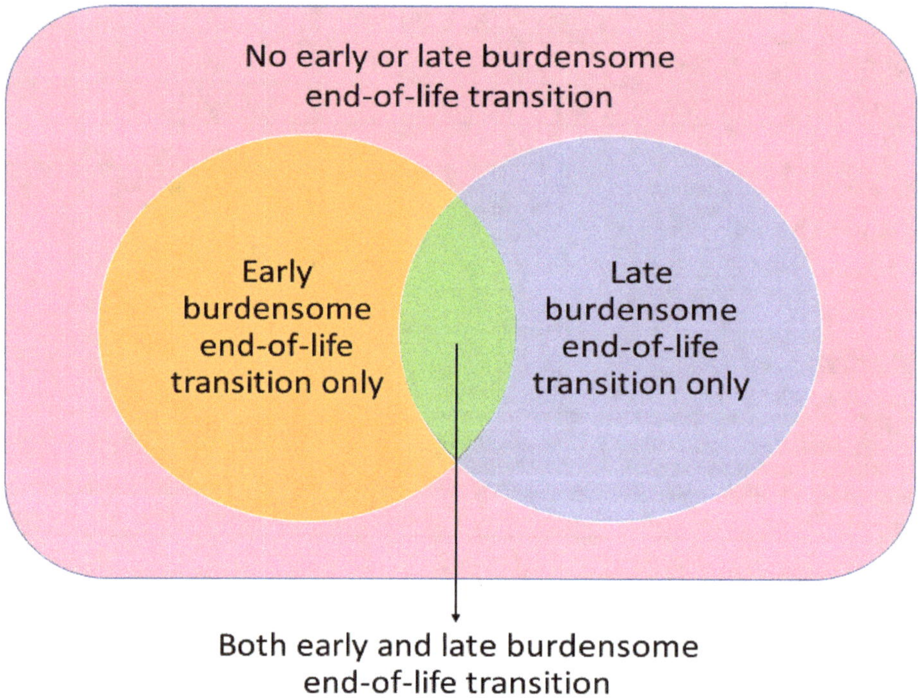

Figure A1. Illustration of people with dementia in different groups with or without burdensome end-of-life transition. In the regression model, the early burdensome transition represents those with early transition only and those with both early and late transition; the late burdensome transition represents those with late transition only.

Table A3. Numbers of cases with burdensome transitions at the end-of-lie and the controls in people with dementia who received home healthcare compared with those who had no home healthcare services.

	Early Burdensome Transition		Late Burdensome Transition	
	Cases	Controls	Cases	Controls
Primary analysis				
No HHC	6255 (71.87)	12755 (73.28)	6475 (73.98)	12,485 (71.33)
HHC	2448 (28.13)	4651 (26.72)	2277 (26.02)	5019 (28.67)
Stratify by age when cohort entry				

Table A3. *Cont.*

	Early Burdensome Transition		Late Burdensome Transition	
	Cases	Controls	Cases	Controls
40–64				
No HHC	477 (81.12)	899 (85.05)	584 (89.02)	893 (82.08)
HHC	111 (18.88)	158 (14.95)	72 (10.98)	195 (17.92)
65–84				
No HHC	3715 (71.77)	7296 (72.80)	3799 (73.68)	7007 (70.74)
HHC	1461 (28.23)	2726 (27.20)	1357 (26.32)	2898 (29.26)
>85				
No HHC	2063 (71.19)	4560 (72.07)	2092 (71.16)	4585 (70.42)
HHC	876 (29.81)	1767 (27.93)	848 (28.84)	1926 (29.58)
Stratify by time from dementia diagnosis to death (years)				
<1				
No HHC	2642 (83.98)	4337 (84.71)	1900 (85.55)	3674 (84.44)
HHC	504 (16.02)	783 (15.29)	321 (14.45)	677 (15.56)
1 to 2				
No HHC	1983 (68.71)	4377 (72.17)	2198 (74.91)	4186 (72.93)
HHC	903 (31.29)	1688 (27.83)	736 (25.09)	1554 (27.07)
3–5				
No HHC	982 (62.59)	2362 (68.31)	1259 (68.65)	2404 (64.42)
HHC	587 (37.41)	1096 (31.69)	575 (31.35)	1328 (35.58)
>5				
No HHC	648 (58.80)	1679 (60.77)	1118 (63.41)	2221 (60.34)
HHC	454 (41.20)	1084 (39.23)	645 (36.59)	1460 (39.66)
Stratify by year of death				
2002–2005				
No HHC	1196 (82.71)	2400 (82.99)	560 (83.71)	1099 (82.14)
HHC	250 (17.29)	492 (17.01)	109 (16.29)	239 (17.86)
2006–2009				
No HHC	2628 (72.20)	5386 (73.98)	2043 (76.40)	3913 (73.17)
HHC	1012 (27.80)	1894 (26.02)	631 (23.60)	1435 (26.83)
2010–2013				
No HHC	2431 (67.21)	4969 (68.69)	3872 (71.58)	7473 (69.08)
HHC	1186 (32.79)	2265 (31.31)	1537 (28.42)	3345 (30.92)
Stratify by stroke happened after cohort entry				
Yes				
No HHC	2007 (56.73)	3632 (56.72)	1631 (56.67)	3715 (55.50)
HHC	1531 (43.27)	2771 (43.28)	1247 (43.33)	2979 (44.50)
No				
No HHC	4248 (82.25)	9123 (82.91)	4844 (82.47)	8770 (81.13)
HHC	917 (17.75)	1880 (17.09)	1030 (17.53)	2040 (18.87)

HHC = home healthcare and ICU = Intensive care unit.

Table A4. Sensitivity test for the influence by the missing data in the urbanisation variable on the risk of burdensome transition at the end-of-lie in people with dementia who received home healthcare compared with those who had no home healthcare services.

	Early Burdensome Transition		Late Burdensome Transition	
	Adjusted OR	**95 % CI**	**Adjusted OR**	**95 % CI**
All people in the matched cases and controls				
No HHC	1	(Reference)	1	(Reference)
HHC	1.14	1.08–1.21	0.89	0.83–0.94
After deleting the people with missing data in urbanisation variable				
No HHC	1	(Reference)	1	(Reference)
HHC	1.10	1.01–1.19	0.87	0.80–0.94

CI = confidence interval, HHC = home healthcare, and OR = odds ratio. In the regression model, the early burdensome transition represents those with early transition only and those with both early and late transition; the late burdensome transition represents those with late transition only. All the analyses were adjusted for age, gender, socioeconomic status, age-adjusted Charlson Comorbidity Index, and comorbidities.

References

1. Sleeman, K.E.; De Brito, M.; Etkind, S.; Nkhoma, K.; Guo, P.; Higginson, I.J.; Gomes, B.; Harding, R. The escalating global burden of serious health-related suffering: Projections to 2060 by world regions, age groups, and health conditions. *Lancet* **2019**, *7*, E883–E892. [CrossRef]
2. Patel, V. *Deaths Registered in England and Wales (Series DR): 2017*; Office for National Statistics: London, UK, 2018.
3. Ellen, A.; Kramarow, B.T.-V. Dementia Mortality in the United States, 2000–2017. *Natl. Vital Stat. Rep.* **2019**, *68*, 1–29.
4. Shepherd, H.; Livingston, G.; Chan, J.; Sommerlad, A. Hospitalisation rates and predictors in people with dementia: A systematic review and meta-analysis. *BMC Med.* **2019**, *17*, 130. [CrossRef]
5. Chen, Y.H.; Ho, C.H.; Huang, C.C.; Hsu, Y.W.; Chen, Y.C.; Chen, P.J.; Chen, G.T.; Wang, J.J. Comparison of healthcare utilization and life-sustaining interventions between elderly patients with dementia and those with cancer near the end of life: A nationwide, population-based study in Taiwan. *Geriatr. Gerontol. Int.* **2017**, *17*, 2545–2551. [CrossRef]
6. Aaltonen, M.; Rissanen, P.; Forma, L.; Raitanen, J.; Jylha, M. The impact of dementia on care transitions during the last two years of life. *Age Ageing* **2012**, *41*, 52–57. [CrossRef]
7. Sleeman, K.E.; Perera, G.; Stewart, R.; Higginson, I.J. Predictors of emergency department attendance by people with dementia in their last year of life: Retrospective cohort study using linked clinical and administrative data. *Alzheimers Dement.* **2018**, *14*, 20–27. [CrossRef]
8. Aaltonen, M.; Raitanen, J.; Forma, L.; Pulkki, J.; Rissanen, P.; Jylha, M. Burdensome transitions at the end of life among long-term care residents with dementia. *J. Am. Med. Dir. Assoc.* **2014**, *15*, 643–648. [CrossRef] [PubMed]
9. Gozalo, P.; Teno, J.M.; Mitchell, S.L.; Sinner, J.; Bynum, J.; Tyler, D.; Mor, V. End-of-life transitions among nursing home residents with cognitive issues. *N. Engl. J. Med.* **2011**. [CrossRef] [PubMed]
10. Leniz, J.; Higginson, I.J.; Stewart, R.; Sleeman, K.E. Understanding which people with dementia are at risk of inappropriate care and avoidable transitions to hospital near the end-of-life: A retrospective cohort study. *Age Ageing* **2019**. [CrossRef] [PubMed]
11. Chen, P.J.; Liang, F.W.; Ho, C.H.; Cheng, S.Y.; Chen, Y.C.; Chen, Y.H.; Chen, Y.C. Association between palliative care and life-sustaining treatments for patients with dementia: A nationwide 5-year cohort study. *Palliat. Med.* **2018**, *32*, 622–630. [CrossRef]
12. Miller, S.C.; Lima, J.C.; Mitchell, S.L. Influence of hospice on nursing home residents with advanced dementia who received Medicare-skilled nursing facility care near the end of life. *J. Am. Geriatr. Soc.* **2012**, *60*, 2035–2041. [CrossRef] [PubMed]

13. Rosenwax, L.; Spilsbury, K.; Arendts, G.; McNamara, B.; Semmens, J. Community-based palliative care is associated with reduced emergency department use by people with dementia in their last year of life: A retrospective cohort study. *Palliat. Med.* **2015**, *29*, 727–736. [CrossRef] [PubMed]
14. De Vleminck, A.; Morrison, R.S.; Meier, D.E.; Aldridge, M.D. Hospice Care for Patients With Dementia in the United States: A Longitudinal Cohort Study. *J. Am. Med. Dir. Assoc.* **2018**, *19*, 633–638. [CrossRef]
15. Sachs, G.A.; Shega, J.W.; Cox-Hayley, D. Barriers to excellent end-of-life care for patients with dementia. *J. Gen. Intern. Med.* **2004**, *19*, 1057–1063. [CrossRef] [PubMed]
16. Miranda, R.; Bunn, F.; Lynch, J.; Van den Block, L.; Goodman, C. Palliative care for people with dementia living at home: A systematic review of interventions. *Palliat. Med.* **2019**, *33*, 726–742. [CrossRef]
17. WHO. *The Growing Need for Home Health Care for the Elderly*; World Health Organization, Regional Office for the Eastern Mediterranean: Cairo, Egypt, 2015.
18. Landers, S.; Madigan, E.; Leff, B.; Rosati, R.J.; McCann, B.A.; Hornbake, R.; MacMillan, R.; Jones, K.; Bowles, K.; Dowding, D.; et al. The Future of Home Health Care: A Strategic Framework for Optimizing Value. *Home Health Care Manag. Pract.* **2016**, *28*, 262–278. [CrossRef]
19. Ritchie, C.S. Population Health and Tailored Medical Care in the Home: The Roles of Home-Based Primary Care and Home-Based Palliative Care. *J. Pain Symptom Manag.* **2018**, *55*, 1041–1046. [CrossRef]
20. Shepperd, S.; Iliffe, S.; Doll, H.A.; Clarke, M.J.; Kalra, L.; Wilson, A.D.; Goncalves-Bradley, D.C. Admission avoidance hospital at home. *Cochrane Database Syst. Rev.* **2016**, *9*, CD007491. [CrossRef]
21. Jennings, L.A.; Turner, M.; Keebler, C.; Burton, C.H.; Romero, T.; Wenger, N.S.; Reuben, D.B. The Effect of a Comprehensive Dementia Care Management Program on End-of-Life Care. *J. Am. Geriatr. Soc.* **2019**, *67*, 443–448. [CrossRef]
22. Mitchell, S.L.; Morris, J.N.; Park, P.S.; Fries, B.E. Terminal care for persons with advanced dementia in the nursing home and home care settings. *J. Palliat. Med.* **2004**, *7*, 808–816. [CrossRef]
23. NHIA. *National Health Insurance Annual Statistical Report, 2018*; National Health Insurance Administration: Taipei City, Taiwan, 2018. Available online: https://www.nhi.gov.tw/english/Content_List.aspx?n=AB41B66610EAC01A&topn=616B97F8DF2C3614 (accessed on 11 April 2020).
24. NHIA. *Integrated Home Healthcare Program, 2016*; National Health Insurance Administration: Taipei City, Taiwan, 2016. Available online: https://www.nhi.gov.tw/Content_List.aspx?n=229E6EBB8F3CF41B&topn=5FE8C9FEAE863B46 (accessed on 11 April 2020).
25. Chang, H.T.; Lai, H.Y.; Hwang, I.H.; Ho, M.M.; Hwang, S.J. Home healthcare services in Taiwan: A nationwide study among the older population. *BMC Health Serv. Res.* **2010**, *10*, 274. [CrossRef] [PubMed]
26. NHIA. Reimbursement Items and Payment Regulations of Healthcare in National Health Insurance. In *Home Health Care Payment Regulations*; National Health Insurance Administration: Taipei, Taiwan, 2015.
27. Charlson, M.; Szatrowski, T.P.; Peterson, J.; Gold, J. Validation of a combined comorbidity index. *J. Clin. Epidemiol.* **1994**, *47*, 1245–1251. [CrossRef]
28. Liu, C.Y.; Hung, Y.T.; Chuang, Y.L.; Chen, Y.J.; Weng, W.S.; Liu, J.S.; Liang, K.Y. Incorporating Development Stratification of Taiwan Townships into Sampling Design of Large Scale Health Interview Survey. *J. Health Manag.* **2006**, *4*, 1–22. [CrossRef]
29. Van den Block, L.; Pivodic, L.; Pardon, K.; Donker, G.; Miccinesi, G.; Moreels, S.; Vega Alonso, T.; Deliens, L.; Onwuteaka-Philipsen, B. Transitions between health care settings in the final three months of life in four EU countries. *Eur. J. Public Health* **2015**, *25*, 569–575. [CrossRef]
30. Lee, Y.H.; Lu, C.W.; Huang, C.T.; Chang, H.H.; Yang, K.C.; Kuo, C.S.; Chang, Y.K.; Hsu, C.C.; Huang, K.C. Impact of a home health care program for disabled patients in Taiwan: A nationwide population-based cohort study. *Medicine (Baltimore)* **2019**, *98*, e14502. [CrossRef] [PubMed]
31. Mondor, L.; Maxwell, C.J.; Hogan, D.B.; Bronskill, S.E.; Gruneir, A.; Lane, N.E.; Wodchis, W.P. Multimorbidity and healthcare utilization among home care clients with dementia in Ontario, Canada: A retrospective analysis of a population-based cohort. *PLoS Med.* **2017**, *14*, e1002249. [CrossRef]
32. Gravelle, H.; Dusheiko, M.; Sheaff, R.; Sargent, P.; Boaden, R.; Pickard, S.; Parker, S.; Roland, M. Impact of case management (Evercare) on frail elderly patients: Controlled before and after analysis of quantitative outcome data. *BMJ* **2007**, *334*, 31. [CrossRef]
33. Huntley, A.L.; Thomas, R.; Mann, M.; Huws, D.; Elwyn, G.; Paranjothy, S.; Purdy, S. Is case management

effective in reducing the risk of unplanned hospital admissions for older people? A systematic review and meta-analysis. *Fam. Pract.* **2013**, *30*, 266–275. [CrossRef]

34. Jee, S.H.; Cabana, M.D. Indices for continuity of care: A systematic review of the literature. *Med. Care Res. Rev.* **2006**, *63*, 158–188. [CrossRef]
35. Amjad, H.; Carmichael, D.; Austin, A.M.; Chang, C.H.; Bynum, J.P. Continuity of Care and Health Care Utilization in Older Adults With Dementia in Fee-for-Service Medicare. *JAMA Intern. Med.* **2016**, *176*, 1371–1378. [CrossRef]
36. Cheng, S.H.; Chen, C.C.; Hou, Y.F. A longitudinal examination of continuity of care and avoidable hospitalization: Evidence from a universal coverage health care system. *Arch. Intern. Med.* **2010**, *170*, 1671–1677. [CrossRef] [PubMed]
37. Chang, C.; Jackson, S.S.; Bullman, T.A.; Cobbs, E.L. Impact of a home-based primary care program in an urban Veterans Affairs medical center. *J. Am. Med. Dir. Assoc.* **2009**, *10*, 133–137. [CrossRef] [PubMed]
38. Huggins, M.; McGregor, M.J.; Cox, M.B.; Bauder, K.; Slater, J.; Yap, C.; Mallery, L.; Moorhouse, P.; Rusnak, C. Advance Care Planning and Decision-Making in a Home-Based Primary Care Service in a Canadian Urban Centre. *Can. Geriatr. J.* **2019**, *22*, 182–189. [CrossRef] [PubMed]
39. Moller, A.D.; Christiansen, D.H.; Bell, C.; Fredberg, U.; Vedsted, P. 24-hour access outpatient clinic for patients with exacerbation of chronic disease: A before-after cohort study of differences in acute healthcare utilisation. *BMC Health Serv. Res.* **2018**, *18*, 663. [CrossRef]
40. Gomes, B.; Calanzani, N.; Curiale, V.; McCrone, P.; Higginson, I.J. Effectiveness and cost-effectiveness of home palliative care services for adults with advanced illness and their caregivers. *Cochrane Database Syst. Rev.* **2013**, *6*, CD007760. [CrossRef]
41. Shepperd, S.; Goncalves-Bradley, D.C.; Straus, S.E.; Wee, B. Hospital at home: Home-based end-of-life care. *Cochrane Database Syst. Rev.* **2016**, *2*, CD009231. [CrossRef]
42. Nakanishi, M.; Ogawa, A.; Nishida, A. Availability of home palliative care services and dying at home in conditions needing palliative care: A population-based death certificate study. *Palliat. Med.* **2020**, *34*, 504–512. [CrossRef]
43. Brian Cassel, J.; Kerr, K.M.; McClish, D.K.; Skoro, N.; Johnson, S.; Wanke, C.; Hoefer, D. Effect of a Home-Based Palliative Care Program on Healthcare Use and Costs. *J. Am. Geriatr. Soc.* **2016**, *64*, 2288–2295. [CrossRef]
44. van der Steen, J.T.; Radbruch, L.; Hertogh, C.M.; de Boer, M.E.; Hughes, J.C.; Larkin, P.; Francke, A.L.; Junger, S.; Gove, D.; Firth, P.; et al. White paper defining optimal palliative care in older people with dementia: A Delphi study and recommendations from the European Association for Palliative Care. *Palliat. Med.* **2014**, *28*, 197–209. [CrossRef]
45. Liao, J.-Y.; Chen, P.-J.; Wu, Y.-L.; Cheng, C.-H.; Yu, S.-J.; Huang, C.-H.; Li, C.-M.; Wang, Y.-W.; Zhang, K.-P.; Liu, I.T.; et al. HOme-based Longitudinal Investigation of the multidiSciplinary Team Integrated Care (HOLISTIC): Protocol of a prospective nationwide cohort study. *BMC Geriatr.* **2020**, *20*, 511. [CrossRef]

2

Ultrastructural and Molecular Analysis of Ribose-Induced Glycated Reconstructed Human Skin

Roberta Balansin Rigon [1,†,‡], Sabine Kaessmeyer [2,†], Christopher Wolff [1], Christian Hausmann [1], Nan Zhang [1], Michaela Sochorová [3], Andrej Kováčik [3], Rainer Haag [4], Kateřina Vávrová [3], Martina Ulrich [5], Monika Schäfer-Korting [1] and Christian Zoschke [1,*]

1 Institute of Pharmacy (Pharmacology & Toxicology), Freie Universität Berlin, Königin-Luise-Str. 2+4, 14195 Berlin, Germany; roberta_rigon@yahoo.com.br (R.B.R.); christopher.wolff@fu-berlin.de (C.W.); christian.hausmann@fu-berlin.de (C.H.); nan.zhang@fu-berlin.de (N.Z.); Monika.Schaefer-Korting@fu-berlin.de (M.S.-K.)

2 Institute of Veterinary Anatomy, Department of Veterinary Medicine, Freie Universität Berlin, Koserstr. 20, 14195 Berlin, Germany; sabine.kaessmeyer@fu-berlin.de

3 Faculty of Pharmacy, Charles University, Akademika Heyrovského 1203, 50005 Hradec Králové, Czech Republic; sochormi@faf.cuni.cz (M.S.); kovacika@faf.cuni.cz (A.K.); katerina.vavrova@faf.cuni.cz (K.V.)

4 Institute of Chemistry and Biochemistry, Freie Universität Berlin, Takustr. 3, 14195 Berlin, Germany; Germany; haag@chemie.fu-berlin.de

5 Collegium Medicum Berlin, Luisenstr. 54, 10117 Berlin, Germany; ulrich@dermatologie-am-regierungsviertel.de

* Correspondence: christian.zoschke@fu-berlin.de

† These authors contributed equally to this work.

‡ Present address: UNESP—Universidade Estadual Paulista "Júlio de Mesquita Filho", Faculdade de Ciências Farmacêuticas, Rodovia Araraquara Jaú, Km 01-s/n, 14800-903 Araraquara, Brazil.

Abstract: Aging depicts one of the major challenges in pharmacology owing to its complexity and heterogeneity. Thereby, advanced glycated end-products modify extracellular matrix proteins, but the consequences on the skin barrier function remain heavily understudied. Herein, we utilized transmission electron microscopy for the ultrastructural analysis of ribose-induced glycated reconstructed human skin (RHS). Molecular and functional insights substantiated the ultrastructural characterization and proved the relevance of glycated RHS beyond skin aging. In particular, electron microscopy mapped the accumulation and altered spatial orientation of fibrils and filaments in the dermal compartment of glycated RHS. Moreover, the epidermal basement membrane appeared thicker in glycated than in non-glycated RHS, but electron microscopy identified longitudinal clusters of the finest collagen fibrils instead of real thickening. The *stratum granulosum* contained more cell layers, the morphology of keratohyalin granules decidedly differed, and the *stratum corneum* lipid order increased in ribose-induced glycated RHS, while the skin barrier function was almost not affected. In conclusion, dermal advanced glycated end-products markedly changed the epidermal morphology, underlining the importance of matrix–cell interactions. The phenotype of ribose-induced glycated RHS emulated aged skin in the dermis, while the two to three times increased thickness of the *stratum granulosum* resembled poorer cornification.

Keywords: advanced glycated end products; aging; diabetes; electron microscopy; nanomedicine; ribose; reconstructed human skin; skin absorption

1. Introduction

Age-related changes in human physiology become increasingly relevant, because life expectancy is rising as fast as the number of geriatric and often multimorbid patients. Aging comprises the functional impairment of cells, tissues, and organs, which promotes diseases like diabetes or cancer [1]. However, drug treatment of elderly patients remains challenging, as drug development mainly focuses on tests in juvenile cells and humans. While drug metabolism and elimination are known to change over lifetime, alterations in the pharmacodynamics of drugs depict a significant knowledge gap—not only in dementia [2].

One hallmark of aging is the accumulation of advanced glycated end-products (AGEs), although increased amounts of AGEs are also found in diabetes and psoriasis [3,4]. Being exclusively removed by protein turn over, AGEs accumulate in proteins with long half-lives. Thus, the collagen half-life of 15 years in skin and 117 years in cartilage fosters the accumulation of AGEs [5]. As products of the non-enzymatic reaction of sugars or aldehydes with proteins, AGEs comprise a heterogeneous group of molecules including pentosidine and *N*-carboxymethyl-lysine (CML).

Several nonclinical models of skin aging tried to emulate the long process of aging in vitro, by exposing juvenile reconstructed human skin (RHS) either to ribose, glyoxal, glyceraldehyde, or specific AGEs [6–10]. As the consequences of extracellular matrix (ECM) glycation depend on the stressor in vitro and strongly deviate among the protocols for RHS glycation, we were intrigued in the unknown effects of AGEs in RHS on epithelial proliferation and differentiation.

Herein, we studied the effects of ECM glycation on the ultrastructure of cellular and extracellular parts of RHS by transmission electron microscopy (TEM) and compared the morphology to juvenile, non-glycated RHS. TEM proved already useful to study subcellular interactions during vascular morphogenesis in 3D cocultures between endothelial cells and fibroblasts [11]. Moreover, we investigated the morphology of ribose-induced glycated RHS by reflectance confocal microscopy, being clinically used for the evaluation of skin cancer and aging [12,13]. Next, we analyzed the protein expression as well as the *stratum corneum* lipid prolife and their spatial orientation. Finally, we studied the effect of collagen glycation on the absorption of reference compounds and the efficacy of an investigative new drug delivery system.

2. Results

2.1. Selection of Glycation Agent

We exposed normal human dermal fibroblasts (NHDF) and keratinocytes (NHK) either to ribose or to glyoxal for 48 h. Next, we tested the efficiency of both glycation agents in producing AGEs in collagen following a three-week exposure to either ribose or glyoxal. The viability of both fibroblasts and keratinocytes markedly declined by up to 87% even in trace concentrations of the reagents (Figure 1a). As ribose and glyoxal induced comparable amounts of AGEs in collagen (Figure 1b), we selected the collagen, glycated with ribose, to build glycated RHS. After three weeks of RHS culture, we still detected 1.4-fold increased levels of *N*-carboxymethyl-lysine (CML), a hallmark AGE, in the dermal compartment of glycated RHS. The accumulation of CML was even higher (1.9-fold increase) in the epidermal compartment, although ribose has been removed from the collagen by dialysis prior to RHS building. Accordingly, the expression of the receptor of AGEs (RAGE) was elevated in the entire glycated RHS (Section 2.5).

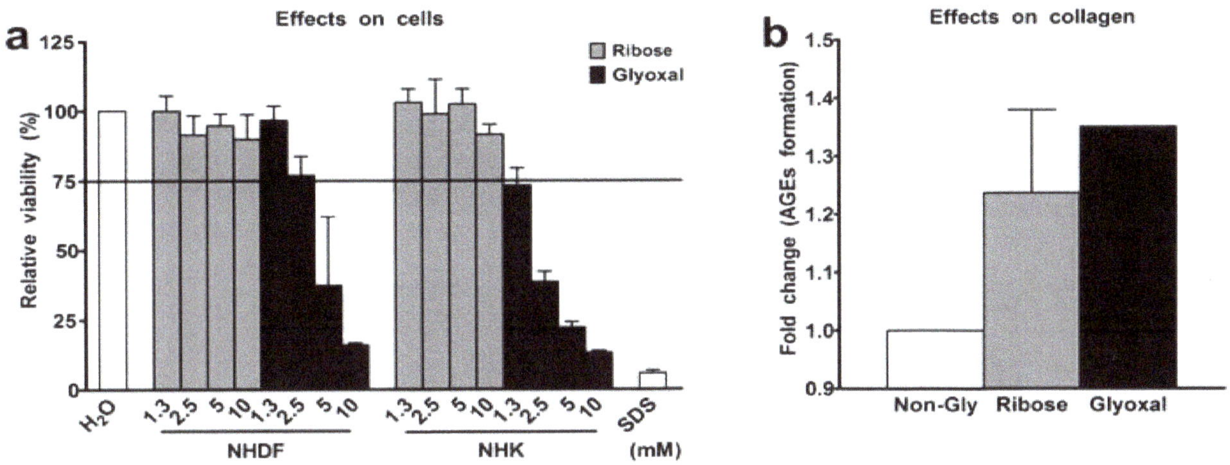

Figure 1. Selection of glycation agent. (**a**) Viability of normal human dermal fibroblasts (NHDF) and normal human keratinocytes (NHK) following exposure to ribose or glyoxal for 48 h. (**b**) Advanced glycation end-products (AGEs) in collagen following the exposure to 10 mM ribose or 10 mM glyoxal. $n = 3$, mean + SD.

2.2. RHS Morphology

Both glycated and non-glycated RHS showed a stratified epidermis, but the epidermal compartment of glycated RHS was 1.3 ± 0.18-fold thicker than the epidermis of non-glycated RHS. Moreover, glycated RHS appeared yellowish during the culture period (Figure 2).

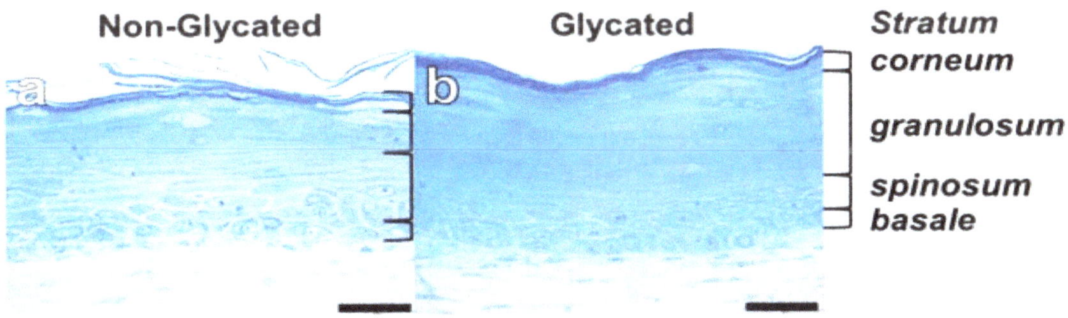

Figure 2. Reconstructed human skin (RHS) morphology. Semi-thin sections of (**a**) non-glycated and (**b**) glycated RHS. Light microscopy, bar = 50 μm.

2.3. Dermal Ultrastructure

Next, we analyzed the dermal morphology of glycated RHS and compared it with non-glycated RHS. The dermal compartment was divided into a *stratum papillare,* connected to the *stratum basale* of the epidermal compartment and the deeper *stratum reticulare.* Reflectance confocal microscopy (RCM) proved a homogenous dermal compartment in non-glycated RHS (Figure 3a) and collagen aggregates (white structures in Figure 3b) in the *stratum papillare* of glycated RHS. These findings were corroborated by TEM, where aggregates appeared as an accumulation of finest fibrils in the *stratum papillare* of glycated RHS. Those fibrils either orientated themselves longitudinally to the basal layer (mimicking a punctually developed basement membrane) or were cross-linked into densely organized ellipsoid structures, comprising an area of approximately 8.4 μm × 5.0 μm (Figure 3d). The fine fibrils within these structures were virtually uniformly parallel and appeared in a wave-like pattern (Figure 3f). Furthermore, areas with a locally higher density of collagen fibrils were identified in both *stratum papillare* and *stratum reticulare* of the glycated RHS. Fibrils of about 38 nm diameter appeared densely-packed while fibrils of about 160 nm were loosely packed. It is noteworthy that the collagen fibrils are aligned parallel to the *stratum basale* in the glycated RHS (Figure 3h,k). In contrast, filaments and collagen fibrils aligned randomly in both parallel and perpendicular directions to the *stratum basale* within *stratum reticulare* of non-glycated RHS (Figure 3g,i). Overall, the fibrils and filaments accumulated locally in the glycated RHS, while they were disseminated in the non-glycated RHS. Interestingly, fibroblasts within both RHS exhibited a spread shape and contained a large amount of rough endoplasmic reticulum. Moreover, on average, fibroblast numbers in the *stratum papillare* exceeded those in the *stratum reticulare* about two-fold in both RHS.

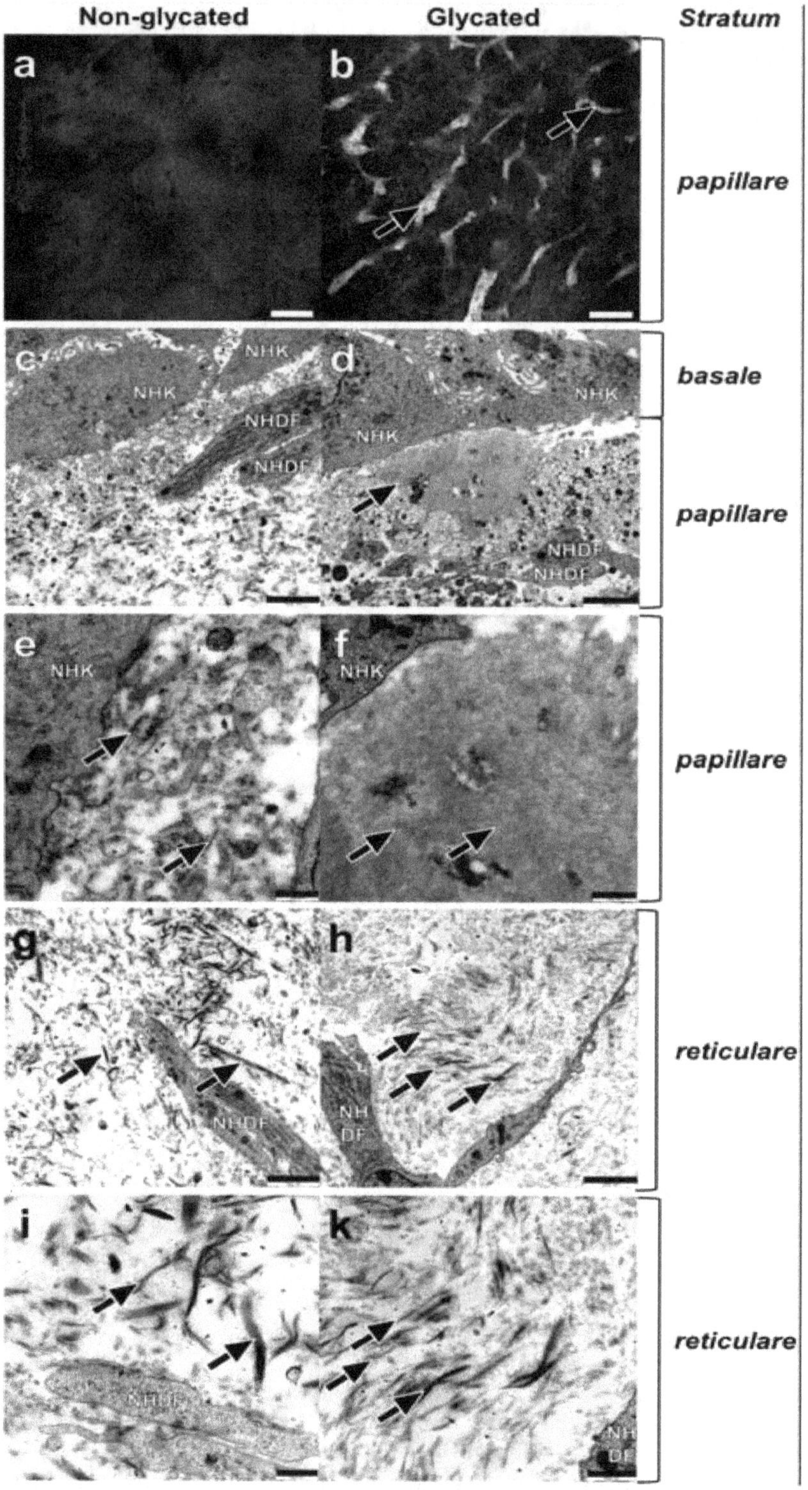

Figure 3. Dermal ultrastructure of (**a**,**c**,**e**,**g**,**i**) non-glycated and (**b**,**d**,**f**,**h**,**k**) glycated RHS. (**a**) Homogenous and (**b**) aggregated collagen in the *stratum papillare*. (**c**–**f**) Ultrastructure of the *stratum papillare*.

Fibroblasts (NHDF), cell fragments, and vesicles, as well as filaments and fibrils of various sizes bordering the keratinocytes (NHK) of the *stratum basale.* (**c**,**e**) Lower concentration of the structural elements in non-glycated dermal compartment filaments with ((**e**) magnification of (**c**)) fibrils of various sizes (arrows). (**d**,**f**) Local accumulations of thin, densely organized structures in glycated RHS, nearby the *stratum basale* (arrow) ((**f**) magnification of (**d**)), finest cross-linked filaments with a wave-like pattern constitute densely organized structures (arrows). (**g**–**k**) Ultrastructure of *stratum reticulare.* (**g**,**i**) Collagen fibers (arrows) show a disorientated pattern in all directions ((**i**) magnification of (**g**)). Collagen fibers with different sizes in non-glycated RHS (arrows). (**h**,**k**) Collagen fibrils axially orientated to the *stratum basale* ((**k**) magnification of (**h**)) the thinner the fibrils, the more densely they are packed. Densely packed fine fibrils and loosely packed thicker fibrils (arrows). (**a**,**b**) Reflectance confocal microscopy, bar = 100 μm; (**c**,**d**,**g**,**h**) transmission electron microscopy (TEM), bar = 2.5 μm; (**e**,**f**,**i**,**k**) TEM, bar = 1.0 μm.

2.4. Epidermal Ultrastructure

TEM analysis of the epidermal compartments revealed striking differences between glycated and non-glycated RHS, especially in the thickness and number of cell layers of the *stratum granulosum* (Figure 4c,d).

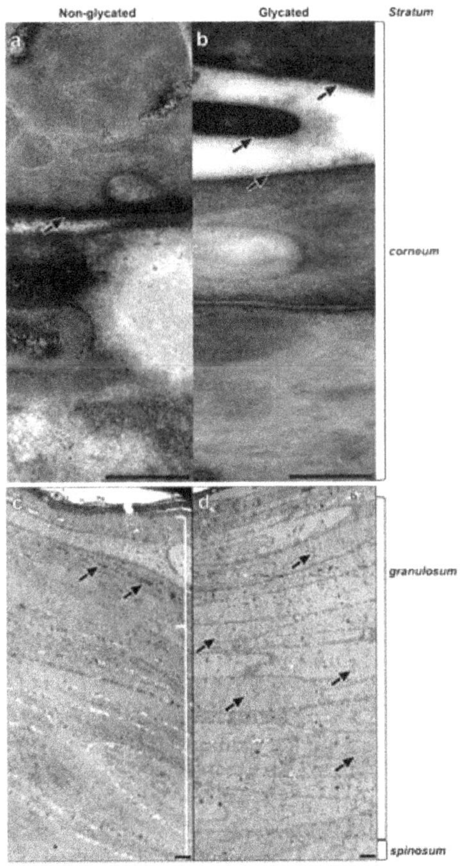

Figure 4. Epidermal ultrastructure of (**a**,**c**) non-glycated and (**b**,**d**) glycated RHS. (**a**) Lipid lamellae within the intercellular space of neighboring corneocytes. (**b**) Fine lines of the intercellular lipids are clearly visible (arrows). (**c**) Packed keratohyalin granule-like structures (arrows) in the upper layers of the viable epidermis, indicating the *stratum granulosum.* (**d**) The *stratum granulosum* dominates the epidermal compartment. Fine electron dense material evenly disseminated within the cytoplasm of the keratinocytes (arrows). Pictures are representative for two batches. (**a**,**b**). TEM, bar = 0.25 μm; (**c**,**d**) TEM, bar = 2.5 μm.

The *stratum spinosum* of non-glycated RHS contained seven layers on average, comprising a decidedly greater proportion of the viable epidermis than in glycated RHS. The *stratum granulosum* of non-glycated RHS constituted on average three layers of tightly packed cells with mitochondria and large, irregularly shaped keratohyalin granules (Figure 4c).

In the glycated RHS, the keratinocytes in the basal layer were columnar and cuboidal shaped. The *stratum spinosum* contained four layers on average, while more than 20 cell layers were designated as *stratum granulosum*, comprising the majority of keratinocytes within the epidermis of glycated RHS. These keratinocytes were increasingly flattened and densely packed. Atypical keratohyalin granules were present as fine, disseminated electron dense material. Although this material slightly differed from the keratohyalin granules in non-glycated RHS, we regarded this material as small keratohyalin granules. Moreover, the number of mitochondria and other cell organelles decreased, especially in the apical parts of the *stratum granulosum* (Figure 4d).

In both constructs, the keratinocytes transformed into flat, tightly packed corneocytes, attaching themselves to each other via corneodesmosomes. *Stratum corneum* of non-glycated RHS consisted of seven layers of corneocytes, which increased to twelve layers in glycated RHS. While a cornified envelope was developed in both types of RHS, the lipids in the glycated models were slightly clearer to visualize and distinguish from the plasma membrane than in non-glycated RHS (Figure 4a,b). This deviating ultrastructure points to different lipid organization in non-glycated and glycated RHS.

2.5. Molecular Analysis

The expressions of the adhesion molecule β1-integrin and laminin-5 slightly increased within the basal layer of the glycated RHS and faded in the suprabasal epidermal layers (Figure 5). In contrast, filaggrin expression markedly decreased and loricrin expression strongly increased in glycated compared with non-glycated RHS.

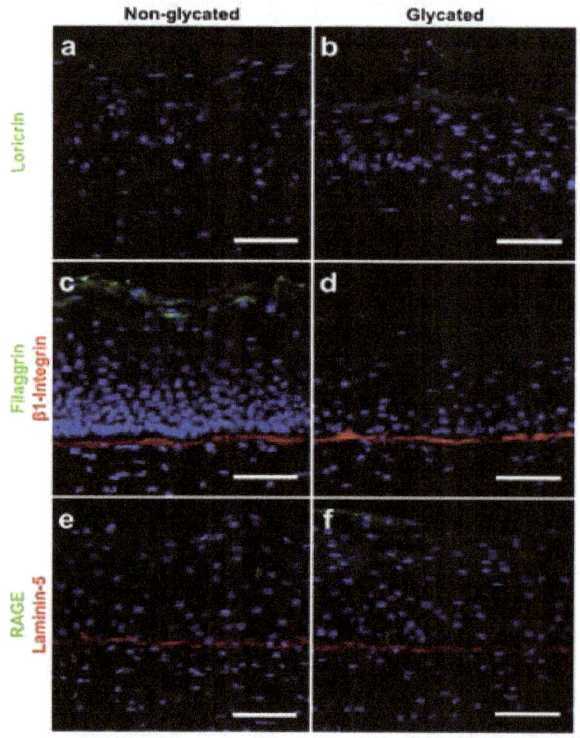

Figure 5. Immunolocalization of proteins in (**a**,**c**,**e**) non-glycated and (**b**,**d**,**f**) glycated RHS. Glycated RHS showed (**a**,**b**) loricrin upregulation, (**c**,**d**) filaggrin downregulation and slight increase in β1-integrin expression, and (**e**,**f**) slight upregulation of both receptor of AGEs (RAGE) and laminin-5 expression compared with non-glycated RHS. Proteins in green or red, cell nuclei (DAPI staining) in blue. Fluorescence microscopy, bar = 100 μm. Pictures are representative for two to four batches.

The arrangement of the intercellular lipids in the *stratum corneum* was probed by Fourier-transform infrared (FT-IR) spectroscopy. The lower wavenumbers of the methylene symmetric stretching vibrations (2851.8 $\pm$ 0.7 cm^{-1} in glycated compared with 2852.8 $\pm$ 1.0 cm^{-1} in non-glycated RHS, $p > 0.05$) indicated a higher proportion of all-trans chain conformers in the chain [14], and thus an improved lipid chain order in glycated RHS (Figure 6a). High performance thin layer chromatography of *stratum corneum* lipids revealed slight compositional differences. The *stratum corneum* lipids in the non-glycated RHS were composed of 7:5:1 FFA/Chol/Cer, while glycated RHS revealed a molar ratio of 5:3:1 (FFA/Chol/Cer). The absolute amounts of free fatty acids (FFA), cholesterol (Chol), and cholesterol sulphate (CholS) apparently decreased in glycated RHS ($p \leq 0.05$), while the levels of the levels of ceramide precursors remained unchanged ($p > 0.05$). The respective values read as follows: FFA, 28.5 $\pm$ 21.0 and 20.9 $\pm$ 14.8 μg/mg *stratum corneum* in non-glycated and glycated RHS; Chol, 19.9 $\pm$ 8.6 and 16.9 $\pm$ 5.5 μg/mg; and CholS, 3.1 $\pm$ 1.4 and 1.8 $\pm$ 0.9 μg/mg ($p = 0.051$). The respective amounts of Cer precursors read sphingomyelin (SM) 8.3 $\pm$ 3.7 and 8.5 $\pm$ 3.7 μg/mg, glucosylceramides (GCer) 5.6 $\pm$ 0.8 and 7.2 $\pm$ 5.4 μg/mg, and phospholipids (PL) 9.9 $\pm$ 6.1 and 11.3 $\pm$ 5.1 μg/mg (Figure 6b). The amounts of ceramides (Cer) subclasses, Cer EO(d)S (0.39 $\pm$ 0.37 and 0.31 $\pm$ 0.15 μg/mg, $p > 0.05$), Cer NP (2.62 $\pm$ 0.71 and 2.69 $\pm$ 0.91 μg/mg, $p > 0.05$), Cer AS+NH (0.90 $\pm$ 0.46 and 0.98 $\pm$ 1.34 μg/mg, $p > 0.05$), and Cer AP+AH (0.68 $\pm$ 0.56 and 0.78 $\pm$ 1.05 μg/mg, $p > 0.05$) did not change. In contrast, the total amounts of Cer (8.7 $\pm$ 4.7 and 12.7 $\pm$ 7.9 μg/mg, $p > 0.05$) and, in particular, Cer N(d)S (4.06 $\pm$ 3.53 and 7.98 $\pm$ 7.18 μg/mg, $p > 0.05$) apparently increased in glycated RHS (Figure 6b,c).

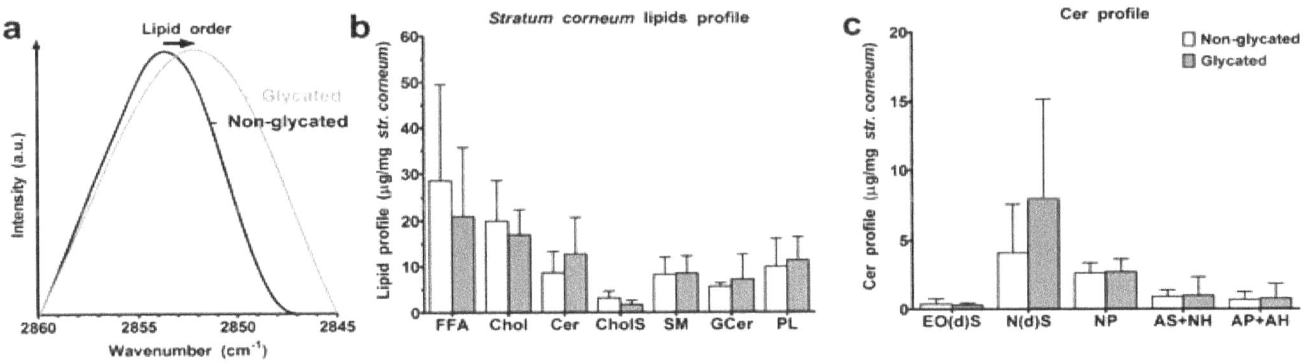

Figure 6. *Stratum corneum* lipids. (**a**) Lipid order. (**b**) *Stratum corneum* lipid profile of non-glycated and glycated RHS for free fatty acids (FFA), cholesterol (Chol), ceramides (Cer), cholesterol sulphate (CholS), sphingomyelin (SM), glucosylceramides (GCer), and phospholipids (PL). (**c**) Ceramide profile, for ceramide nomenclature, see Figure 8; $n = 3–4$, mean + SD.

2.6. Skin Barrier Function

Next, we studied the barrier function of glycated RHS. We found comparable caffeine permeation over 6 h (Figure 7a), with apparent permeability (P_{app}) values of 7.6 and 6.6 $\times$ 10^{-6} cm/s ($p > 0.05$) in non-glycated and glycated RHS, respectively. The lag-time increased from 26 min in non-glycated to 44 min in ribose-induced glycated RHS. However, this trend was not statistical significant.

Finally, we evaluated the delivery of the fluorescent drug surrogate Bodipy, either in base cream or loaded to dendritic core-multishell (CMS) nanotransporters into RHS (Figure 7b–g). Bodipy and CMS nanotransporters penetrated the *stratum corneum* of both glycated and non-glycated RHS. While Bodipy readily penetrated viable epidermal layers in the non-glycated RHS, this uptake appeared slightly reduced in glycated RHS (Figure 7c,f). However, Bodipy uptake was enhanced by CMS nanotransporters compared with cream in both non-glycated and glycated RHS (Figure 7b,c,e,f).

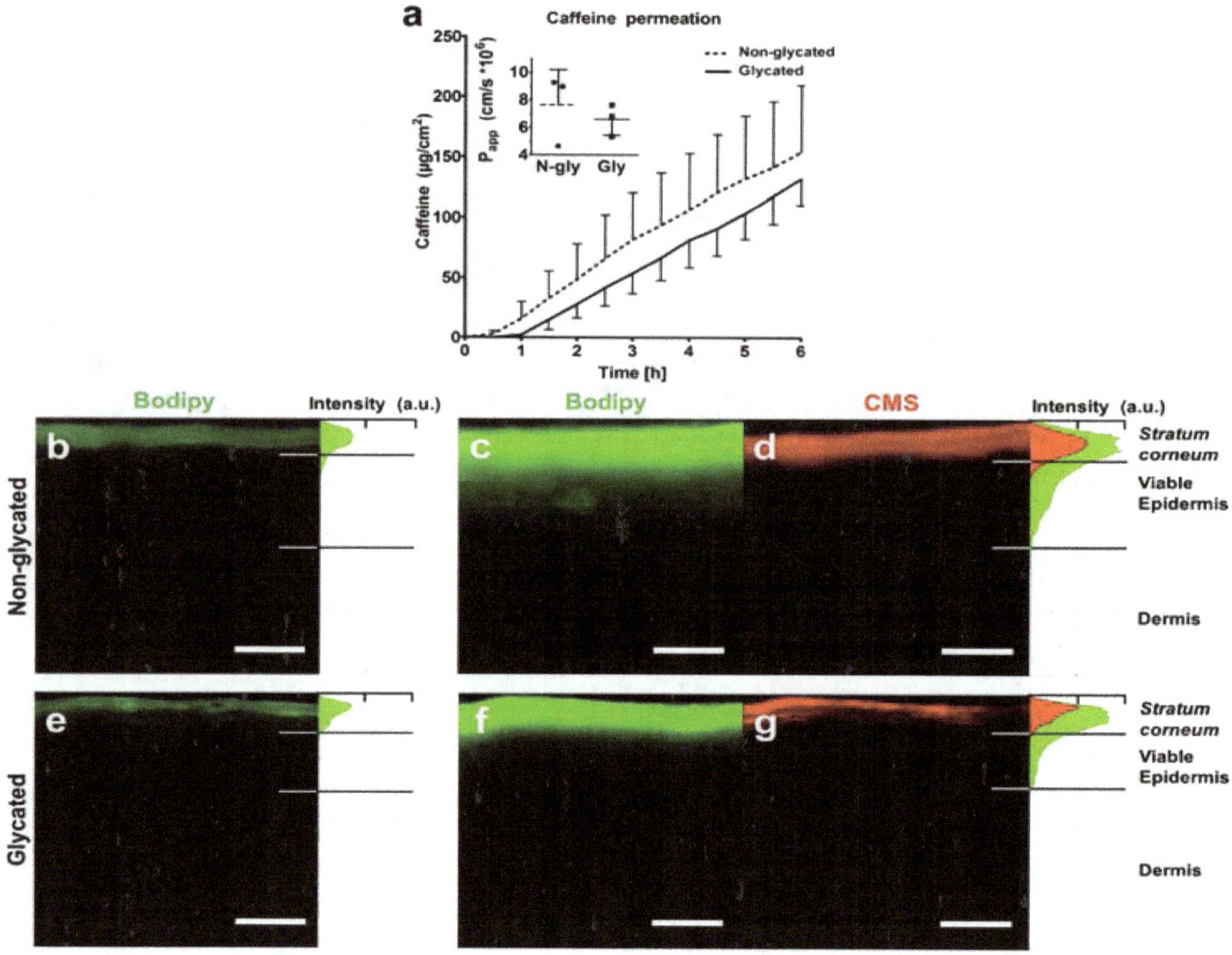

Figure 7. Skin barrier function. (**a**) Caffeine permeation through non-glycated and glycated RHS. The inset shows the respective P_{app} values. (**b**) Penetration of Bodipy cream and (**c**,**d**) Bodipy-core-multishell (CMS) into non-glycated RHS. (**e**) Penetration of Bodipy cream and (**f**,**g**) Bodipy-CMS into glycated RHS. (**c**,**d**,**f**,**g**) CMS labelled with red fluorescent indocarbocyanine. Fluorescence microscopy, bar = 100 µm, $n = 3$, mean ± SD.

3. Discussion

The complex and heterogeneous nature of skin aging challenges the relevant and reliable emulation of ageing hallmarks in vitro. However, RHS proved to be a powerful tool to mimic at least some important features of skin diseases like atopic dermatitis, psoriasis, and non-melanoma skin cancer [15–17]. In order to mimic aged skin, the ECM of juvenile RHS was exposed to either ribose glyoxal or specific AGEs. These artificial glycation stimuli are necessary to speed up the slow amino carbonylation by glucose. We selected ribose because of its biocompatibility and its glycation efficiency (Figure 1). In contrast to glyoxal, ribose did not affect the viability of skin cells. Moreover, ribose not only produces structurally similar AGEs [18], but also reacts faster than glucose [19]. Nevertheless, the effects of glycation appear to depend on the glycation agent; with ribose and glyoxal being the most frequently used compounds [8,9,20]. Granted that aged skin is sufficiently perfused in vivo, the oxidative environment should favor glycation by sugars [21].

The increased stiffness of the dermal ECM by collagen cross-linking depicts one hallmark of aged skin [22]. Ribose glycation reliably mimicked this morphology as reflectance confocal microscopy showed collagen aggregates and the ultrastructural analysis revealed the altered alignment and higher amounts of collagen fibers and fibrils in glycated RHS (Figure 3). Moreover, we proved the interdependency between fibril diameter and packing, as well as a hierarchy of fiber accumulation. While densely packed fibrils are smaller in diameter, loosely packed collagen fibrils showed larger diameters (Figure 3). The overall architecture of the dermal compartment in glycated RHS showed more or less axially orientated collagen fibrils. Cross-linking of the fibrils resulted in their dissociation to finer structures. Accumulations of increasingly finer cross-linked fibrils in densely packed structures resembled stiffly plaques within the skin. These changes in ECM also explain the lost dermal flexibility in diabetic patients [3] and are not limited to skin, but apply also to glycated vascular walls or tendons. In accordance, glycation in vivo increases fibril packing density, the range of fibril diameters, and the fusion of fibrils in tendons of diabetes patients [4].

The effects of dermal collagen glycation go beyond the mechanical alterations of dermal ECM. This is particular intriguing, as epidermal changes are induced either by traces of ribose (despite of the extensive dialysis to eliminate the glycation agent) or by AGEs or by altered paracrine signaling between fibroblasts and keratinocytes in glycated RHS. We argue for the latter, because the mechanical separation of glycated ECM and the epidermal compartments did not impair the effects of AGEs on keratinocytes [23]. Moreover, the constant paracrine signaling likely transduces stress signals from fibroblasts to keratinocytes [24].

In particular, the basement membrane appeared thicker in glycated RHS, although RHS in general lacks the sub-basal laminae of the basement membrane [25]. This alteration is well in accordance with the increased collagen-IV expression in glycated RHS [23], but the ultrastructural analysis identified longitudinal clusters of finest collagen fibrils to mimic a thick *lamina fibroreticularis* (fibroblast derived) of the basement membrane (Figure 3). Increased laminin-5 expression (Figure 4) nicely supports this hypothesis. As one of the principal structural elements of the basement membrane, laminin establishes networks with other proteins like collagens and determines the basement membranes common structure [26]. It is tempting to speculate that these structures emulate the age-specific reduplication of the lamina densa and its associated anchoring fibril complex as observed in vivo [27].

Moreover, we observed enhanced keratinocyte proliferation in glycated RHS, indicated by the increase in total epidermal thickness (Figures 2 and 4). In our study, more than 20 cell layers corresponded to the *stratum granulosum*, containing disseminated electron dense material, which we interpreted as atypical keratohyalin granules. Absent keratohyalin and increased *stratum granulosum* height were described in particular types of psoriatic epidermis [28,29]. The increased thickness of the *stratum granulosum* indicates defective differentiation of the transitional located keratinocytes of the *stratum granulosum* and thus resembles parakeratotic psoriatic skin. The increased expression of loricrin was well in accordance with the abundant fine granula in the epidermal compartment of glycated RHS (Figure 5) [30]. In fact, keratinocytes with atypical keratohyalin granules dominated the epidermal compartment as "*stratum intermedium*" of glycated RHS. Furthermore, we observed changes in the intercellular space of the *stratum corneum* (Figure 4), which intrigued us to investigate the *stratum corneum* lipid order and profile.

We found an apparent, although not statistically significant, trend to increased Cer amounts in glycated RHS, being accompanied by the significantly improved lipid order (Figure 6). The apparent increase in Cer levels without a change in the SM and GCer concentrations suggests enhanced Cer synthesis de novo, with similar activities of sphingomyelinase and β-glucocerebrosidase. The improved chain order of barrier lipids would explain the trend to reduced permeability of glycated RHS as the membranes with fully stretched all-trans lipid chains would provide a stronger barrier to permeating substances than that with more fluid mobile lipids. This was applied to small molecules like caffeine, a recommended test compound for percutaneous absorption experiments by the Organisation for Economic Co-operation and Development, as well as to Bodipy 493/503, which shares the physicochemical properties of glucocorticoids. As with non-glycated RHS, macromolecules like CMS nanotransporters do not surmount the *stratum corneum* (Figure 7). This is well in accordance with previous models with intact skin barrier and suggests a penetration enhancing effect of CMS nanotransporters beyond simply carrying their cargo [31].

Our results are well in accordance with previous ribose-based approaches, but are not in line with glyoxal induced effects [6,32]. Moreover, we found a deviating *stratum corneum* lipid profile from glycated reconstructed human epidermis [7]. These changes might be attributed to the glycation method or the fact that reconstructed human epidermis lack the cross-talk between fibroblasts and keratinocytes. Even glyoxal impaired the skin barrier function in excised murine skin only after 72 h of direct exposure [7]. Culturing reconstructed human epidermis on a basement membrane surrogate, glycated by glyceraldehyde, resulted in decreased filaggrin expression and skin barrier function [10]. Although we found similar changes in the protein expressions, we could not confirm an impaired barrier function due to collagen glycation. In fact, neither caffeine (M_r 194; log*P* 0.08), Bodipy (M_r 262.1; log*P* 3.5), nor CMS nanotransporter (M_r 74,000) were absorbed better into glycated RHS compared with non-glycated RHS. As fluorescence readings provide only a first insight, further studies on the trans-epidermal resistance of glycated human skin ex vivo might explain these deviating results. Taking into account the cytotoxic effects of aldehydes on keratinocytes, the constructs in both aldehyde-based studies might overestimate the impaired barrier function due to glycation.

Glycation induced aged or diabetic phenotypes in the dermis, while the glycated dermal ECM did not cause these phenotypes in the epidermal compartment of RHS. The increased epidermal thickness with incomplete differentiation resembles a psoriasis-like epidermal morphology. Correlating to increased granulocyte-macrophage colony-stimulating factor and interleukin-6 expression, the reduced filaggrin expression hinted towards an inflammatory RHS phenotype [33,34]. Moreover, keratinocytes in the level of *stratum granulosum* also lacked normal keratohyalin granules and pointed to a disturbed keratinization process with defective tonofibrillar differentiation—similar to psoriatic skin [35]. Nevertheless, glycation alone would not be suitable to emulate psoriatic skin, because neither immune cells nor Th-17 cytokines were added to the culture. Moreover, glycated RHS did not show the impaired barrier function of psoriatic skin [36]. Nevertheless, a clinical study proved increased amounts of AGEs in patients with severe psoriasis [3], and AGEs appeared to fuel cutaneous inflammation [37].

In conclusion, our study adds several missing links to the effects of AGEs on the cutaneous morphology and skin barrier function. Based on our results, glycation of the ECM markedly affects epithelial differentiation, and thus should be considered when emulating (skin) diseases like diabetes, psoriasis, and skin cancer. The better understanding of the interactions between matrix and cells will help to improve the pharmacological treatment of these diseases. Finally, the ultrastructural analysis proved indispensable, especially for matrix effects, and should be used complementarily with molecular analyses in the characterization of human cell-based models.

4. Materials and Methods

4.1. Collagen Glycation

Collagen was glycated as described previously [9]. In brief, collagen G (4 mg bovine collagen per mL; Biochrom, Berlin, Germany) was incubated with 10 mM D-ribose (Sigma Aldrich, München, Germany) in phosphate-buffered saline (PBS) at room temperature for three weeks and protected against light. Moreover, collagen G was incubated with PBS only as negative control and with 10 mM glyoxal (Sigma Aldrich, München, Germany) for comparison. Subsequently, glycated collagen was extensively dialyzed in sterile water at 4 °C for 48 h, using Spectra/Por® 4 Dry Standard RC Dialysis Tubing, 12–14 kD molecular weight cut-off, 32 mm flat width, 100 ft length (132703; Spectrum, Henderson, NV, USA). The sterile water was changed every 12 h. Following the dialysis, we subjected the samples to fluorescence analysis (Hitachi F-4500; Hitachi, Tokyo, Japan) to detect AGEs. Therefore, 1.5 mL glycated collagen was digested by pepsin (1 mg pepsin in 5 mL of 0.5 M acetic acid) at 37 °C overnight. The solution was centrifuged at 10,000× *g* for 5 min, the supernatant, containing the digested collagen, was measured at λ_{ex} 370 nm/λ_{em} 440 nm for total AGEs [9].

4.2. Cell Culture and Viability

Cell viability was assessed by 3-(4,5-dimethylthiazol-2-yl)-2,5 diphenyltetrazolium bromide (MTT; Sigma Aldrich, München, Germany) reduction as previously described [38]. In brief, NHK (passage 3) and NHDF (passage 3) were isolated from therapeutically indicated circumcision with permission (ethical approval EA1/081/13). Cell culture was performed according to standard operating procedures, and referring to good cell culture practice. We used 0.005% [*w*/*v*] sodium dodecyl sulphate (SDS) as positive control and 10% [*v*/*v*] double distilled, sterile water as solvent control.

4.3. Reconstructed Human Skin (RHS)

RHS was built in three steps [15]. First, 1 mL acellular collagen G or a 1:1 mixture of collagen G and glycated collagen G was poured into a cell-culture insert (Corning, Corning, NY, USA) and incubated for 2 h to form a gel. Second, fibroblasts (0.8×10^6 cells per construct) were added to 3 mL collagen G or a 1:1 mixture of collagen G and glycated collagen G, poured onto the acellular collagen, and incubated for 24 h. The dermal equivalents were submerse cultured for seven days in construct growth medium (CGM: Dulbecco's modified eagle's medium /F12 + GlutaMax supplemented with 10% fetal calf serum, 1% Pen/Strep, adenine HCl monohydrate 40 μM, amphotericin B 30 μg/L, choleratoxin 0.1 nM, epidermal growth factor 10 μg/L, hydrocortisone 3.5 mg/L, insulin 4.4 mg/L, non-essential amino acids 0.5%, transferrin 4.4 mg/L, triiodothyronine 2 nM). Third, NHK (3.0×10^6 per construct) were seeded onto the dermal compartment at day 8. RHS were raised to the air–liquid interface at day 10 and cultured in construct differentiation medium (CDM: CGM supplemented with ascorbic acid 0.25 mM, calcium chloride 2 mM). The culture medium was changed three times a week. At day 21, the constructs were subjected to further analyses as described below.

4.4. Reflectance Confocal Microscopy (RCM) and Immunolocalization of Proteins

RCM was performed with VivaScope® 3000 (MAVIG; München, Germany). Subsequently, the constructs were snap frozen, sectioned into 7 μm slices (Leica CM 1510S; Wetzlar, Germany), and analyzed by immunofluorescence staining [15]. Antibodies against the following antigens were purchased from Abcam (Cambridge, UK): filaggrin (1:1000; ab81468), carboxymethyl lysine (1:100; ab27684), human integrin beta 1 (1:100; ab3167); and from Thermo Fisher Scientific (Darmstadt, Germany): loricrin (1:500; PA5-34945). Immunofluorescence staining was performed according to standard protocols. Pictures were taken with a fluorescence microscope (BZ-8000, Keyence; Keyence, Neu-Isenburg, Germany) and analyzed with BZAnalyzer and ImageJ software. Five individual measurements per construct were performed observer-blinded (RBR, CH, CW, CZ).

4.5. Transmission Electron Microscopy (TEM)

RHS was fixed in Karnovsky solution (7.5% glutaraldehyde and 3% paraformaldehyde in phosphate buffered saline) for 4 h, then washed in 0.1 M cacodylate buffer (cacodylic acid sodium salt trihydrate; Roth, Karlsruhe, Germany) and incubated in 1% osmium tetroxide (Chempur; Karlsruhe, Germany) for 120 min. Dehydration was performed in an ascending series of ethanol. Finally, the models were washed in the intermedium propylene oxide (1,2 Epoxypropan; VWR, Darmstadt, Germany).

Embedding of RHS was performed in a mixture of agar 100 (epoxy resin), DDSA (softener), Epoxy embedding medium (hardener), and DMP 30 (catalyst) (all: Agar Scientific, Stansted, UK), followed by polymerization at 45 °C and 55 °C, each for 24 h. Semi- and ultrathin sections were cut using an ultra-microtome Reichert Ultracut S (Leica, Wetzlar, Germany) and the semi-thin sections (0.5 μm) were stained with modified Richardson solution [39] for 45 s at 80 °C.

Semi-thin sections were examined under light microscopy Olympus CX21 (Olympus, Stuttgart, Germany). Next, ultrathin (80 nm) sections were mounted on nickel-grids (Agar Scientific). The RHS morphology was assessed with an electron microscope (ZeissEM109, Oberkochen, Germany). Images were taken and processed using Adobe® Photoshop® (Adobe® Systems, San José, CA, USA).

4.6. Carboxymethyl Lysine Quantification

RHS was separated into epidermal and dermal compartments and dissected. Thereafter, constructs were transferred to tubes containing 300 μL (epidermis) or 700 μL (dermis) PBS and a 5 mm stainless steel bead and immediately disintegrated using Tissue Lyser II (Qiagen, Hilden, Germany) at 25 Hz for 5 min. The lysed suspensions were analyzed for *N*-carboxymethyl-lysine content by OxiSelect™ ELISA (Cell Biolabs; San Diego, CA, USA) according to the manufacturers' instructions.

4.7. Stratum Corneum Lipid Analysis

The *stratum corneum* of RHS was isolated, and subjected to infrared spectroscopy using a Nicolet 6700 spectrometer (Thermo Fisher Scientific, Waltham, MA, USA) equipped with a single-reflection MIRacle attenuated total reflectance ZnSe crystal (PIKE technologies, Madison, WI, USA) at 23 °C. The spectra were generated by co-addition of 256 scans collected at 4 cm^{-1} resolution and analyzed with the Bruker OPUS software. The exact peak positions were determined from second derivative spectra. The lipids were then extracted and analyzed by high performance thin layer chromatography (HPTLC; [40]). Briefly, the analysis was performed on silica gel 60 HPTLC plates (20 × 10 cm, Merck, Darmstadt, Germany). Cer subclasses, FFA, and Chol were separated using $CHCl_3$/MeOH/acetic acid 190:9:1.5 (*v*/*v*/*v*) mobile phase twice to the top of the plate, whereas GCer, SM, PL, and CholS were separated using $CHCl_3$/MeOH/acetic acid/H_2O 65:25:6:3. The lipids were visualized by dipping in a derivatization reagent (7.5% $CuSO_4$, 8% H_3PO_4, 10% MeOH in water) for 10 s, heating at 160 °C for 30 min, and quantitated by densitometry using TLC scanner 3 and WinCats software (Camag, Muttenz, Switzerland). For the used standard lipids and their calibration curve ranges, see Table 1; for ceramide nomenclature, see Figure 8. Cer and GCer were purchased from Avanti Polar Lipids (Alabaster, AL, USA). All other chemicals, including lignoceric acid, Chol, CholS, SM, and PL, were purchased from Sigma Aldrich (München, Germany). Non-commercially available Cer EOS and NH standards were synthesized according to previously published methods [41,42].

Table 1. Calibration curve ranges of lipid standards used for high performance thin layer chromatography (HPTLC) analysis. FFA—free fatty acid.

Lipid Standard		Calibration Curve Range [μg]
FFA	Lignoceric acid	0.5–12.5
Chol	Cholesterol	0.5–12.5
Cer	Ceramide EOS	0.05–1.25
	Ceramide NS	0.2–5
	Ceramide NP	0.4–9.5
	Ceramide AS	0.1–2.5
	Ceramide NH	0.15–4
	Ceramide AP	0.1–2.5
CholS	Cholesterol sulphate	0.105–2.474
SM	Sphingomyelin	0.211–4.947
GCer	Glucosylceramide	0.263–6.184
PL	Phospholipid	0.421–9.895

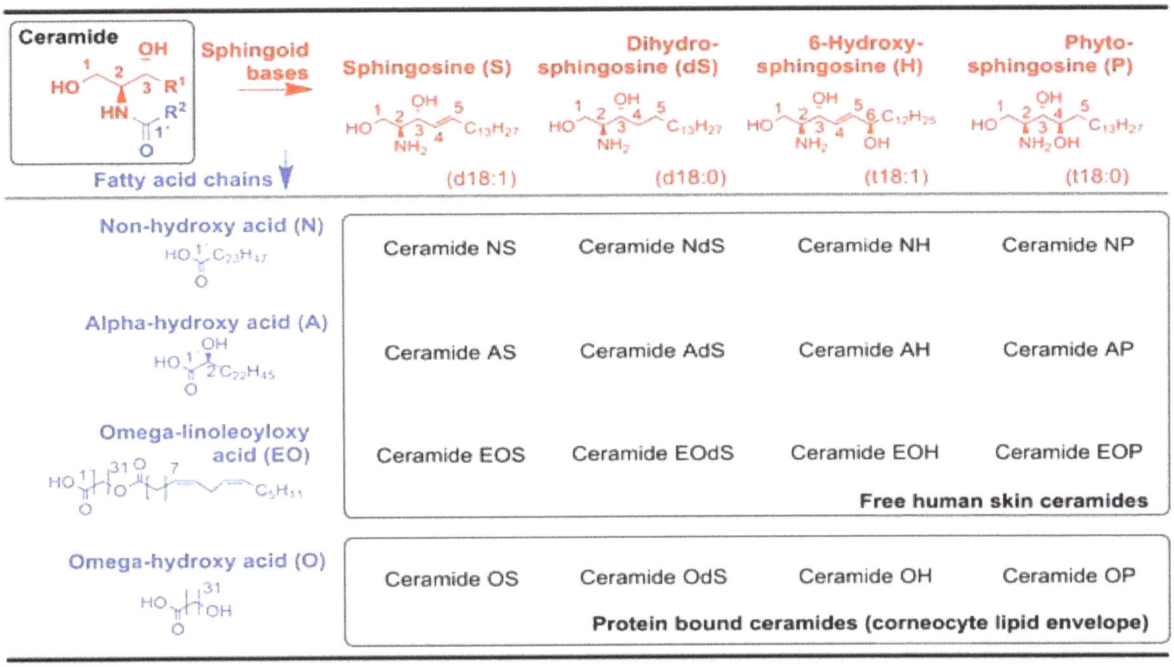

Figure 8. Ceramide nomenclature. Reprinted from the literature [15], Copyright 2016, with permission from Elsevier.

4.8. Skin Permeation

The permeation of radiolabeled [1-methyl^{14}C]caffeine (M_r 194; log$P$ 0.08; PerkinElmer, Waltham, MA, USA) was studied according to the validation study on the use of skin models for skin absorption testing [39]. In brief, tissue integrity of RHS was evaluated prior to mounting RHS in static Franz cells (∅ = 15 mm, with receptor chamber volume = 12 cm^3; PermeGear, Bethlehem, PA, USA). The stratum corneum was placed facing the air and the dermal compartment of RHS was in contact with the supporting membrane and the receptor medium PBS. The receptor medium was kept at a constant temperature of 33.5 ± 0.5 °C using a temperature-controlled water jacket, and stirred with a magnetic bar at 500 rpm. The absence of air bubbles was monitored throughout the experiment. Then, 281.4 μg/cm^2 caffeine was applied in aqueous solution onto the RHS surface. The opening of the Franz cell was covered by Parafilm® and the caffeine permeation was quantified from the receptor medium by radiochemical detection (Hidex 300 SL liquid scintillation counter; HIDEX, Turku, Finland).

4.9. Penetration of Bodipy Loaded Dendritic Core-Multishell Nanotransporters (Bodipy-CMS)

Bodipy 493/503 (λ_{ex} 493 nm; λ_{em} 503, M_r 262.1, log$P$ 3.5, Thermo Fisher Scientific; Darmstadt, Germany) was dispersed in base cream (13.6 mg/L Bodipy; 40.0% purified water, 25.5% white vaseline; 10.0% propylenglycol; 7.5% medium chain triglycerides; 7.0% macrogol-1000-glycerol monostearate; 6.0% cetyl alcohol; and 4.0% glycerol monostearate 60). Additionally, CMS nanotransporters [43] were labelled with indocarbocyanine and loaded with Bodipy (13.6 mg/L). Then, 30 μL/cm^2 of test formulations was applied onto the RHS surface and remained there for 6 h according to a previously published protocol [31]. Pictures were taken with a fluorescence microscope (BZ-8000, Keyence; Keyence, Neu-Isenburg, Germany) and analyzed with ImageJ software. Five individual measurements per construct were performed observer-blinded (RBR, CW, CZ).

4.10. Statistical Analysis

Data are presented as the mean ± SD from two to four independent experiments. The Mann–Whitney test or Kruskal–Wallis test with Dunn's Post hoc test was used to indicate statistically significant differences ($p \leq 0.05$).

Author Contributions: Conceptualization, R.B.R. and C.Z.; Methodology, R.B.R. S.K., and C.Z.; Formal Analysis, R.B.R., S.K., K.V., M.U., and C.Z.; Investigation, R.B.R., S.K., C.W., C.H., N.Z., M.S., A.K., and M.U.; Resources, R.H. and M.S.-K.; Writing—Original Draft Preparation, R.B.R., S.K., and C.Z.; Writing—Review & Editing, R.B.R., S.K., M.S.-K., and C.Z.; Visualization, R.B.R., S.K., C.W., and C.Z.; Supervision, C.Z.; Project Administration, C.Z.; Funding Acquisition, R.B.R., C.H., K.V., M.S.-K., and C.Z.

Acknowledgments: We thank Verena Eckert-Funke, Franziska Ermisch, and Carola Kapfer for excellent technical assistance.

Abbreviations

AGEs	Advanced Glycated End-products
CML	N-CarboxyMethyl-Lysine
CMS	Dendritic Core-Multishell
DAPI	4′,6-DiAmidino-2-PhenylIndole
ECM	ExtraCellular Matrix
HPTLC	High-Performance Thin-Layer Chromatography
NHDF	Normal Human Dermal Fibroblast
NHK	Normal Human Keratinocytes
PBS	Phosphate-Buffered Saline
RAGE	Receptor of AGEs
RHS	Reconstructed Human Skin
SDS	Sodium Dodecyl Sulphate
TEM	Transmission Electron Microscopy

References

1. López-Otín, C.; Blasco, M.A.; Partridge, L.; Serrano, M.; Kroemer, G. The hallmarks of aging. *Cell* **2013**, *153*, 1194–1217. [CrossRef] [PubMed]
2. Reeve, E.; Trenaman, S.C.; Rockwood, K.; Hilmer, S.N. Pharmacokinetic and pharmacodynamic alterations in older people with dementia. *Expert Opin. Drug Metab. Toxicol.* **2017**, *13*, 651–668. [CrossRef] [PubMed]
3. Papagrigoraki, A.; Del Giglio, M.; Cosma, C.; Maurelli, M.; Girolomoni, G.; Lapolla, A. Advanced Glycation End Products are Increased in the Skin and Blood of Patients with Severe Psoriasis. *Acta Derm.-Venereol.* **2017**, *97*, 782–787. [CrossRef] [PubMed]
4. Lima, A.L.; Illing, T.; Schliemann, S.; Elsner, P. Cutaneous Manifestations of Diabetes Mellitus: A Review. *Am. J. Clin. Dermatol.* **2017**, *18*, 541–553. [CrossRef] [PubMed]
5. Verzijl, N.; DeGroot, J.; Thorpe, S.R.; Bank, R.A.; Shaw, J.N.; Lyons, T.J.; Bijlsma, J.W.; Lafeber, F.P.; Baynes, J.W.; TeKoppele, J.M. Effect of collagen turnover on the accumulation of advanced glycation end products. *J. Biol. Chem.* **2000**, *275*, 39027–39031. [CrossRef] [PubMed]
6. Pageon, H.; Zucchi, H.; Dai, Z.; Sell, D.R.; Strauch, C.M.; Monnier, V.M.; Asselineau, D. Biological Effects Induced by Specific Advanced Glycation End Products in the Reconstructed Skin Model of Aging. *BioRes. Open Access* **2015**, *4*, 54–64. [CrossRef] [PubMed]
7. Yokota, M.; Tokudome, Y. The Effect of Glycation on Epidermal Lipid Content, Its Metabolism and Change in Barrier Function. *Skin Pharmacol. Physiol.* **2016**, *29*, 231–242. [CrossRef] [PubMed]
8. Cadau, S.; Leoty-Okombi, S.; Pain, S.; Bechetoille, N.; Andre-Frei, V.; Berthod, F. In vitro glycation of an endothelialized and innervated tissue-engineered skin to screen anti-AGE molecules. *Biomaterials* **2015**, *51*, 216–225. [CrossRef] [PubMed]
9. Pennacchi, P.C.; de Almeida, M.E.; Gomes, O.L.; Faiao-Flores, F.; de Araujo Crepaldi, M.C.; Dos Santos, M.F.; de Moraes Barros, S.B.; Maria-Engler, S.S. Glycated Reconstructed Human Skin as a Platform to Study the Pathogenesis of Skin Aging. *Tissue Eng. Part A* **2015**, *21*, 2417–2425. [CrossRef] [PubMed]
10. Morimoto, H.; Gu, L.; Zeng, H.; Maeda, K. Amino Carbonylation of Epidermal Basement Membrane Inhibits Epidermal Cell Function and Is Suppressed by Methylparaben. *Cosmetics* **2017**, *4*, 38. [CrossRef]

11. Käßmeyer, S.; Sehl, J.; Khiao In, M.; Merle, R.; Richardson, K.; Plendl, J. Subcellular interactions during vascular morphogenesis in 3D cocultures between endothelial cells and fibroblasts. *Int. J. Mol. Sci.* **2017**, *18*, 2590. [CrossRef] [PubMed]
12. Longo, C.; Casari, A.; De Pace, B.; Simonazzi, S.; Mazzaglia, G.; Pellacani, G. Proposal for an in vivo histopathologic scoring system for skin aging by means of confocal microscopy. *Skin Res. Technol.* **2013**, *19*, e167–e173. [CrossRef] [PubMed]
13. Ulrich, M.; Lange-Asschenfeldt, S.; Gonzalez, S. Clinical applicability of in vivo reflectance confocal microscopy in dermatology. *G. Ital. Dermatol. Venereol.* **2012**, *147*, 171–178. [PubMed]
14. Lewis, R.N.; McElhaney, R.N. Fourier transform infrared spectroscopy in the study of lipid phase transitions in model and biological membranes: Practical considerations. *Methods Mol. Biol.* **2007**, *400*, 207–226. [CrossRef] [PubMed]
15. Zoschke, C.; Ulrich, M.; Sochorova, M.; Wolff, C.; Vavrova, K.; Ma, N.; Ulrich, C.; Brandner, J.M.; Schafer-Korting, M. The barrier function of organotypic non-melanoma skin cancer models. *J. Control. Release* **2016**, *233*, 10–18. [CrossRef] [PubMed]
16. van den Bogaard, E.H.; Tjabringa, G.S.; Joosten, I.; Vonk-Bergers, M.; van Rijssen, E.; Tijssen, H.J.; Erkens, M.; Schalkwijk, J.; Koenen, H.J. Crosstalk between keratinocytes and T cells in a 3D microenvironment: A model to study inflammatory skin diseases. *J. Investig. Dermatol.* **2014**, *134*, 719–727. [CrossRef] [PubMed]
17. Danso, M.O.; van Drongelen, V.; Mulder, A.; van Esch, J.; Scott, H.; van Smeden, J.; El Ghalbzouri, A.; Bouwstra, J.A. TNF-alpha and Th2 cytokines induce atopic dermatitis-like features on epidermal differentiation proteins and stratum corneum lipids in human skin equivalents. *J. Investig. Dermatol.* **2014**, *134*, 1941–1950. [CrossRef] [PubMed]
18. Khalifah, R.G.; Todd, P.; Booth, A.A.; Yang, S.X.; Mott, J.D.; Hudson, B.G. Kinetics of nonenzymatic glycation of ribonuclease A leading to advanced glycation end products. Paradoxical inhibition by ribose leads to facile isolation of protein intermediate for rapid post-Amadori studies. *Biochemistry* **1996**, *35*, 4645–4654. [CrossRef] [PubMed]
19. Luers, L.; Rysiewski, K.; Dumpitak, C.; Birkmann, E. Kinetics of advanced glycation end products formation on bovine serum albumin with various reducing sugars and dicarbonyl compounds in equimolar ratios. *Rejuv. Res.* **2012**, *15*, 201–205. [CrossRef] [PubMed]
20. Pageon, H.; Techer, M.P.; Asselineau, D. Reconstructed skin modified by glycation of the dermal equivalent as a model for skin aging and its potential use to evaluate anti-glycation molecules. *Exp. Gerontol.* **2008**, *43*, 584–588. [CrossRef] [PubMed]
21. Brings, S.; Fleming, T.; Freichel, M.; Muckenthaler, M.; Herzig, S.; Nawroth, P. Dicarbonyls and Advanced Glycation End-Products in the Development of Diabetic Complications and Targets for Intervention. *Int. J. Mol. Sci.* **2017**, *18*, 984. [CrossRef] [PubMed]
22. Rinnerthaler, M.; Streubel, M.K.; Bischof, J.; Richter, K. Skin aging, gene expression and calcium. *Exp. Gerontol.* **2015**, *68*, 59–65. [CrossRef] [PubMed]
23. Pageon, H.; Bakala, H.; Monnier, V.M.; Asselineau, D. Collagen glycation triggers the formation of aged skin in vitro. *Eur. J. Dermatol.* **2007**, *17*, 12–20. [CrossRef] [PubMed]
24. Maas-Szabowski, N.; Szabowski, A.; Stark, H.J.; Andrecht, S.; Kolbus, A.; Schorpp-Kistner, M.; Angel, P.; Fusenig, N.E. Organotypic cocultures with genetically modified mouse fibroblasts as a tool to dissect molecular mechanisms regulating keratinocyte growth and differentiation. *J. Investig. Dermatol.* **2001**, *116*, 816–820. [CrossRef] [PubMed]
25. Löwa, A.; Vogt, A.; Kaessmeyer, S.; Hedtrich, S. Generation of full-thickness skin equivalents using hair follicle-derived primary human keratinocytes and fibroblasts. *J. Tissue Eng. Regener. Med.* **2018**, *12*, e2134–e2146. [CrossRef] [PubMed]
26. Breitkreutz, D.; Koxholt, I.; Thiemann, K.; Nischt, R. Skin basement membrane: The foundation of epidermal integrity—BM functions and diverse roles of bridging molecules nidogen and perlecan. *BioMed Res. Int.* **2013**, *2013*, 179784. [CrossRef] [PubMed]
27. Candiello, J.; Cole, G.J.; Halfter, W. Age-dependent changes in the structure, composition and biophysical properties of a human basement membrane. *Matrix Biol.* **2010**, *29*, 402–410. [CrossRef] [PubMed]
28. Wolberink, E.A.; van Erp, P.E.; Teussink, M.M.; van de Kerkhof, P.C.; Gerritsen, M.J. Cellular features of psoriatic skin: Imaging and quantification using in vivo reflectance confocal microscopy. *Cytom. Part B Clin. Cytom.* **2011**, *80*, 141–149. [CrossRef] [PubMed]

29. Brody, I. The ultrastructure of the epidermis in psoriasis vulgaris as revealed by electron microscopy. 1. The dermo-epidermal junction and the stratum basale in parakeratosis without keratohyalin. *J. Ultrastruct. Res.* **1962**, *6*, 304–323. [CrossRef]
30. Steven, A.C.; Bisher, M.E.; Roop, D.R.; Steinert, P.M. Biosynthetic pathways of filaggrin and loricrin—Two major proteins expressed by terminally differentiated epidermal keratinocytes. *J. Struct. Biol.* **1990**, *104*, 150–162. [CrossRef]
31. Alnasif, N.; Zoschke, C.; Fleige, E.; Brodwolf, R.; Boreham, A.; Rühl, E.; Eckl, K.M.; Merk, H.F.; Hennies, H.C.; Alexiev, U.; et al. Penetration of normal, damaged and diseased skin—An in vitro study on dendritic core-multishell nanotransporters. *J. Control. Release* **2014**, *185c*, 45–50. [CrossRef] [PubMed]
32. Pageon, H.; Asselineau, D. An in vitro approach to the chronological aging of skin by glycation of the collagen: The biological effect of glycation on the reconstructed skin model. *Ann. N. Y. Acad. Sci.* **2005**, *1043*, 529–532. [CrossRef] [PubMed]
33. Turksen, K.; Kupper, T.; Degenstein, L.; Williams, I.; Fuchs, E. Interleukin 6: Insights to its function in skin by overexpression in transgenic mice. *Proc. Natl. Acad. Sci. USA* **1992**, *89*, 5068–5072. [CrossRef] [PubMed]
34. Sakai, T.; Hatano, Y.; Zhang, W.; Fujiwara, S.; Nishiyori, R. Knockdown of either filaggrin or loricrin increases the productions of interleukin (IL)-1alpha, IL-8, IL-18 and granulocyte macrophage colony-stimulating factor in stratified human keratinocytes. *J. Dermatol. Sci.* **2015**, *80*, 158–160. [CrossRef] [PubMed]
35. Brody, I. The ultrastructure of the epidermis in psoriasis vulgaris as revealed by electron microscopy: 4. Stratum corneum in parakeratosis without keretohyalin. *J. Ultrastruct. Res.* **1962**, *6*, 354–367. [CrossRef]
36. Gould, A.R.; Sharp, P.J.; Smith, D.R.; Stegink, A.J.; Chase, C.J.; Kovacs, J.C.; Penglis, S.; Chatterton, B.E.; Bunn, C.L. Increased permeability of psoriatic skin to the protein, plasminogen activator inhibitor 2. *Arch. Dermatol. Res.* **2003**, *295*, 249–254. [CrossRef] [PubMed]
37. Papagrigoraki, A.; Maurelli, M.; del Giglio, M.; Gisondi, P.; Girolomoni, G. Advanced Glycation End Products in the Pathogenesis of Psoriasis. *Int. J. Mol. Sci.* **2017**, *18*, 2471. [CrossRef] [PubMed]
38. Gerecke, C.; Edlich, A.; Giulbudagian, M.; Schumacher, F.; Zhang, N.; Said, A.; Yealland, G.; Lohan, S.B.; Neumann, F.; Meinke, M.C.; et al. Biocompatibility and characterization of polyglycerol-based thermoresponsive nanogels designed as novel drug-delivery systems and their intracellular localization in keratinocytes. *Nanotoxicology* **2017**, *11*, 267–277. [CrossRef] [PubMed]
39. Richardson, K.C.; Jarett, L.; Finke, E.H. Embedding in epoxy resins for ultrathin sectioning in electron microscopy. *Stain Technol.* **1960**, *35*, 313–323. [CrossRef] [PubMed]
40. Vavrova, K.; Henkes, D.; Struver, K.; Sochorova, M.; Skolova, B.; Witting, M.Y.; Friess, W.; Schreml, S.; Meier, R.J.; Schafer-Korting, M.; et al. Filaggrin deficiency leads to impaired lipid profile and altered acidification pathways in a 3D skin construct. *J. Investig. Dermatol.* **2014**, *134*, 746–753. [CrossRef] [PubMed]
41. Opálka, L.; Kováčik, A.; Sochorová, M.; Roh, J.; Kuneš, J.; Lenčo, J.; Vávrová, K. Scalable synthesis of human ultralong chain ceramides. *Org. Lett.* **2015**, *17*, 5456–5459. [CrossRef] [PubMed]
42. Kováčik, A.; Opálka, L.; Šilarová, M.; Roh, J.; Vávrová, K. Synthesis of 6-hydroxyceramide using ruthenium-catalyzed hydrosilylation-protodesilylation. Unexpected formation of a long periodicity lamellar phase in skin lipid membranes. *RSC Adv.* **2016**, *6*, 73343–73350. [CrossRef]
43. Radowski, M.R.; Shukla, A.; von Berlepsch, H.; Bottcher, C.; Pickaert, G.; Rehage, H.; Haag, R. Supramolecular aggregates of dendritic multishell architectures as universal nanocarriers. *Angew. Chem. Int. Ed. Engl.* **2007**, *46*, 1265–1269. [CrossRef] [PubMed]

Aging and Intermittent Fasting Impact on Transcriptional Regulation and Physiological Responses of Adult *Drosophila* Neuronal and Muscle Tissues

Sharon Zhang [1,2,3], Eric P. Ratliff [1,3], Brandon Molina [1,3], Nadja El-Mecharrafie [1,3], Jessica Mastroianni [1,3], Roxanne W. Kotzebue [1,3], Madhulika Achal [1], Ruth E. Mauntz [1], Arysa Gonzalez [1,3], Ayeh Barekat [1,3], William A. Bray [1,3,4], Andrew M. Macias [1,3], Daniel Daugherty [5], Greg L. Harris [3], Robert A. Edwards [2,3] and Kim D. Finley [1,3,*]

[1] Donald P. Shiley BioScience Center, San Diego State University, San Diego, CA 92182, USA; sharonzh10@yahoo.com (S.Z.); epratliff@hotmail.com (E.P.R.); Brandonrm.16@gmail.com (B.M.); nadjaelm@outlook.com (N.E.-M.); jmfmastroianni@yahoo.com (J.M.); rkotzebue@gmail.com (R.W.K.); madhulika.achal@gmail.com (M.A.); rmauntz@gmail.com (R.E.M.); gonzalez.arysa@gmail.com (A.G.); ayeh.sdsu@gmail.com (A.B.); yossarianassyrian@gmail.com (W.A.B.); maciasandrew01@gmail.com (A.M.M.)

[2] Biological and Medical Informatics Research Center, San Diego State University, San Diego, CA 92182, USA; redwards@sdsu.edu

[3] Department of Biology, San Diego State University, San Diego, CA 92182, USA; gharris@sdsu.edu

[4] Sanford Consortium for Regenerative Medicine, 2880 Torrey Pines Scenic Dr., La Jolla, CA 92037, USA

[5] The Salk Institute for Biological Studies, Cellular Neurobiology, 10010 North Torrey Pines Road, La Jolla, CA 92037, USA; ddaugherty@salk.edu

* Correspondence: kfinley@sdsu.edu

Abstract: The progressive decline of the nervous system, including protein aggregate formation, reflects the subtle dysregulation of multiple functional pathways. Our previous work has shown intermittent fasting (IF) enhances longevity, maintains adult behaviors and reduces aggregates, in part, by promoting autophagic function in the aging *Drosophila* brain. To clarify the impact that IF-treatment has upon aging, we used high throughput RNA-sequencing technology to examine the changing transcriptome in adult *Drosophila* tissues. Principle component analysis (PCA) and other analyses showed ~1200 age-related transcriptional differences in head and muscle tissues, with few genes having matching expression patterns. Pathway components showing age-dependent expression differences were involved with stress response, metabolic, neural and chromatin remodeling functions. Middle-aged tissues also showed a significant increase in transcriptional drift-variance (TD), which in the CNS included multiple proteolytic pathway components. Overall, IF-treatment had a demonstrably positive impact on aged transcriptomes, partly ameliorating both fold and variance changes. Consistent with these findings, aged IF-treated flies displayed more youthful metabolic, behavioral and basal proteolytic profiles that closely correlated with transcriptional alterations to key components. These results indicate that even modest dietary changes can have therapeutic consequences, slowing the progressive decline of multiple cellular systems, including proteostasis in the aging nervous system.

Keywords: aging; aging-delaying interventions; metabolism; cellular proteostasis; neural degeneration; intermittent fasting; RNA-sequencing; *Drosophila*

1. Introduction

Both human and model organism studies have shown even modest dietary modifications can have a significant positive influence on longevity and the health of aging individuals [1–7]. Existing research into the molecular mechanisms that underpin such improved health and longevity metrics indicates that the long-term function of multiple cellular systems is essential [3,5,8–10]. Indeed, numerous genetic studies have shown that a diverse range of regulatory, metabolic and clearance pathways are required for the healthy aging of the nervous system [8,11–13]. In addition, a wide range of environmental factors, especially modified diets, have consistently shown a positive influence on the age-related decline of select tissues as well as the overall functional health and performance of older individuals [2,10,14,15].

We have recently characterized a mild intermittent fasting (IF) protocol that promotes longevity and neural function of middle-aged adult *Drosophila* strains from divergent genetic backgrounds [1,16,17]. The beneficial effects of this fasting protocol included a delay in the progressive decline of locomotor behaviors and a reduction in neural aggregate levels [1,16,17]. This was associated with improvements in the acute and long-term functions of the autophagy pathway within middle-aged fly neurons [1,16,17]. Multiple studies have established that this pathway plays a central role in stress responses and in promoting healthy aging, partly through facilitating the clearance of protein aggregates and damaged cellular components [13,18,19]. At the mechanistic level, autophagy represents a downstream effector pathway, the activity of which is tightly regulated by multiple upstream factors that control and coordinate complex cellular responses [1,16,17,19,20]. The impact of IF-treatment on the aging CNS could reflect the alteration to multiple signaling and metabolic pathways that in turn influence pathway function, and as a result, the long-term maintenance of the aging nervous system [1,16,17,19,20].

Most organisms show well-defined aging phenotypes, which can reflect tissue-specific alterations to numerous molecular and metabolic pathways [15,21–23]. Taken together, these changes precede and eventually lead, to the functional decline (behavior, metabolism, stress responses), and the eventual death of an individual. Both genetic and drug-based studies using in vivo model systems have shown that the different genetic backgrounds and treatment regimens, which promote health and longevity, are often linked to basal changes to gene expression profiles [2,14,15,23,24]. Of note, a recent RNA-sequencing (RNA-seq) study that examined changes to the acult *C. elegans* transcriptome profiles, characterized a novel age-related phenomenon termed "transcriptional drift-variance" (TD), which reflects the progressive dysregulation of mRNA expression patterns [23]. In older worms, TD was significantly increased between replicate transcriptomes, which was partially suppressed in matching cohorts following exposure to the anti-aging compound, mianserin [23,25]. The analysis of transcriptome profiles from a range of mouse and human frontal cortex tissues samples also indicated that TD was an evolutionary conserved feature of aging [23]. A recent report examining the neural physiology of middle-age senescence-accelerated prone (SAMP8) mice also showed elevated TD levels in neural tissues. Following treatment with the neural protective compound, J147, TD levels were significantly reduced in mice and the average lifespan of adult *Drosophila* increased [26]. The implications from these studies are that environmental interventions that promote longevity, including IF-treatment, could facilitate more youthful mRNA expression patterns and variance profiles [1,2,5,26–28].

In this report, we examined the impact that aging and IF-treatment have upon the transcriptome profiles (non-fasted) in the adult *Drosophila* neural (head) and muscle (thorax) tissues [1,2,23,26]. Our analyses revealed that, by 4-week of age, both fly tissues showed significant basal changes to expression levels, with IF-treatment promoting more youthful global expression profiles. Both tissues exhibited the age-dependent phenomenon of transcriptional drift-variance, providing further evidence that the progressive disruption of transcriptional regulation also occurs in middle-aged flies [23,25,26]. Transcripts demonstrating fold changes and TD differences involved a wide array of genes representing a number of functional groups and pathways. In several cases, the age and IF-dependent changes were consistent with unique tissue-specific phenotypes and functional changes that included metabolic, behavioral and epigenetic systems [26]. Of particular interest were the dynamic variance changes, in neural tissues that occurred to multiple proteolytic pathway components, including members of the ubiquitin-proteasome system (UPS) and autophagy–lysosomal pathway. Globally these results indicate that even modest dietary manipulations could improve basal transcriptomic and phenotypic trends, which are themselves associated with partial suppression of several cellular processes linked to impaired cellular aging [23,26,29].

2. Results

2.1. Global Expression Differences Due to Age or IF-Treatment

To elaborate upon our original investigation into the impact of intermittent fasting (IF) on neuronal autophagy and aging, high throughput RNA-sequencing was used to examine global changes to the gene expression profiles in adult male *Drosophila* tissues. Examined were fly body segments that represented regions highly enriched with either neuronal (head) or skeletal muscle (thorax) tissues. Triplicate mRNA pools from adult heads were isolated from 1-week (1W), 4-week (4W) to 4-week IF-treated (4W-IF) male flies [1,20]. Matching thoracic mRNA pools (duplicates) were also isolated and used as reference non-neuronal control tissue set. Individual cDNA libraries were generated for each tissue and condition and then sequenced using Illumina HiSeq2000 technology [2,24,27,30]. Sequencing read mapping and alignments were done using the *Drosophila* reference genome (UCSC) and Genome Browser (genome.ucsc.edu, Santa Cruz, CA, USA), with sequence alignments and internal read mapping generated using TopHat and Bowtie (see Methods and Materials) [2,23,29]. Comparisons between annotated library sequences found that most reads (~80%) aligned with the reference transcriptome and represented ~94% exon-only sequences (Table S1).

As part of the predictive modeling of global transcriptome profiles, the high-dimensional variable analysis provided by the AltAnalyze analytical pipeline (Available online: https://www.altanalyze.org), was used to characterize the heterogeneity between individual RNA-seq datasets. This included performing principal component analyses (PCA) on total reads per kilobase of transcript, per million mapped reads (RPKM) values, which reduced the dimensionality of each expression dataset into two principal components (Figure 1) [23,29]. The PCA comparison of head transcriptomes demonstrated the close alignment between replicate samples as well as the expression differences that could largely be attributed to aging or IF-treatment (X axis, 98.9%, Figure 1A). PC analysis of head and thoracic datasets found distinct non-overlapping transcriptome profiles between the two tissues (PCA1 89.7%, Figure S1A), though both showed comparable shifts in global expression due to age or IF-treatment (PCA2 3.9%, Figure S1A). Interestingly, the head 4W-IF transcriptomes showed a significant tread toward more youthful patterns and had reduced TD variability when compared to matching non-fasted 4W controls (Figure 1A). Hierarchical clustering plots further highlighted the similarities between replicate samples as well as the impact that aging (4W) and IF-treatment (4W-IF) have upon global transcriptome trends (Figure 1B and Fgure S1B) [29,30]. The average RPKM values for transcripts typically expressed in muscle, neural or glial cell types were examined for both sets of tissues. In general, muscle specific genes were enriched in all thoracic samples ($n = 6$), while genes typically expressed in neural or glial cell types were preferentially detected across all RNA-seq samples from adult heads ($n = 9$, Table S2). This indicated that the transcriptome patterns from each body segment in large part reflected the expected tissue-specific expression profiles [2,29].

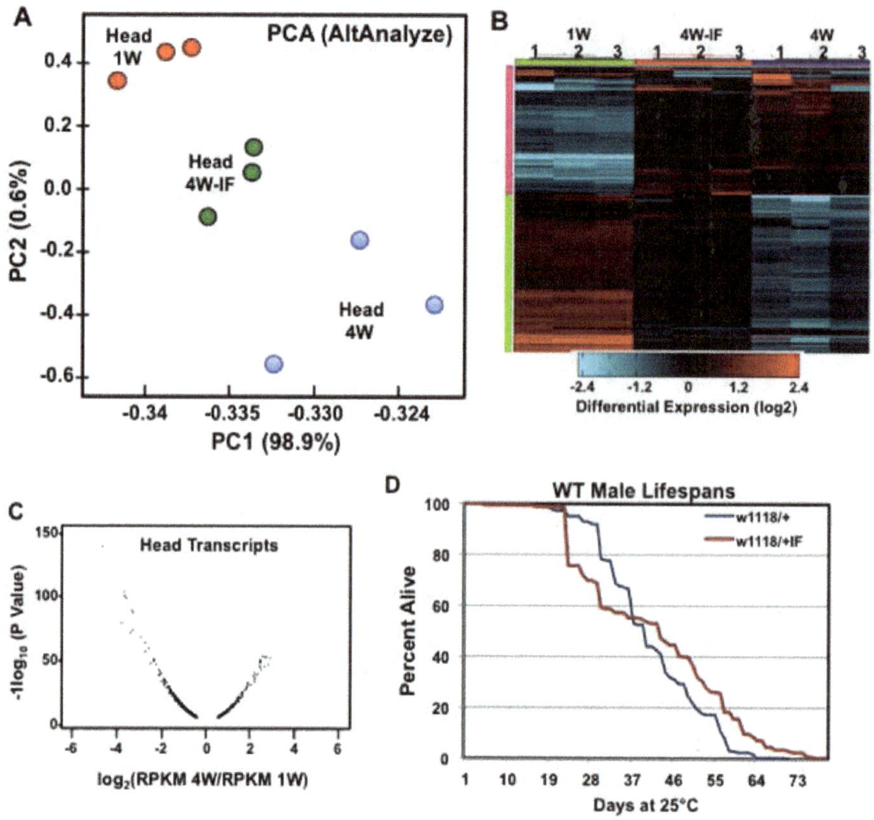

Figure 1. Principal component analysis (PCA) and expression clustering profiles of head transcriptomes. (**A**) The AltAnalyze software was used to compare PCA values for individual RNA-seq transcriptomes isolated from 1-week (1W), 4-week (4W) to IF-treated (4W-IF) male flies (n = 3). (**B**) AltAnalyzer was also used to establish the individual expression clustering profiles for head (n = 9) transcriptomes at different ages and treatment conditions. (**C**) Volcano plot showing significant message fold directional (±) changes in the CNS that occurs as a function of age (4W/1W, negative log10 of p-values as a function of log2). (**D**) Kaplan–Meier survival curves of male flies ($w^{1118}/+$) maintained on *ad libitum* or IF conditions starting at 1-week of age (25 °C) [1].

2.2. Age and IF-Dependent Changes in Transcriptome Profiles

The global assessment of neural profiles indicated that significant basal expression changes were occurring both as a consequence of aging and the IF-treatment regimen. Anticipating relatively modest changes to basal gene expression, the average fold change to each mRNA cohort was then examined, with significant cutoffs for aging set at >1.4 ± fold (4W/1W), and for IF-dependent changes, at >1.3 ± fold (4W/4W-IF) [2,29]. By 4-weeks, a similar number of genes from head (1197) and thoracic (1347) tissues showed substantial expression differences (Table 1). Age-related transcriptional changes in the fly head tended toward a broader deregulation of mRNA profiles (Figure 1C; Table 1), though the relative amplitude of such changes were more pronounced in 4W thoracic tissues (Figure S2A) [2,23]. In contrast, a larger number of neural transcripts showed a significant global response to IF-exposure when heads were compared to thoracic samples (294 versus 102 genes, Table 1). Further analysis of dynamic expression differences determined there was minimal gene overlap between fly head and thoracic tissues due to aging (Figure S2B; Table 1). Tissue-specific differences were also reflected in the IF-dependent responses, with neural tissues showing a significant shift toward more youthful expression patterns in 4W-IF cohorts, relative to those in the thorax (221 versus 58 genes, Table 1). The positive impact that

IF-treatment has on progressive transcriptional changes in both tissues was consistent with the more general phenotype of enhanced longevity, which was demonstrated in our previous studies for male flies from several genotypes (Figure 1D) [1].

Table 1. Genes with Fold Changes due to Aging and Intermittent Fasting.

Tissue	Change with Age	Age Down	Age Up	Change with IF	Age Down IF Up	Age Up IF Down	IF More Youthful
Thorax	1347	790	557	102	22	36	58
Head	1197	806	391	294	178	43	221

2.3. Gene Ontology (GO) or DAVID Analysis of Functional Pathway Changes

To assess the functional classification of genes or pathways influenced by age or IF-treatment, the DAVID bioinformatics program was used to identify functional clusters of genes with tissue-specific expression differences (Figure 2B; Table 1) [2,29]. For each condition, the transcriptome profiles from neural tissues showed a greater number of annotated functional groups with altered patterns of expression relative to thoracic tissues (Table S3). The largest functional gene clusters that showed dynamic age and youthful IF-dependent expression trends in the adult fly CNS were metabolic-related (Figure 2). Generally, these components are associated with longevity and lipid, carbohydrate (arrows) and mitochondrial related functions (Figure 2A). To confirm RNA-seq expression trends, quantitative RT-PCR (qRT-PCR) analysis of the *Tobi*, *Lps2* and *Sodh-1* genes was undertaken in neural tissues [31,32]. This indicated that the relative expression profiles of each gene matched the age and IF-dependent fluctuations detected by RNA-seq (Figure 2B–D). All three proteins have well-established metabolic functions and expression patterns that are influenced by aging, diet or alterations to the insulin-signaling pathway [31,32]. In thoracic tissues, the *Tobi* transcript also showed pronounced changes in expression due to aging and IF-treatment, albeit in the opposing directions (arrow, Figure S2C).

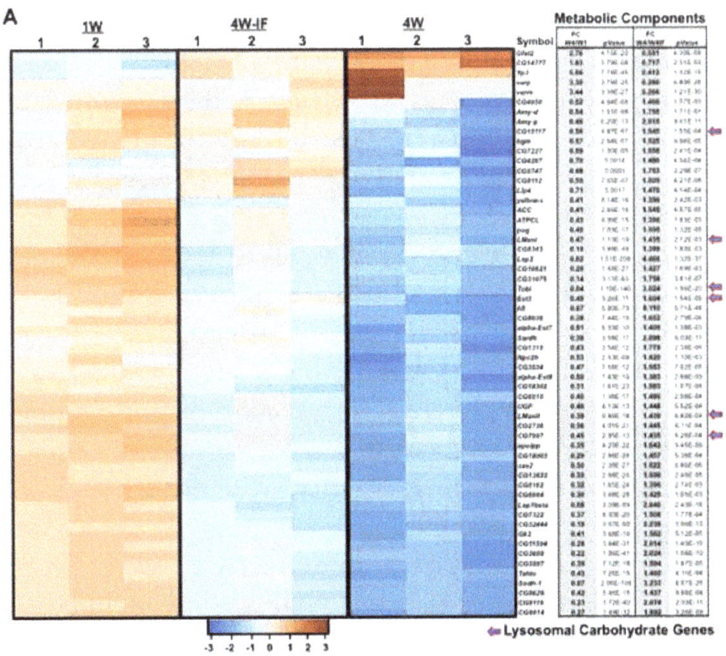

Figure 2. *Cont.*

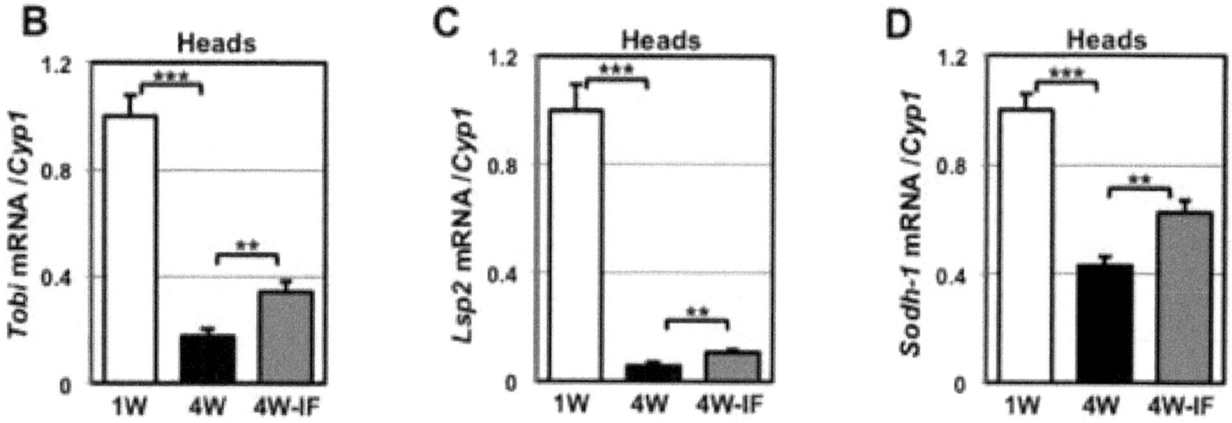

Figure 2. Age and IF-dependent fold changes (FC) to the expression profiles of metabolic pathway components in adult *Drosophila* heads. Quantitative RNA-sequencing and DAVID analysis identified metabolic genes that showed age and IF-dependent differences in expression levels. (**A**) Heatmap and corresponding table represents hierarchical clustering of scaled gene expression profiles and the respective fold change (FC) and p values between 4W/1W and 4W/4W-IF cohorts. Scaled expression values (z-score) were plotted in red–blue color scale with red indicating high expression and blue indicating low expression levels. Arrows highlight lysosomal proteins involved with carbohydrate metabolism. (**B–D**) qRT-PCR of expression changes to the *Tobi, Lsp2* and *Sodh-1* genes in neural tissues. ** $p \leq 0.01$, *** $p \leq 0.001$.

2.4. *Age and IF-Dependent Neuronal and Behavioral Changes*

Previously, we determined that IF-treated flies have lower insoluble protein aggregate profiles in neural tissues, which was linked to the preservation of adult climbing behaviors [1]. This was consistent with other modified diet studies that also detect a positive impact on the long-term function of neural tissues [1,33–37]. DAVID analysis revealed genes involved with a wide range of neural functions, including olfaction, had dynamic changes in expression patterns (Figure 3A). We had previously demonstrated that older male flies develop a marked increase in nighttime activity that was linked with the dysregulation of odorant binding protein (*Obp*) gene expression profiles and olfactory-based courtship behaviors [16]. In this study, elevated expression of *Atg8a* in neuronal tissues maintained both *Obp* expression patterns and suppressed the changes to courtship behaviors [16]. To determine whether IF-treatment could similarly alter nighttime activity profiles, 1W, 4W and 4W-IF treated male flies ($w^{1118}/+$) were placed in group-housed conditions (10 flies/tube) and examined using 12-h light:dark (LD) cycling conditions for 48-h (LAM system). The 24-h activity profiles showed normal behavior patterns for young males (1W), including typical morning and evening peaks of activity, with extended mid-day and mid-dark rest periods (ZT15-21, Figure 3B,C) [16]. Middle-aged males (4W) demonstrated the normal increase in nighttime activity, which was largely suppressed in IF-treated cohorts (Figure 3B,C). Similar to transgenic enhancement of neuronal *Atg8a* levels, these results indicated that even modest dietary manipulations can protect the progressive dysregulation of this and other behaviors, further indicating the preservation of neural function in aged animals [1,16,17,19].

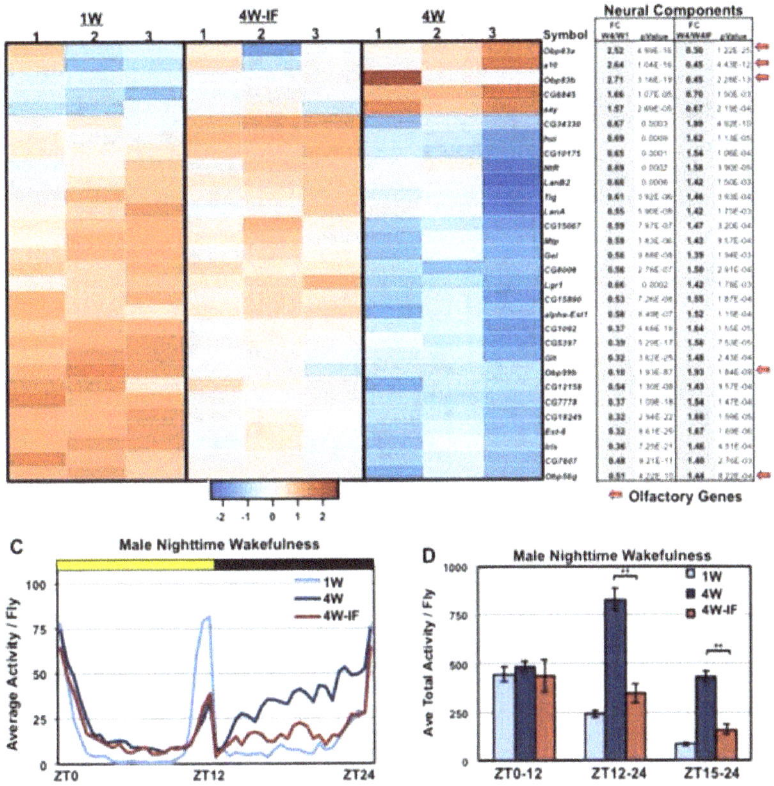

Figure 3. Age and IF-dependent expression changes to adult neuronal pathway components and adult olfactory-based behaviors. DAVID analysis identified genes with neuronal functions that demonstrated age and IF-dependent fluctuations in expression levels. (**A**) Heatmap and corresponding table represents hierarchical clustering of scaled gene expression profiles and fold change (FC) and p values between 4W/1W and 4W/4W-IF RNA-seq cohorts. Scaled expression values (Z-score) of RPKM expression levels were plotted in red (high) versus blue (low) color scale. Arrows indicate olfactory binding genes that are linked to behavioral defects. (**B**,**C**) Average 24 h activity profiles of grouped housed 1W, 4W and 4W IF male fly cohorts (n = 16 groups of 10 flies) and (**D**) Activity levels during light (ZT0 to 12) dark (ZT12 to 24) and mid-dark (ZT15 to 24) time periods. ** $p \leq 0.01$.

2.5. Altered Expression Patterns of Stress Response and Epigenetic Pathway Components

DAVID analysis of thoracic samples identified significant fluctuations to the expression profiles of regulatory, proteolytic, vesicle transport and structural pathway components (Figure S3A–C). The fly CNS also demonstrated significant age and IF dependent fold changes to the expression levels of several stress response pathway components (Figure 4A). This included the *Drosophila Hsp22* transcript (mitochondrial heat shock protein), which in both head and thoracic tissues showed an age-dependent increase and IF-related decrease in expression levels (Figure 4B). Changes to *Hsp22* mRNA values were confirmed using quantitative (qRT-PCR) analyses (n = 16, Figure 4C), with expression patterns becoming highly variable in aged thorax samples (4W, Figure 4B,C). The age-related increase in expression variance for this gene suggested that transcription drift variance (TD) was occurring in older *Drosophila* tissues [23,26]. It also suggested that upstream transcription factors that regulated downstream expression and variance profiles could be influenced by protective dietary conditions [23,26]. Comparing the two tissues identified significant FC to the expression pattern of epigenetic pathway components, although there was minimal specific overlap between head and muscle samples (Figure 5A,B). For example the *CoRest* and *Df31* genes showed opposing response to aging IF exposure (blue arrows, Figure 5A,B). Taken together, our data suggests that both age and modified diets can produce unique tissue-specific changes to epigenetic pathway components in concert with the broader regulatory differences seen in the adult *Drosophila* transcriptome [38,39].

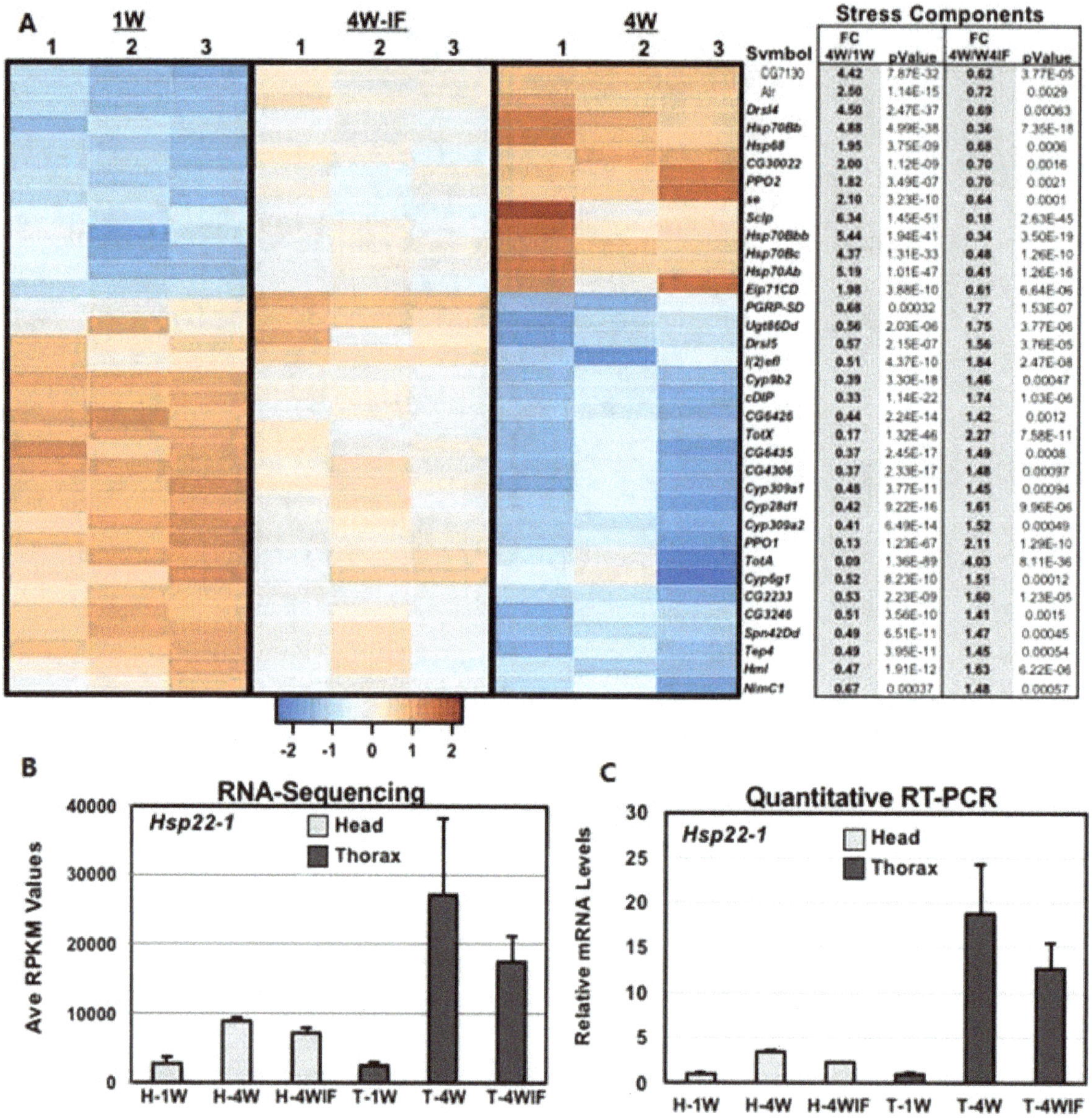

Stress Components

Svmbol	FC 4W/1W	pValue	FC 4W/W4IF	pValue
CG7130	4.42	7.87E-32	0.62	3.77E-05
Alr	2.50	1.14E-15	0.72	0.0029
Drsl4	4.50	2.47E-37	0.69	0.00063
Hsp70Bb	4.88	4.99E-38	0.36	7.35E-18
Hsp68	1.95	3.75E-09	0.68	0.0006
CG30022	2.00	1.12E-09	0.70	0.0016
PPO2	1.82	3.49E-07	0.70	0.0021
se	2.10	3.23E-10	0.64	0.0001
Sclp	6.34	1.45E-51	0.18	2.63E-45
Hsp70Bbb	5.44	1.94E-41	0.34	3.50E-19
Hsp70Bc	4.37	1.31E-33	0.48	1.26E-10
Hsp70Ab	5.19	1.01E-47	0.41	1.26E-16
Eip71CD	1.98	3.88E-10	0.61	6.64E-06
PGRP-SD	0.68	0.00032	1.77	1.53E-07
Ugt86Dd	0.56	2.03E-06	1.75	3.77E-06
Drsl5	0.57	2.15E-07	1.56	3.76E-05
l(2)efl	0.51	4.37E-10	1.84	2.47E-08
Cyp9b2	0.39	3.30E-18	1.46	0.00047
cDIP	0.33	1.14E-22	1.74	1.03E-06
CG6426	0.44	2.24E-14	1.42	0.0012
TotX	0.17	1.32E-46	2.27	7.58E-11
CG6435	0.37	2.45E-17	1.49	0.0008
CG4306	0.37	2.33E-17	1.48	0.00097
Cyp309a1	0.48	3.77E-11	1.45	0.00094
Cyp28d1	0.42	9.22E-16	1.61	9.96E-06
Cyp309a2	0.41	6.49E-14	1.52	0.00049
PPO1	0.13	1.23E-67	2.11	1.29E-10
TotA	0.09	1.36E-89	4.03	8.11E-36
Cyp6g1	0.52	8.23E-10	1.51	0.00012
CG2233	0.53	2.23E-09	1.60	1.23E-05
CG3246	0.51	3.56E-10	1.41	0.0015
Spn42Dd	0.49	6.51E-11	1.47	0.00045
Tep4	0.49	3.95E-11	1.45	0.00054
Hml	0.47	1.91E-12	1.63	6.22E-06
NimC1	0.67	0.00037	1.48	0.00057

Figure 4. Age and IF associated changes to stress and inflammation pathway components in adult neural tissues. RNA-Seq and DAVID analysis of *Drosophila* head transcriptomes identified multiple genes in stress and inflammation related pathways that demonstrated both an age and IF-dependent difference in expression levels. (**A**) The heatmap and corresponding table represents the clustering of scaled gene expression profiles and includes the respective fold change in expression (FC, *p* values) that occur between 4W/1W and 4W/4W-IF tissue cohorts. Scaled expression values (*z*-scores) were plotted using a red–blue color scale represented dynamic differences expression differences to individual genes. Red indicates relative elevated expression and blue indicates relative reduced expression levels. The mRNA expression levels of *Hsp22-1* in head (**H**) and thorax (**T**) tissues measured in RPKM values by (**B**) RNA-seq or (**C**) qRT-PCR analyses. The relative mRNA expression of 1W flies (w^{1118}/+) was set to 1.0 and subsequent RNA values were also normalized to the housekeeping *CXba* transcript.

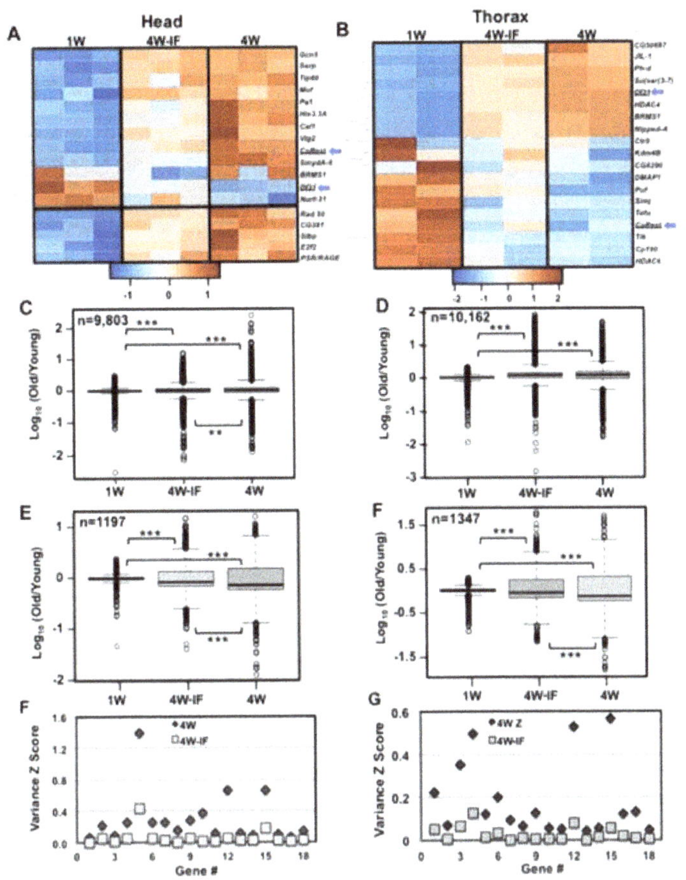

Figure 5. Age and IF-dependent changes to epigenetic pathway components and tissue specific transcriptional drift-variance profiles. Heatmaps of chromatin remodeling pathway components, showing dynamic FC to expression levels in aged (**A**) head or (**B**) thoracic tissue samples (n = number of genes). Arrows highlight the *Df31* and *CoRest* transcripts (blue arrows) that have significant but opposing tissue specific FC to expression profiles. Representative drift-plots showing the global variance changes or VC (~10,000 genes) to (**C**) head or (**D**) thorax tissue transcriptomes, isolated from 1-week 1W, 4W to 4W-IF adult cohorts. Drift plots representing (**E**) head and (**F**) thoracic transcripts (~1200 genes) that showed significant age-dependent FC to expression levels. *** $p \leq 0.001$. See Table 2 for additional details. DAVID analyses were used to determine the functional pathways of head and thoracic genes that demonstrated elevated variance Z scores (4W/4W-IF VC > 3.75). (**G**) The scaled variance Z scores (SD/Ave) for individual transcripts involved with neuronal function were used to generate scatter plots of 4W (◆) and 4W-IF (■) head cohorts. (**H**) The scaled variance Z scores (SD/Ave) for lipid metabolic genes were plotted for 4W (◆) and 4W-IF (■) thoracic transcriptome samples.

2.6. Age and IF-Dependent Changes to Transcriptional Drift

Neural PCA values (4-week, Figure 1A) and muscle *Hsp22* mRNA profiles (Figure 4B,C) suggested that middle-aged fly tissues showed an increased variability between matching replicate transcriptomes [23]. Therefore, the impact of aging and IF-treatment on transcriptional drift variance (TD) was assessed for both tissues. The global variance differences were examined for those genes with replicate RNA-seq values of >1.0 RPKM across all datasets for a particular tissues. The corrected log-fold change in expression variance was determined for each transcriptional cohort, using the 1W transcriptomes as 'young' reference values ($\log_{10}$[old/young reference$_{1W}$]) [23,26,40]. Global TD profiles for head (9803) and thorax (10,163) mRNA cohorts are outlined in Table 2 and illustrated as drift-plots (Figure 5C–F, www.r-project.org) [23,26]. When compared to young flies (1W), total transcriptome profiles from aged cohorts (4W, 4W-IF) demonstrated a significant increase in expression variance or TD (Figure 5C,D) [23]. However, when the two aged profiles were compared, global TD levels were suppressed in 4W-IF neural samples (Figure 5C, Table S4). When a subset of genes that had age-dependent FCs in expression was examined, IF-treatment reduced the variance levels for both tissues (Figure 5E,F, Table S4). This analysis indicated that expression variance significantly increased in middle-aged *Drosophila,* while IF-treatment promoted more youthful TD or variance change (VC) profiles for both tissues, suggestive of alteration in global transcriptional regulation [23,26].

Table 2. Variance Changes * with Age and IF.

Variance > 3.75	4W/1W	4W/4W-IF	1W/4W-IF
Thorax genes	1457	1592	1441
Head genes	1156	1322	520

* Based on replicate RPKM values and corrected Z scores (SD/Ave).

Further characterization of mRNA fold changes suggested that differences in expression patterns could be classified in terms of variability between replicate mRNA samples. Therefore, gene variance Z scores (**VZ**) from normalized replicate RNA-seq values were generated (VZ = SD/Ave RPKM). Comparisons were made between the different age (4W/1W) and treatment (4W/4W-IF) cohorts for both tissues, and individual genes with fold VCs were identified. Nearly 1300 neural and 1600 thoracic transcripts demonstrated a significant reduction in variance profiles following IF-exposure (4W/4W-IF VC > 3.75, Table 2). Often, gene specific FC to message levels did not coincide with VCs, which itself may reflect a heretofore-underappreciated feature of aging. DAVID analysis was performed on those transcripts in both tissues with high VC levels (4W), and that were suppressed in 4W-IF cohorts. In the aging CNS, genes with both FC and VC differences included odorant-binding and synaptic proteins and key components of the circadian pathway (*tim, per*) (Figure 5G, Table S5) [2,16]. Together with the age-dependent behavioral changes (Figure 3B,C), these finding suggest that examining both FC and VC differences could serve to clarify the genes and functional pathways that have malleable expression patterns that can be influenced by aging, diets or other modifying factors [23,26,29,41].

DAVID analysis was also performed on thoracic genes demonstrating age-related TD or expression variance patterns (4W/4W-IF). Several lipid pathway components showed substantial VCs that were significantly reduced following IF-exposure (Figure 5H), while the FC to expression levels remained largely unchanged (Table S6). As previously reported, basal and acute autophagy responses are influenced by age and IF-treatment, suggesting that whole animal fasting responses and rates of metabolic catabolism may also be similarly altered [1,2,32,42]. Therefore, the global starvation responses of 1W, 4W and 4W-IF treated flies were examined. Male flies were placed on fasting media (1% agar) and the number of dead flies counted every 8 h [43]. Middle-aged adults showed a heightened sensitivity to starvation that was partly suppressed in age matched IF-treated cohorts (Figure S4A,B). Since aged thoraces showed both substantial fold and variance changes to metabolic pathways, we examined the global catabolism rates of stored metabolites. Young (1W) and middle-aged (4W, 4W-IF) flies were fasted for 0 or 8 h, flash frozen and tissue homogenates used to determine whole body triglyceride (TG), glycogen and glucose levels (mg/mg protein, Figure S4C–H) [8,42]. Young flies had the highest basal stores and catabolism rates for all three metabolites (Figure S4C–H). Interestingly, older adults (4W) showed similar TG levels but lower consumption rates following and 8-h fast (14% decrease). In fasted 4W-IF cohorts, the TG catabolism profiles were more youthful (27.5% decrease, Figure S4C,D), while turnover of carbohydrate stores showed different profiles (Figure S4E–H) [42,44]. Together, this suggests that age and IF-dependent changes that are reflected as FC and VC expression differences in thoracic tissues have functional consequences in metabolic and survival responses in older individuals (Figure S4) [8,42].

2.7. Altered Proteolytic Pathways and Protein Aggregate Profiles in Aging Fly Tissues

Using a sequential detergent extraction and Western analysis, we have consistently shown that under normal culturing conditions that by middle-age, adult flies have a significant buildup of insoluble ubiquitinated protein (IUP) aggregates in neural tissues [1,16,17,19,45]. We have also demonstrated that the rate at which protein aggregates increase (IUP, Ref(2)P) closely correlates with the tissue specific decline in autophagic capacity, which can be manipulated by genetic, transgenic and dietary factors [1,16,17,19,45]. Close examinations of FCs found relatively few proteolytic pathway components with significant expression differences in either head or thoracic tissues (Figure S3B). In sharp contrast, DAVID analysis of neural genes with altered variance scores identified multiple elements in proteolytic pathways that became hyper-variable with age (4W), which were largely suppressed by IF-treatment (4W/4W-IF ratio > 3.5, Tables S7 and S8). Individually, this included proteasomal (18), lysosomal (21), autophagy (7) and ubiquitin (7) pathway components, which in neural samples had remained undetected due to minimal FCs to message levels (Figure 6A; Tables S7 and S8). Following IF-treatment (4W-IF) there was substantial suppression of variance profiles for the same set of genes (Figure 6A) [23,26,43,45,46]. In matching thoracic samples, these genes showed minimal FC or VC differences, indicating proteolytic pathway components were largely unaffected by aging or dietary conditions in muscle tissues (Figure 6B; Tables S7 and S8).

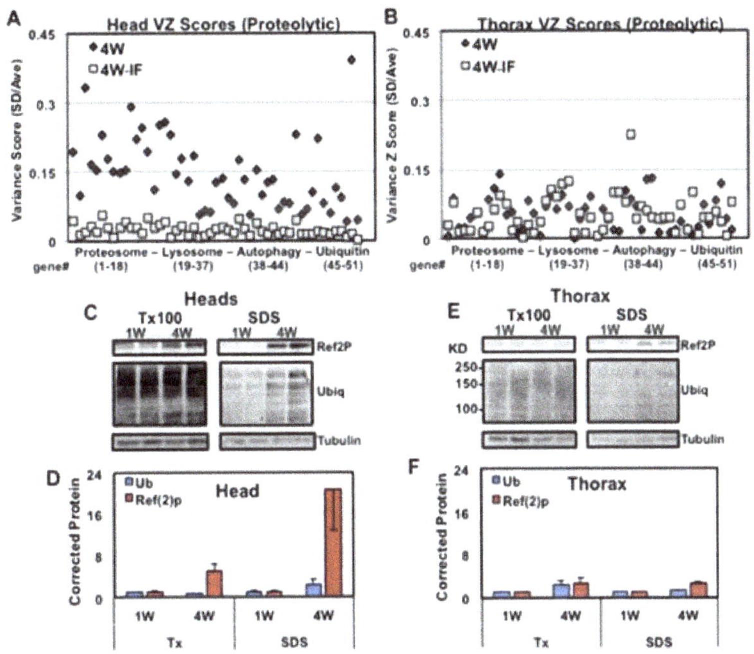

Figure 6. Age and IF-dependent tissue specific changes to proteolytic pathway variance and aggregate profiles. DAVID analysis was performed on neural transcripts that showed an age-related elevation and IF-reduction in TD variance scores (4W/4W-IF, >3.75). (**A**) Scatter plot of scaled variance Z scores (SD/Ave) of proteolytic pathway components from 4W (◆) to 4W-IF (■) head transcriptomes. (**B**) The scaled variance Z scores (SD/Ave) for the same cohort of genes from replicate 4W (◆) to 4W-IF (■) thoracic transcriptomes. See Tables S7 and S8 for individual gene information. Head and thoracic tissues from 1W to 4W flies underwent sequential detergent fractionation before Western analyses. Blots containing the Triton-X100 and SDS soluble protein fractions were probed with ant-UB, anti-Ref(2)P and anti-Tubulin antibodies and corrected protein levels quantified for both (**C**,**D**) head and (**E**,**F**) thoracic tissues. At 4 weeks of age, neural tissues demonstrated the buildup of protein aggregates, which is limited in age-matched thoracic samples.

Given the marked tissue-specific differences in proteolytic expression patterns, the age-dependent buildup of aggregate profiles between head and thoracic tissue samples was directly compared. Sequential Triton-X100 (1%) and SDS (2%) detergent protein extracts were isolated from replicate 1W to 4W old fly heads and thoraxes and Westerns probed to establish protein aggregate profiles (Figure 6C–F). In neural tissues, Western blots of the SDS soluble protein fractions showed the normal age-dependent buildup of neural protein aggregates (4W) (Figure 6C,D). Age-matched thoracic samples showed minimal IUP and Ref(2)P level differences (Figure 6E,F). Together this was consistent with our studies showing the timeline and tissue specific development of protein aggregates in the aging fly CNS, which also coincides with altered transcriptional regulation for proteolytic pathway components [1]. These results also underscored the concept that therapeutic changes, including modified diets, can have a positive influence on a diverse array of tissue-specific cellular processes including proteolysis [1,23,26,29]. The transcriptional changes observed with the intermittent fasting based diet also appears to reflect the long-term positive consequences for aged individuals in terms of global and tissue-specific expression patterns and physiological responses [38,39].

3. Discussion

The progressive changes to multiple interconnected cellular systems has been mechanistically linked to the aging [1,8,16,39]. It has consequently been challenging to separate the primary cause(s) leading to the progressive deterioration of cells and tissues from the downstream or secondary collateral effects of aging [3,8,9]. Both genetic and environmental studies have established that multiple cellular pathways are involved with and can influence the normal aging process as well as long-term maintenance and function of the nervous system [1,12,16,25,34]. The implications from other longevity studies are that net positive changes due to diet likely involved subtle alterations to signaling, epigenetic, mitochondrial and proteolytic based pathways [2,3,25,28,31,47]. In this report, we have used RNA-seq analysis to continue our investigation into the dynamic expression and phenotypic changes that occur in adult *Drosophila* as a consequence of aging and exposure to intermittent fasting [1]. Previously, we have demonstrated that IF-treatment had a positive impact on middle-aged flies by slowing the progression of several global and neurodegenerative phenotypes [1]. This included longer average lifespans, the preservation of adult behaviors (geotaxis), lower neural aggregate profiles (IUP, Ref(2)P) and enhance basal and acute autophagic responses in the aging fly nervous system [1]. This implied that even modest dietary changes could have a significant impact on the regulation of cellular pathways and that are essential for the long-term functional maintenance of adult tissues.

For this study, the selection of mRNA samples (time, treatment, tissue) was based on well-defined age-dependent alterations to the behavioral and physiological profiles of wild type adult flies [1,17,45]. The over primary goal of these studies was to identify early changes to transcriptome profiles that could serve as the nexus to assess early changes to molecular mechanisms involved with progressive age-related defects, and to highlight cellular pathways that are responsive to environmental treatments [1,2,8]. Our initial comparisons of PCA and expression clustering profiles for individual RNA-sequenced transcriptomes confirmed the similarities between replicate samples, and highlighted the dynamic tissue-specific changes occurring to basal expression profiles as consequence of aging or IF-treatment (Figure 1 and Figures S1 and S2; Tables 1 and 2) [29]. Further analysis confirmed that adult head and thoracic tissues have unique expression profiles that are selectively enriched for genes normally produced in neural, glial, or muscle cell types (Table S2). Global tissue-specific responses also included a relatively higher fold expression for thoracic transcripts, though neural tissues showed a larger number of genes responding to IF-treatment (4W/1W, Table 1). The relative number of genes that showed significant age-dependent FC and VC differences were similar between the two tissue types, although relatively few genes showed matching mRNA fluctuation patterns (Figure S2B).

IF-treatment may have a greater impact on the regulation of the adult head transcriptome profiles in part due to the level of tissue heterogeneity found within this *Drosophila* body segment. The majority of the adult thorax represents a relatively homogenous tissue, primarily comprised of flight and jump skeletal muscle cell type (see Table S2). Conversely, the adult fly head is comprised of diverse neural and glial cells, which have multiple functions and unique tissue specific transcriptional responses as a result of aging or IF exposure. The difference in the number of replicate transcriptome data sets used in our analysis of head (n = 3) and thorax (n = 2) tissues could have resulted in an under representation of expression differences between the two tissue types. However, the PCA and expression clustering analyses (Figure 1A,B and Figure S1) confirmed replicate sample similarities as well as the divergence expression trends that occurred as a result of age or dietary conditions for each tissue type. In addition, the relatively uniform number of genes showing age and IF-dependent changes between the two tissues (Tables 1 and 2) suggested that analysis of duplicate RNA-seq data sets, while not optimal could be used to identify significant fold and variance changes to individual transcripts.

From these initial studies, non-directed DAVID analysis identified multiple functional groups and pathways that demonstrated unique tissue-specific FC in expression that could be attributed to both aging and nutritional conditions (Figures 2–5 and Figures S2 and S3; Table 1 and Table S7) [23,29]. Each tissue showed unique age or IF-dependent changes to multiple pathway components, with only few genes demonstrating similar expression trends. One notable exception was the *Hsp22* gene, which in *Drosophila* serves as a chaperone protein involved with mitochondrial homeostasis, ROS detoxification and longevity-based functions [15,21]. Previously, fly tissues showed a basal age-dependent FC to *Hsp22* message and protein levels that closely correlates with enhanced longevity and stress resistance [15,21]. Consistent with these findings, RNA-seq and qRT-PCR analysis for both tissues showed an aged-dependent increase (4W) and IF-dependent reduction in the *Hsp22* message (Figure 4B,C). Together with elevated variance profiles in thoracic tissues (4W), this data suggests that IF-treatment reduces endogenous levels of cellular stress and may improve mitochondrial function in 4W-IF flies [15,21].

Recent studies examining the impact that aging and therapeutic compounds have on the regulation of adult *C. elegans* and murine transcriptome profiles, has highlighted the occurrence of transcriptional drift-variance in model organism [23,26]. This work has strengthened the concept that along with average FCs to mRNA levels, there exists an age-dependent increase in global expression drift-variance, likely reflecting the dysregulation of transcriptional stoichiometry [23,26]. Treatment with the drug mianserin (serotonergic pathway inhibitor) promoted longevity in adult *C. elegans* and resulted in a dose dependent reduction in TD and more youthful serotonergic pathway function [23,25]. Older mice exposed to the neural protective compound J147 also showed suppressed TD in neural tissues as well as the reduction in plasma metabolomics drift profiles [26]. Further, detecting TD variance in tissue transcriptome profiles from older human tissues suggests this is a conserved phenomenon, likely to involve progressive changes to epigenetic regulatory pathways [23,38,48,49]. In this study, we determined that tissue-specific changes to chromatin-remodeling pathway components (Figure 5A,B), closely correlated with the significant increase in TD profiles (4W) and the partial suppression of both following IF-treatment (Figure 5C–H). While both head and thoracic tissues showed a similar number of transcripts with an age-dependent increase in TD variance, the individual components were tissue-specific and largely did not overlap (Table 2). In addition, neural tissues appeared to have a greater response to IF-treatment and lower global expression variance profiles (4W-IF) than those found for matching thoracic transcriptome profiles (>3.75, Figure 5C–F; Table 2).

Since middle-aged *Drosophila* tissues showed unique VC transcriptional patterns DAVID analysis was used to characterized genes and functional pathways influenced by aging with IF-treatment and restored to more youthful pattern following IF exposure. In neural tissues genes showing lower VC have circadian (*tim, per*), olfactory (*Obp99a*), and neural (*neur, mnb, Fmr1, Sap47*) functions (Figure 5G; Table S5). The increase in TD profiles coincided with neuronal FC differences and the progressive decline and partial rescue of adult behaviors (Figure 3) [1,16]. For thoracic tissues, DAVID analyses revealed a very different set of genes showing dynamic FC and VC differences (Figure 5B,H and Figure 6B; Tables S6–S8). This included proteins involved with metabolism (Figures S2C and S4) as well as significant VCs to lipid homeostatic components (Figure 5H; Table S6) [32,42]. The functional potential impact of aging and IF-treatment on metabolic-based FC and VC in expression patterns closely correlated with improved starvation responses (Figure S4A,B) and more youthful catabolism rates for lipids (TG) in fasting 4W-IF flies (Figure S4C,D) [1,42]. Overall, the metabolic differences seen in IF-treated flies were consistent with previous dietary studies showing improved metabolic and physiological metrics in aged animals [2,32].

Along with age-related changes to key neuronal systems, the decline in CNS function is often associated with progressive proteostasis defects that include functional changes to the ubiquitin-proteasome and autophapy-lysosomal systems [1,16,17,25,34,50]. Indeed, the age-dependent formation of protein inclusions is often closely associated with the decline of motor behaviors, sensory perception (olfaction), sleep/circadian patterns and cognition [1,16,29,34]. Human studies and work using model systems have shown modified diets can slow the functional decline of the nervous system and may promote synaptic plasticity and neurogenesis in older adults [3,37,50]. In previous studies, we demonstrated that middle-aged flies exposed to IF-treatment demonstrated improved autophagy profiles including basal and acute fasting responses [1]. Consistent with this finding was the pronounced VC detected for multiple proteolytic components within the proteasome (*Rpn1,*), ubiquitin (*UBE4A*), lysosomal (*Cath-L*), and autophagy (*Atg16L2*, *PI3K59F*) pathways (Figure 6A; Tables S7 and S8). This appeared to be dynamic neural-specific VC, which was primarily not detected in matching thoracic samples (Figure 6B; Tables S7 and S8) [43,45,46,51]. Of particular note are key components involved with regulating proteostasis by the proteasome (subunits *Rpt*, *Rpn*) [46] and autophagy (*PI3K59F*, *Atg16L2*) [51], which showed significant VC and minimal FC in expression in contrasting transcriptome samples from aged fly cohorts (4W/4W-IF, Figure 6A; Tables S7 and S8). Taken together, the selective neuronal increase in proteolytic VC profiles was consistent with tissue-specific disparities observed in the timing and relative level of ubiquitinated protein aggregate accumulation (Figure 6C–F).

Overall this study indicates that conditions that alter in vivo aging phenotypes can be closely linked to expression difference to pathway components associated with individual functions. In addition, this analysis can also be used to identify upstream regulatory factors that coordinate the expression of key downstream functional components [39]. Therefore, observing the suppression of FC and TD profiles by select treatment conditions could not only highlight "sensitive" gene targets but also identify the cellular mechanisms that facilitate or promote their long-term regulation. This could include individual changes to signaling systems, transcription factors or epigenetic pathway components. In this study, IF-associated basal changes to expression patterns primarily highlighted differences to epigenetic components for both adult *Drosophila* tissues (Figure 5A,B). This implies that individual treatments or environmental conditions that alter aging phenotypes may be reflected as unique tissue-specific transcriptional "fingerprints" that are impacted by nucleosome and heterochromatin modifications [18,38,39,52]. In terms of healthy human aging, there is a growing appreciation that modest dietary interventions may be an effective method to preserve more youthful transcription patterns and facilitate the treatment of chronic progressive disorders [27,34,53,54]. The overarching goal for this type of treatment would be to maximize the benefit, while minimizing the side effects and compliance issues associated with harsher dietary regimens, including caloric restriction [34,54,55]. Given these attributes, applying targeted dietary modifications to aging population may have a lasting beneficial effect upon disorders linked to the functional decline of the nervous system [6,37,47,56–58].

4. Material and Methods

4.1. Drosophila Stocks, Culturing Conditions and Starvation Responses

Canton-S (CS) and w^{1118} fly stocks (Bloomington *Drosophila* Stock Center, Bloomington, IN, USA), crosses and F1 offspring have been previously described and were originally obtained from the Bloomington Stock center (Bloomington, IN, USA) [1]. Flies used for each study represented F1 offspring generated from crosses between CS virgin females and w^{1118} males (w^{1118}/+) [16]. Adult male flies were collected within four hours of eclosion and maintained on standard fly media (25 per vial) and culturing conditions (25 °C, 65% humidity, 12-h light:dark, LD cycle) [1,16]. For IF-treatment studies, flies were maintained using standard conditions and media until 1-week of age, then were exposed to either IF or *ad libitum* culturing conditions [1]. IF-treated flies were turned onto fasting vials (1% agar) three times per week from 9:00 a.m. to 5:00 p.m. (8-h) [1]. For all studies, IF-treated flies were placed on *ad libitum* conditions for two full days prior to being used for behavioral and starvation studies or being flash frozen in liquid nitrogen for subsequent tissue isolation [1]. Flies were stored at −80 °C for before tissues were isolated and processed for mRNA, protein or metabolic analyses [1].

4.2. RNA Isolation, Library Construction, RNA-Sequencing and Bioinformatics Analyses

F1 fly cohorts ($w^{1118}/+$) exposed to IF-treatment or *ad libitum* conditions for three weeks were collected and flash frozen at 1-week or at 4-week of age. *Drosophila* tissue processing, RNA isolation and cDNA library construction are outlined in Supplemental Information [16]. Libraries were sequenced using the Illumina HiSeq2000 technology (Illumina, Inc., San Diego, CA, USA) for single-end 100-bp format (7-base index). Briefly, staff at The Scripps Research Institute Sequencing Core Facility (La Jolla, CA, USA) processed sequencing data to generate FASTQ files demultiplexed based on index sequences [2,24]. Sequenced reads were mapped to a *Drosophila* reference genome (UCSC Genome and Browser (vmm9.gtf, UCSC, Santa Cruz, CA, USA) and alignments generated using TopHat (v2.0.9) and Bowtie 2 (v2.1.0, John Hopkins University, Baltimore, MD, USA) software., Cufflinks (http://cufflinks.cbcb.umd.edu/) was used to assemble sequence reads for individual transcripts [2,24,29]. For each sequenced library, the number of reads per gene was normalized and reported as RPKM values as an estimation of expression levels. To determine the fold changes, both the average RPKM and $\log_2$ RPKM scaled values for each gene was determined from replicate reads (FC = Ave log2 RPKM 4W/Ave log2 RPKM 1W). Significant expression differences due to aging were set at >1.4 (4W/1W) and IF-treatment at >1.3 (4W/4W-IF). In addition, normalized RPKM values used to generate heat maps (fold), variance fold changes and drift-variance plots (box plots) from different transcript cohorts and are further detailed in Supplemental Information. The AltAnalyse software (v2.1.0, Cincinnati Children's Hospital, Cincinnati, OH, USA) was used for PCA analysis and to generate expression-clustering profiles for each RNA-seq data set. The DAVID bioinformatics program (https://david.ndifcrf.gov) was used to identify functional gene clusters and associations for transcripts showing fold or variance differences due to age or IF. A custom designed Python program (Python 3.6.4, Copyright© 2001–2018 Python Software Foundation, https://www.python.org/psf/) was used to refine functional pathway gene lists that were used to generate heatmaps, expression tables and variance scatter plots. Methods used to normalize values for heatmaps, transcriptional drift and drift-variance profiles and normalized drift-variance values are further detailed in Supplemental Information.

4.3. 24-h Activity Profiles of Aged Group-Housed Male Flies

Outcrossed male flies were collected within 4 h of eclosion and aged in cohorts of 25 using standard husbandry and IF conditions. Flies were entrained using 12-h light and 12-h dark conditions (LD), with lights-on starting at 8:00 a.m. and lights-off at 8:00 p.m. [16,20]. The activity profiles of group-housed male flies were examined using the LAM25 systems (Trikinetics Inc., Waltham, MA, USA) and established protocols [16]. The LAM25 system detects fly movement (infrared beam breaks) and activity events were detected using the DAM System3 program (Trikinetics Inc., Waltham, MA, USA) [16]. Following an overnight recovery, the activity profiles of 1W, 4W and 4W-IF male fly groups (10 per vial) were monitored for 48 consecutive hours, using 12-h LD conditions [16]. Collected data sets were further analyzed using a custom-designed Python program (https://www.python.org/psf/, Python v3.6.4, Copyright © 2001-2018 Python Software Foundation) and Microsoft Excel software (Microsoft Office®, Mac 2011 v14.7.1) to generate activity graphs during the 12-light (ZT0–12), 12-dark (ZT12–24) and 6-h mid-dark (ZT15–21) time periods [16].

4.4. Quantitative RT-PCR

Flies from different ages and treatment conditions were collected, flash frozen and stored at −80 °C. Head and thoracic tissues were isolated, cDNA libraries generated quantitative Real-Time PCR studies performed using established technique [16,20]. The relative mRNA expression of 1W WT flies (w^{1118}/+) was set to 1.0 and subsequent RNA values were also normalized to the housekeeping *CXba* transcript [1,16,19]. Primer sequences will be provided upon request and additional methods details are included in Supplemental Information.

4.5. Metabolite Profiles

Adult male flies from 1W, 4W, or 4W-IF conditions were fasted for 0-h, 4-h or 8-h on 1% agar prior to final collection, flash freezing and storage at −80 °C. See Supplemental Information for additional detailed methods used to determine whole body triglyceride, glycogen and glucose levels and Figure S4 for results [1,42,43].

4.6. Western Blot Analysis

Outcrossed male flies were aged, collected and flash frozen at 1 and 3-week of age. Adult heads and thoraces were collected and individual tissues homogenized using standardized reagents and techniques. [1,16,20]. See Supplemental Information for detailed methods.

4.7. Statistical Analysis

Quantified Western blot, activity profiles, and metabolic graphs were generated using Microsoft Excel and figures assembled in PowerPoint (Microsoft Office®, Mac 2011 v14.7.1) [16]. Unless otherwise stated statistical analyses between groups were performed using the GraphPad software (https://www.graphpad.com/) and Student's *t*-test (two-tailed, unpaired). All values are reported as mean values ± SEM [16,20].

5. Conclusions

This and previous studies have demonstrated that even modest dietary modifications can have a significant beneficial impact on the cellular processes and physiological responses of aging worms, flies, mice and humans [1–3,5,47]. Along with promoting longevity and healthy neural aging, we have shown that IF-treatment can have a net positive impact on the progressive decline of several additional phenotypes that are reflected by the tissue-specific fluctuations to adult *Drosophila* transcriptome profiles [1,2]. This includes more youthful metabolic responses, the maintenance of olfactory-based courtship behavior, and the neural specific buildup of proteins aggregates [1,3,4,7,16,34]. The work detailed in this study indicates that even modest dietary changes can have a significant impact on progression of aging phenotypes, which in turn is reflected by significant differences in basal expression patterns. Our results indicate that protein homeostasis and clearance pathways in neural tissues are influenced and that changes to upstream epigenetic factors may be mediating these responses [59,60].

Acknowledgments: We would like to thank Steven Head and other members of the Next Generation Sequencing Core facility at The Scripps Research Institute (TSRI). We would also like to thank Michael Petrascheck (TSRI) for helpful discussions regarding the analysis and modeling of transcriptional drift-variance in *Drosophila* tissues. This work was supported by grants from NIH/NIA including: R21AG030187, R01AG039628 and R44AG033427.

Author Contributions: Eric P. Ratliff, Roxanne W. Kotzebue, Sharon Zhang, Kim D. Finley conceived of these studies. Eric P. Ratliff, Sharon Zhang, Brandon Molina, Ruth E. Mauntz, Arysa Gonzalez, Madhulika Achal, Nadja El-Mecharrafie, Roxanne W. Kotzebue, Ayeh Barekat, Kim D. Finley carried out the analyses of expression data (RNA sequencing, qRT-PCR) as well as experiments involving Western analysis, behaviors and metabolic experiments. Sharon Zhang, Daniel Daugherty, Eric P. Ratliff, Ruth E. Mauntz, Madhulika Achal, Robert A. Edwards, Kim D. Finley conducted bioinformatics analysis and interpretation of data sets. Sharon Zhang,

Andrew M. Macias, Eric P. Ratliff, Greg L. Harris, Jessica Mastroianni, William A. Bray, Kim D. Finley prepared the manuscript.

References

1. Ratliff, E.P.; Kotzebue, R.W.; Molina, B.; Mauntz, R.E.; Gonzalez, A.; Barekat, A.; El-Mecharrafie, N.; Garza, S.; Gurney, M.A.; Achal, M.; et al. Assessing Basal and Acute Autophagic Responses in the Adult *Drosophila* Nervous System: The Impact of Gender, Genetics and Diet on Endogenous Pathway Profiles. *PLoS ONE* **2016**, *11*, e0164239. [CrossRef] [PubMed]
2. Gill, S.; Le, H.D.; Melkani, G.C.; Panda, S. Time-restricted feeding attenuates age-related cardiac decline in *Drosophila*. *Science* **2015**, *347*, 1265–1269. [CrossRef] [PubMed]
3. Brandhorst, S.; Choi, I.Y.; Wei, M.; Cheng, C.W.; Sedrakyan, S.; Navarrete, G.; Dubeau, L.; Yap, L.P.; Park, R.; Vinciguerra, M.; et al. A Periodic Diet that Mimics Fasting Promotes Multi-System Regeneration, Enhanced Cognitive Performance, and Healthspan. *Cell Metab.* **2015**, *22*, 86–99. [CrossRef] [PubMed]
4. Hansen, M.; Chandra, A.; Mitic, L.L.; Onken, B.; Driscoll, M.; Kenyon, C. A role for autophagy in the extension of lifespan by dietary restriction in *C. elegans*. *PLoS Genet.* **2008**, *4*, e24. [CrossRef] [PubMed]
5. Longo, V.D.; Antebi, A.; Bartke, A.; Barzilai, N.; Brown-Borg, H.M.; Caruso, C.; Curiel, T.J.; de Cabo, R.; Franceschi, C.; Gems, D.; et al. Interventions to Slow Aging in Humans: Are We Ready? *Aging Cell* **2015**, *14*, 497–510. [CrossRef] [PubMed]
6. Longo, V.D.; Panda, S. Fasting, Circadian Rhythms, and Time-Restricted Feeding in Healthy Lifespan. *Cell Metab.* **2016**, *23*, 1048–1059. [CrossRef] [PubMed]
7. Min, K.J.; Tatar, M. Restriction of amino acids extends lifespan in *Drosophila melanogaster*. *Mech. Ageing Dev.* **2006**, *127*, 643–646. [CrossRef] [PubMed]
8. Wang, L.; Karpac, J.; Jasper, H. Promoting longevity by maintaining metabolic and proliferative homeostasis. *J. Exp. Biol.* **2014**, *217*, 109–118. [CrossRef] [PubMed]
9. Hansen, M.; Kennedy, B.K. Does Longer Lifespan Mean Longer Healthspan? *Trends Cell Biol.* **2016**, *26*, 565–568. [CrossRef] [PubMed]
10. Sala, A.J.; Bott, L.C.; Morimoto, R.I. Shaping proteostasis at the cellular, tissue, and organismal level. *J. Cell Biol.* **2017**, *216*, 1231–1241. [CrossRef] [PubMed]
11. Grandison, R.C.; Wong, R.; Bass, T.M.; Partridge, L.; Piper, M.D. Effect of a standardised dietary restriction protocol on multiple laboratory strains of *Drosophila melanogaster*. *PLoS ONE* **2009**, *4*, e4067. [CrossRef] [PubMed]
12. Hwangbo, D.S.; Gershman, B.; Tu, M.P.; Palmer, M.; Tatar, M. *Drosophila* dFOXO controls lifespan and regulates insulin signalling in brain and fat body. *Nature* **2004**, *429*, 562–566. [CrossRef] [PubMed]
13. Yamamoto, R.; Tatar, M. Insulin receptor substrate chico acts with the transcription factor FOXO to extend *Drosophila* lifespan. *Aging Cell* **2011**, *10*, 729–732. [CrossRef] [PubMed]
14. Stegeman, R.; Weake, V.M. Transcriptional Signatures of Aging. *J. Mol. Biol.* **2017**. [CrossRef] [PubMed]
15. Tower, J.; Landis, G.; Gao, R.; Luan, A.; Lee, J.; Sun, Y. Variegated expression of Hsp22 transgenic reporters indicates cell-specific patterns of aging in *Drosophila* oenocytes. *J. Gerontol. A Biol. Sci. Med. Sci.* **2014**, *69*, 253–259. [CrossRef] [PubMed]
16. Ratliff, E.P.; Mauntz, R.E.; Kotzebue, R.W.; Gonzalez, A.; Achal, M.; Barekat, A.; Finley, K.A.; Sparhawk, J.M.; Robinson, J.E.; Herr, D.R.; et al. Aging and Autophagic Function Influences the Progressive Decline of Adult *Drosophila* Behaviors. *PLoS ONE* **2015**, *10*, e0132768. [CrossRef] [PubMed]
17. Bartlett, B.J.; Isakson, P.; Lewerenz, J.; Sanchez, H.; Kotzebue, R.W.; Cumming, R.C.; Harris, G.L.; Nezis, I.P.; Schubert, D.R.; Simonsen, A.; et al. p62, Ref(2)P and ubiquitinated proteins are conserved markers of neuronal aging, aggregate formation and progressive autophagic defects. *Autophagy* **2011**, *7*. [CrossRef]
18. Wood, J.G.; Hillenmeyer, S.; Lawrence, C.; Chang, C.; Hosier, S.; Lightfoot, W.; Mukherjee, E.; Jiang, N.; Schorl, C.; Brodsky, A.S.; et al. Chromatin remodeling in the aging genome of *Drosophila*. *Aging Cell* **2010**, *9*, 971–978. [CrossRef] [PubMed]
19. Simonsen, A.; Cumming, R.C.; Brech, A.; Isakson, P.; Schubert, D.R.; Finley, K.D. Promoting basal levels of autophagy in the nervous system enhances longevity and oxidant resistance in adult *Drosophila*. *Autophagy* **2008**, *4*, 176–184. [CrossRef] [PubMed]

20. Barekat, A.; Gonzalez, A.; Mauntz, R.E.; Kotzebue, R.W.; Molina, B.; El-Mecharrafie, N.; Conner, C.J.; Garza, S.; Melkani, G.C.; Joiner, W.J.; et al. Using *Drosophila* as an integrated model to study mild repetitive traumatic brain injury. *Sci. Rep.* **2016**, *6*, 25252. [CrossRef] [PubMed]
21. Morrow, G.; Tanguay, R.M. *Drosophila melanogaster* Hsp22: A mitochondrial small heat shock protein influencing the aging process. *Front. Genet.* **2015**, *6*, 103. [CrossRef] [PubMed]
22. Ivanisevic, J.; Stauch, K.L.; Petrascheck, M.; Benton, H.P.; Epstein, A.A.; Fang, M.; Gorantla, S.; Tran, M.; Hoang, L.; Kurczy, M.E.; et al. Metabolic drift in the aging brain. *Aging* **2016**, *8*, 1000–1020. [CrossRef] [PubMed]
23. Rangaraju, S.; Solis, G.M.; Thompson, R.C.; Gomez-Amaro, R.L.; Kurian, L.; Encalada, S.E.; Niculescu, A.B., 3rd; Salomon, D.R.; Petrascheck, M. Suppression of transcriptional drift extends *C. elegans* lifespan by postponing the onset of mortality. *Elife* **2015**, *4*, e08833. [CrossRef] [PubMed]
24. Landis, G.N.; Salomon, M.P.; Keroles, D.; Brookes, N.; Sekimura, T.; Tower, J. The progesterone antagonist mifepristone/RU486 blocks the negative effect on life span caused by mating in female *Drosophila*. *Aging* **2015**, *7*, 53–69. [CrossRef] [PubMed]
25. Rangaraju, S.; Solis, G.M.; Andersson, S.I.; Gomez-Amaro, R.L.; Kardakaris, R.; Broaddus, C.D.; Niculescu, A.B., 3rd; Petrascheck, M. Atypical antidepressants extend lifespan of Caenorhabditis elegans by activation of a non-cell-autonomous stress response. *Aging Cell* **2015**, *14*, 971–981. [CrossRef] [PubMed]
26. Goldberg, J.; Currais, A.; Prior, M.; Fischer, W.; Chiruta, C.; Ratliff, E.; Daugherty, D.; Dargusch, R.; Finley, K.; Esparza-Molto, P.B.; et al. The mitochondrial ATP synthase is a shared drug target for aging and dementia. *Aging Cell* **2018**. [CrossRef] [PubMed]
27. Schafer, M.J.; Dolgalev, I.; Alldred, M.J.; Heguy, A.; Ginsberg, S.D. Calorie Restriction Suppresses Age-Dependent Hippocampal Transcriptional Signatures. *PLoS ONE* **2015**, *10*, e0133923. [CrossRef] [PubMed]
28. Min, K.J.; Yamamoto, R.; Buch, S.; Pankratz, M.; Tatar, M. *Drosophila* lifespan control by dietary restriction independent of insulin-like signaling. *Aging Cell* **2008**, *7*, 199–206. [CrossRef] [PubMed]
29. Currais, A.; Goldberg, J.; Farrokhi, C.; Chang, M.; Prior, M.; Dargusch, R.; Daugherty, D.; Armando, A.; Quehenberger, O.; Maher, P. A comprehensive multiomics approach toward understanding the relationship between aging and dementia. *Aging* **2015**, *7*, 937–955. [CrossRef] [PubMed]
30. Tariq, M.A.; Kim, H.J.; Jejelowo, O.; Pourmand, N. Whole-transcriptome RNAseq analysis from minute amount of total RNA. *Nucleic Acids Res.* **2011**, *39*, e120. [CrossRef] [PubMed]
31. Buch, S.; Melcher, C.; Bauer, M.; Katzenberger, J.; Pankratz, M.J. Opposing effects of dietary protein and sugar regulate a transcriptional target of *Drosophila* insulin-like peptide signaling. *Cell Metab.* **2008**, *7*, 321–332. [CrossRef] [PubMed]
32. Chatterjee, D.; Katewa, S.D.; Qi, Y.; Jackson, S.A.; Kapahi, P.; Jasper, H. Control of metabolic adaptation to fasting by dILP6-induced insulin signaling in *Drosophila* oenocytes. *Proc. Natl. Acad. Sci. USA* **2014**, *111*, 17959–17964. [CrossRef] [PubMed]
33. Fann, D.Y.; Santro, T.; Manzanero, S.; Widiapradja, A.; Cheng, Y.L.; Lee, S.Y.; Chunduri, P.; Jo, D.G.; Stranahan, A.M.; Mattson, M.P.; et al. Intermittent fasting attenuates inflammasome activity in ischemic stroke. *Exp. Neurol.* **2014**, *257*, 114–119. [CrossRef] [PubMed]
34. Halagappa, V.K.; Guo, Z.; Pearson, M.; Matsuoka, Y.; Cutler, R.G.; Laferla, F.M.; Mattson, M.P. Intermittent fasting and caloric restriction ameliorate age-related behavioral deficits in the triple-transgenic mouse model of Alzheimer's disease. *Neurobiol. Dis.* **2007**, *26*, 212–220. [CrossRef] [PubMed]
35. Lee, S.; Notterpek, L. Dietary restriction supports peripheral nerve health by enhancing endogenous protein quality control mechanisms. *Exp. Gerontol.* **2013**, *48*, 1085–1090. [CrossRef] [PubMed]
36. Mattson, M.P. Lifelong brain health is a lifelong challenge: From evolutionary principles to empirical evidence. *Ageing Res. Rev.* **2015**, *20*, 37–45. [CrossRef] [PubMed]
37. Murphy, T.; Dias, G.P.; Thuret, S. Effects of diet on brain plasticity in animal and human studies: Mind the gap. *Neural Plast.* **2014**, *2014*, 563160. [CrossRef] [PubMed]
38. Xia, B.; Gerstin, E.; Schones, D.E.; Huang, W.; Steven de Belle, J. Transgenerational programming of longevity through E(z)-mediated histone H3K27 trimethylation in *Drosophila*. *Aging* **2016**, *8*, 2988–3008. [CrossRef] [PubMed]
39. Sierra, M.I.; Fernandez, A.F.; Fraga, M.F. Epigenetics of Aging. *Curr. Genom.* **2015**, *16*, 435–440. [CrossRef] [PubMed]

40. Anders, S.; McCarthy, D.J.; Chen, Y.; Okoniewski, M.; Smyth, G.K.; Huber, W.; Robinson, M.D. Count-based differential expression analysis of RNA sequencing data using R and Bioconductor. *Nat. Protoc.* **2013**, *8*, 1765–1786. [CrossRef] [PubMed]
41. Currais, A.; Fischer, W.; Maher, P.; Schubert, D. Intraneuronal protein aggregation as a trigger for inflammation and neurodegeneration in the aging brain. *FASEB J.* **2017**, *31*, 5–10. [CrossRef] [PubMed]
42. Walls, S.M., Jr.; Attle, S.J.; Brulte, G.B.; Walls, M.L.; Finley, K.D.; Chatfield, D.A.; Herr, D.R.; Harris, G.L. Identification of sphingolipid metabolites that induce obesity via misregulation of appetite, caloric intake and fat storage in *Drosophila*. *PLoS Genet.* **2013**, *9*, e1003970. [CrossRef] [PubMed]
43. Simonsen, A.; Cumming, R.C.; Finley, K.D. Linking lysosomal trafficking defects with changes in aging and stress response in *Drosophila*. *Autophagy* **2007**, *3*, 499–501. [CrossRef] [PubMed]
44. Zirin, J.; Nieuwenhuis, J.; Perrimon, N. Role of autophagy in glycogen breakdown and its relevance to chloroquine myopathy. *PLoS Biol.* **2013**, *11*, e1001708. [CrossRef] [PubMed]
45. Simonsen, A.; Cumming, R.C.; Lindmo, K.; Galaviz, V.; Cheng, S.; Rusten, T.E.; Finley, K.D. Genetic modifiers of the *Drosophila* blue cheese gene link defects in lysosomal transport with decreased life span and altered ubiquitinated-protein profiles. *Genetics* **2007**, *176*, 1283–1297. [CrossRef] [PubMed]
46. Tsakiri, E.N.; Sykiotis, G.P.; Papassideri, I.S.; Terpos, E.; Dimopoulos, M.A.; Gorgoulis, V.G.; Bohmann, D.; Trougakos, I.P. Proteasome dysfunction in *Drosophila* signals to an Nrf2-dependent regulatory circuit aiming to restore proteostasis and prevent premature aging. *Aging Cell* **2013**, *12*, 802–813. [CrossRef] [PubMed]
47. Longo, V.D.; Mattson, M.P. Fasting: Molecular mechanisms and clinical applications. *Cell Metab.* **2014**, *19*, 181–192. [CrossRef] [PubMed]
48. Tower, J. Mitochondrial maintenance failure in aging and role of sexual dimorphism. *Arch. Biochem. Biophys.* **2015**, *576*, 17–31. [CrossRef] [PubMed]
49. Lapierre, L.R.; Kumsta, C.; Sandri, M.; Ballabio, A.; Hansen, M. Transcriptional and epigenetic regulation of autophagy in aging. *Autophagy* **2015**, *11*, 867–880. [CrossRef] [PubMed]
50. Van Praag, H.; Fleshner, M.; Schwartz, M.W.; Mattson, M.P. Exercise, energy intake, glucose homeostasis, and the brain. *J. Neurosci.* **2014**, *34*, 15139–15149. [CrossRef] [PubMed]
51. Lipinski, M.M.; Zheng, B.; Lu, T.; Yan, Z.; Py, B.F.; Ng, A.; Xavier, R.J.; Li, C.; Yankner, B.A.; Scherzer, C.R.; et al. Genome-wide analysis reveals mechanisms modulating autophagy in normal brain aging and in Alzheimer's disease. *Proc. Natl. Acad. Sci. USA* **2010**, *107*, 14164–14169. [CrossRef] [PubMed]
52. Jiang, N.; Du, G.; Tobias, E.; Wood, J.G.; Whitaker, R.; Neretti, N.; Helfand, S.L. Dietary and genetic effects on age-related loss of gene silencing reveal epigenetic plasticity of chromatin repression during aging. *Aging* **2013**, *5*, 813–824. [CrossRef] [PubMed]
53. Hanzen, S.; Vielfort, K.; Yang, J.; Roger, F.; Andersson, V.; Zamarbide-Fores, S.; Andersson, R.; Malm, L.; Palais, G.; Biteau, B.; et al. Lifespan Control by Redox-Dependent Recruitment of Chaperones to Misfolded Proteins. *Cell* **2016**, *166*, 140–151. [CrossRef] [PubMed]
54. Huffman, D.M.; Schafer, M.J.; LeBrasseur, N.K. Energetic interventions for healthspan and resiliency with aging. *Exp. Gerontol.* **2016**, *86*, 73–83. [CrossRef] [PubMed]
55. Rogina, B.; Helfand, S.L. Sir2 mediates longevity in the fly through a pathway related to calorie restriction. *Proc. Natl. Acad. Sci. USA* **2004**, *101*, 15998–16003. [CrossRef] [PubMed]
56. Wang, H.B.; Loh, D.H.; Whittaker, D.S.; Cutler, T.; Howland, D.; Colwell, C.S. Time-Restricted Feeding Improves Circadian Dysfunction as well as Motor Symptoms in the Q175 Mouse Model of Huntington's Disease. *eNeuro* **2018**, *5*. [CrossRef] [PubMed]
57. Schumacher, B.; van der Pluijm, I.; Moorhouse, M.J.; Kosteas, T.; Robinson, A.R.; Suh, Y.; Breit, T.M.; van Steeg, H.; Niedernhofer, L.J.; van Ijcken, W.; et al. Delayed and accelerated aging share common longevity assurance mechanisms. *PLoS Genet.* **2008**, *4*, e1000161. [CrossRef] [PubMed]
58. Melkani, G.C.; Panda, S. Time-restricted feeding for prevention and treatment of cardiometabolic disorders. *J. Physiol.* **2017**, *595*, 3691–3700. [CrossRef] [PubMed]
59. Pal, S.; Tyler, J.K. Epigenetics and aging. *Sci. Adv.* **2016**, *2*, e1600584. [CrossRef] [PubMed]
60. Wood, J.G.; Jones, B.C.; Jiang, N.; Chang, C.; Hosier, S.; Wickremesinghe, P.; Garcia, M.; Hartnett, D.A.; Burhenn, L.; Neretti, N.; et al. Chromatin-modifying genetic interventions suppress age-associated transposable element activation and extend life span in *Drosophila*. *Proc. Natl. Acad. Sci. USA* **2016**, *113*, 11277–11282. [CrossRef] [PubMed]

4

Quiescence Entry, Maintenance and Exit in Adult Stem Cells

Karamat Mohammad, Paméla Dakik, Younes Medkour, Darya Mitrofanova and Vladimir I. Titorenko *

Department of Biology, Concordia University, 7141 Sherbrooke Street, West, SP Building, Room 501-13, Montreal, QC H4B 1R6, Canada; karamat.mohammad@concordia.ca (K.M.); pameladakik@gmail.com (P.D.); writetoyounes@gmail.com (Y.M.); mitrofanova_darya@hotmail.com (D.M.)

* Correspondence: vladimir.titorenko@concordia.ca

Abstract: Cells of unicellular and multicellular eukaryotes can respond to certain environmental cues by arresting the cell cycle and entering a reversible state of quiescence. Quiescent cells do not divide, but can re-enter the cell cycle and resume proliferation if exposed to some signals from the environment. Quiescent cells in mammals and humans include adult stem cells. These cells exhibit improved stress resistance and enhanced survival ability. In response to certain extrinsic signals, adult stem cells can self-renew by dividing asymmetrically. Such asymmetric divisions not only allow the maintenance of a population of quiescent cells, but also yield daughter progenitor cells. A multistep process of the controlled proliferation of these progenitor cells leads to the formation of one or more types of fully differentiated cells. An age-related decline in the ability of adult stem cells to balance quiescence maintenance and regulated proliferation has been implicated in many aging-associated diseases. In this review, we describe many traits shared by different types of quiescent adult stem cells. We discuss how these traits contribute to the quiescence, self-renewal, and proliferation of adult stem cells. We examine the cell-intrinsic mechanisms that allow establishing and sustaining the characteristic traits of adult stem cells, thereby regulating quiescence entry, maintenance, and exit.

Keywords: cell cycle; cellular quiescence; mechanisms of quiescence maintenance; mechanisms of quiescence entry and exit; adult stem cells; metabolism; mitochondria; reactive oxygen species; cell signaling; proteostasis

---

1. Introduction

Cellular quiescence is a reversible state of a temporary cell cycle arrest that can be induced in both metazoans and unicellular eukaryotes as a response to some anti-mitogenic factors [1–4]. These factors include cell-nonautonomous, extrinsic environmental cues and cell-autonomous, intrinsic regulatory mechanisms [1–4]. In mammals, the temporary cell cycle arrest and quiescence entry occur before cells reach the growth factor-dependent "restriction" (R) point of the G_1 phase [5,6]. In the budding yeast *Saccharomyces cerevisiae*, the nutrient-dependent "START A" point at the G_1 phase of the cell cycle is believed to be evolutionarily related to the R point in mammals [6–8]. Notably, under certain conditions some unicellular and multicellular cells, eukaryotic organisms can undergo a temporary cell cycle arrest and enter the quiescent state not only from the G_1 phase of the cell cycle, but also from the S, G_2, or M phase [9–19]. Studies in budding yeast suggest that this is because the entry into quiescence is controlled not by (or not only by) the cell cycle regulation machinery, but by (or also by) the metabolic status of the cell at a certain cell cycle phase [17,18]. Once the cell cycle is arrested at the R or START A point, cells enter a reversible G_0 phase of the cell cycle and become quiescent. In budding yeast and mammals, this reversible G_0 state of quiescence is also called the "quiescence cycle" of cell oscillation between at least two functional states [1–4,20].

The entry of cells into the reversible G_0 state of quiescence prevents their entry into the irreversible G_0 state of senescence or the irreversible G_0 state of terminal differentiation [2–4]. Of note, some "irreversibly arrested" senescent or terminally differentiated cells retain an intact (although silenced) mechanism for cell cycle re-entry, as they can resume proliferation in response to certain cell-extrinsic and cell-intrinsic factors [21–25]. Quiescent cells in the reversible G_0 state do not divide, but rather retain the ability to re-enter the cell cycle and resume proliferation in response to certain pro-mitogenic factors, which include cell-extrinsic environmental signals and cell-intrinsic regulatory mechanisms [2,4]. Cellular quiescence is actively maintained by complex multiprotein networks and represents a collection of heterogeneous states in both multicellular and unicellular eukaryotes [2–4,26–32].

Populations of unicellular eukaryotic organisms (such as various yeast species) in the wild are always able to undergo a reversible switch between the states of cellular quiescence and proliferation; such a switch is controlled by nutrient availability and some other environmental factors [3,8,19,33–36]. Adult organisms in "lower" metazoan organisms (such as nematodes and fruit flies) and in "higher" metazoans (such as plants, mammals, and humans) contain several distinct types of quiescent cells; adult stem cells are among these quiescent cells in mammals and humans [2,37–44].

Quiescent adult stem cells in different mammalian tissues are long-lived [2,29,45,46]. This is because they can actively support their resistance to various stresses and toxicities [2,29,45,46]. This is also because, when stimulated, quiescent adult stem cells can often self-renew by dividing infrequently and asymmetrically to form a new quiescent stem cell and an actively dividing daughter progenitor cell; then, the daughter progenitor cell can advance through a hierarchically organized and tightly controlled series of events that yield one or more types of terminally differentiated cells [2,47–51]. Of note, quiescent adult stem cells can also sometime undergo two types of symmetric divisions, either a proliferation division (which yields two identical quiescent stem cells) or a differentiation division (which yields two differentiated cells) [49,52–60].

A body of evidence indicates that the abilities of quiescent adult stem cells to resist stresses, self-renew, and produce fully differentiated cells are crucial for tissue repair and regeneration, and are vital for the growth, development, and health of the adult body [2,19,48,61–64]. The number of quiescent adult stem cells and the efficiencies with which they resist stresses, self-renew, and produce fully differentiated cells declines with age [29,31,32,45,46,61,62,64–81]. Such an age-related numerical and functional decline of quiescent adult stem cells impairs their ability to balance quiescence with proliferation activity, and has been implicated in the pathophysiology of cancer and other aging-associated diseases in mammals and humans [19,29,31,32,45,46,48,61,62,64,66,67,69,70,72–77,79–84]. Some genetic, dietary, and pharmacological interventions can delay cellular and organismal aging and postpone the onset of aging-associated diseases by decelerating an age-related decline in the number and/or functionality of quiescent adult stem cells [2,19,29,31,32,45,46,48,61,62,64–84]. Aging-associated changes in the specialized cellular neighborhoods of adult stem cells, which are known as the stem cell niches, provide an essential contribution to an age-related decline in the abilities of adult stem cells to sustain quiescence, proliferation capacity, and differentiation potential [85–91]. This is because the stem cell niches in diverse tissues produce and release certain short-range molecular signals that are indispensable for maintaining the quiescence, self-renewal, proliferation capacity, differentiation potential, and functionality of neighboring adult stem cells [2,91–93]. Since the efficiencies with which the stem cell niches produce and release such transmissible molecular signals are either enhanced or weakened with age, the cell-nonautonomous mechanisms orchestrated by these niches critically contribute to the age-related weakening of various aspects of stem cell functionality [85–91].

Here, we examine the characteristic metabolic, signal transduction, gene expression, epigenetic, stress survival, and cell cycle regulation features of quiescent adult stem cells in mammals and humans. We explore cell-intrinsic mechanisms regulating quiescence entry, maintenance, and exit in these cells.

2. Common Traits of Quiescent Adult Stem Cells and Cell-Intrinsic Mechanisms That in These Cells Control Quiescence Entry, Maintenance, and Exit

Quiescent adult stem cells residing in different tissues share a discrete set of metabolic, signal transduction, gene expression, epigenetic, stress survival, and cell cycle regulation traits, all of which are distinct from those of the fully differentiated progeny of such cells [94–97]. Many of these common traits are actively maintained by quiescent adult stem cells and define their stress resistance, self-renewal potential, and regulated proliferation and differentiation routes; thus, adult stem cells have developed cell-autonomous, intrinsic regulatory mechanisms for quiescence entry, maintenance, and exit [28,94–99]. These traits and mechanisms are outlined below and schematically depicted in Figures 1–6.

2.1. Common Metabolic Traits of Quiescent Adult Stem Cells Define Their Fate

Quiescent adult stem cells metabolize glucose and other carbohydrates mainly through aerobic glycolysis that yields pyruvate; instead of being transported to mitochondria, converted to acetyl-CoA, and incorporated into the mitochondrial tricarboxylic acid (TCA) cycle, this pyruvate is then transformed to lactate in the cytosol of these cells [28,43,97,98,100–103]. This metabolic signature of quiescent adult stem cells is actively sustained by the following processes and features that are characteristic of these cells: (1) the transcription factor hypoxia-inducible factor 1α (HIF-1α)-dependent upregulation of levels of many glycolytic enzymes (such as hexokinase, phosphofructokinase, glyceraldehyde 3-phosphate dehydrogenase, phosphoglycerate kinase, and enolase) and lactate dehydrogenase A (an enzyme involved in the formation of lactate from pyruvate) in the cytosol; (2) a downregulation of the MPC1 subunit of the pyruvate carrier complex in mitochondria; (3) a HIF-1α-dependent upregulation of the mitochondrial pyruvate dehydrogenase kinases PDK2 and PDK4, both of which inhibit the pyruvate dehydrogenase complex-driven conversion of pyruvate to acetyl CoA in mitochondria; (4) a dynamin-related protein 1 (DRP1)-dependent fragmentation of the mitochondrial network into globular and immature mitochondria with underdeveloped cristae; (5) an increased abundance of the mitochondrial membrane uncoupling protein UCP2 that uncouples and lowers oxidative phosphorylation (OXPHOS) in mitochondria; (6) an elevated concentration of the ATPase inhibitory factor 1 (IF1) that suppresses mitochondrial adenosine triphosphate (ATP) synthase activity; (7) an upregulation of the mitochondrial carrier homolog 2 (MTCH2), a negative regulator of mitochondrial OXPHOS that induces mitochondrial depolarization; (8) an HIF-2α-dependent upregulation of the primary antioxidant enzymes involved in the detoxification of reactive oxygen species (ROS); among these enzymes are catalase (CAT) in peroxisomes and mitochondria, glutathione peroxidase type 1 (GPX1) in peroxisomes and mitochondria, copper/zinc superoxide dismutase (SOD1) in the cytosol, mitochondria, and peroxisomes, and manganese superoxide dismutase (SOD2) in mitochondria; and (9) a decline in the extent of ROS-inflicted apoptotic cell death (Figure 1) [27,43,94,96,97,100,103–112].

A body of evidence supports the notion that the common features of adult stem cells are to metabolize carbohydrates mainly through aerobic glycolysis in the cytosol, to suppress carbohydrate oxidation in mitochondria, to fragment mitochondrial network into globular and immature mitochondria with underdeveloped cristae, and to stimulate ROS detoxification in several cellular locations are essential for the maintenance of quiescence, identity, high number, regulated proliferation, and controlled differentiation of these cells [43,71,94–97,100,101,110,113]. Specifically, the HIF-1α, HIF-2α, and transcription factor Meis1 (myeloid ecotropic viral insertion site 1)-dependent program of an intensified glycolytic flow, a weakened mitochondrial OXPHOS, and an enhanced ROS detoxification within hematopoietic stem cells residing in a hypoxic niche is essential for the maintenance of their quiescent state and number (Figure 1) [28,109,110,114–121]. An increased glycolytic flow and a decreased mitochondrial OXPHOS are also required for the quiescent state maintenance and number preservation in mesenchymal stromal cells that are known to reside within the hypoxic environment of the bone marrow niche [28,122].

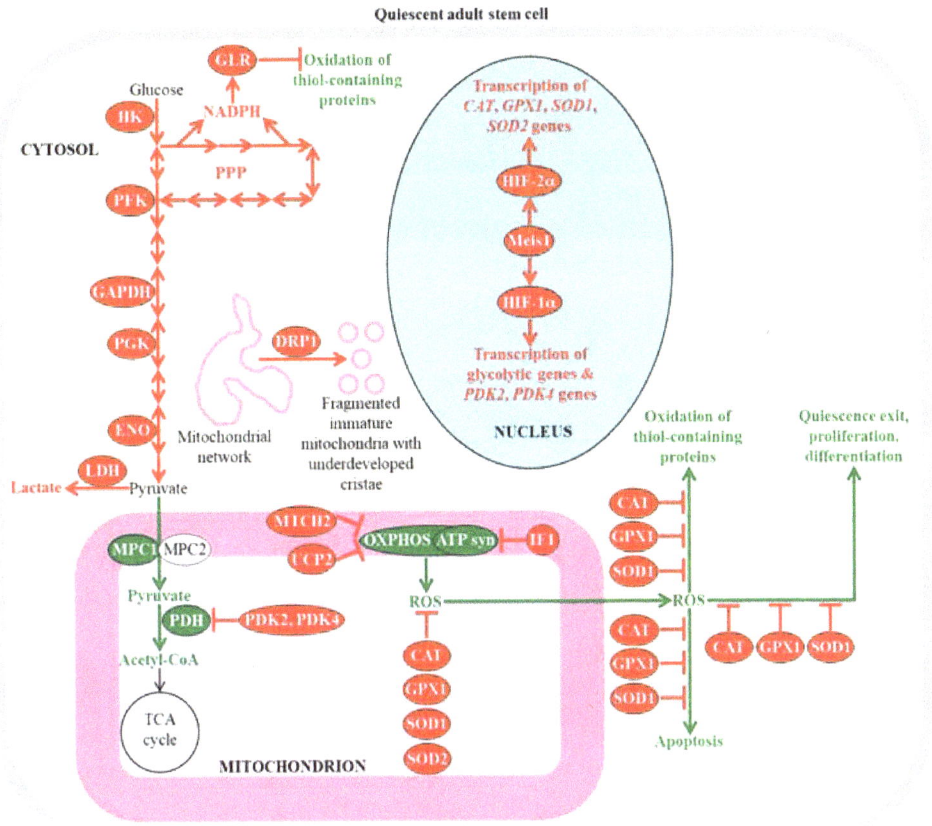

Figure 1. Some common metabolic features of adult stem cells are essential for the maintenance of their quiescence, number, proliferation potential, and differentiation ability. Among these metabolic features are carbohydrate metabolism mainly through aerobic glycolysis in the cytosol, suppressed carbohydrate oxidation in mitochondria, mitochondrial network fragmentation into globular and immature mitochondria with underdeveloped cristae, and stimulated ROS detoxification in several cellular locations. Enzymes, metabolites and processes whose activities, concentrations and rates are increased or decreased in quiescent adult stem cells (as compared to their fully differentiated progeny) are displayed in red or green color, respectively. The red one-way arrows and the red two-way arrows define irreversible and reversible (respectively) chemical reactions whose rates are increased in quiescent adult stem cells. The red inhibitory bars define inhibitory effects whose intensities are increased in quiescent adult stem cells. The green arrows define chemical reactions or processes whose rates or intensities are decreased in quiescent adult stem cells. The black arrow defines the irreversible chemical reaction whose rate is not changed in quiescent adult stem cells. See text for more details. Abbreviations: ATP syn, ATP synthase; CAT, catalase; DRP1, dynamin-related protein 1; ENO, enolase; GAPDH, glyceraldehyde 3-phosphate dehydrogenase; GLR, glutathione reductase; GPX1, glutathione peroxidase type 1; HIF-1α and HIF-2α, transcription factor hypoxia-inducible factors 1α and 2α, respectively; HK, hexokinase; IF1, inhibitory factor 1; LDH, lactate dehydrogenase; Meis1, myeloid ecotropic viral insertion site 1; MPC1 and MPC2, mitochondrial pyruvate carrier subunits 1 and 2; MTCH2, mitochondrial carrier homolog 2; OXPHOS, oxidative phosphorylation; PDH, pyruvate dehydrogenase; PDK2 and PDK4, pyruvate dehydrogenase kinases 2 and 4 (respectively); PFK, phosphofructokinase; PGK, phosphoglycerate kinase; PPP, pentose phosphate pathway; ROS, reactive oxygen species; SOD1 and SOD2, superoxide dismutases 1 and 2 (respectively); UCP2, uncoupling protein 2.

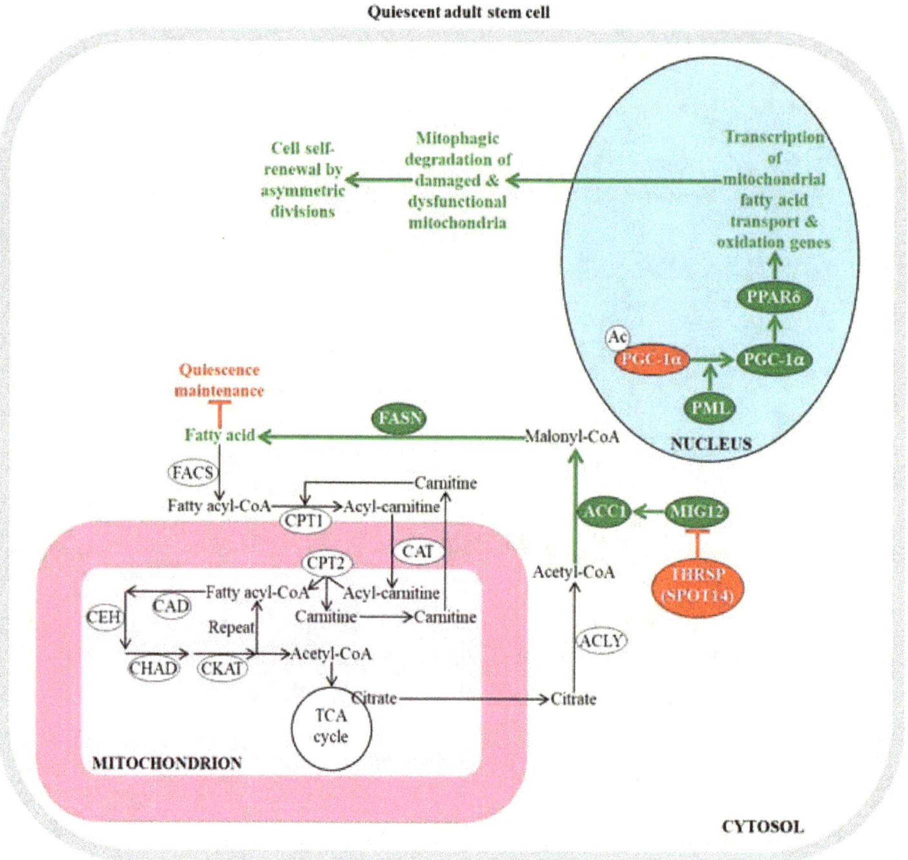

Figure 2. Mitochondrial β-oxidation of fatty acids and their synthesis in the cytosol of adult stem cells control the efficiency with which these cells can sustain quiescence or self-renew by asymmetric divisions. An inhibition of fatty acid synthesis in the cytosol is needed to sustain the quiescent state of adult neural stem cells. An activation of the transcription of nuclear genes that are involved in mitochondrial fatty acid transport and β-oxidation within adult stem cells is essential for the self-renewal of these cells by asymmetric divisions; such divisions lead to the formation of a new quiescent stem cell and an actively dividing daughter progenitor cell. Enzymes, metabolites, and processes whose activities, concentrations, and rates must be increased to maintain the quiescence of adult stem cells are displayed in red. Enzymes, metabolites, and processes whose activities, concentrations, and rates need be decreased to promote the self-renewal of adult stem cells by asymmetric divisions are displayed in green. The back arrows define chemical reactions whose rates are not essential for the maintenance of quiescence by adult stem cells. The green arrows define chemical reactions or processes whose rates or intensities must be decreased to maintain the quiescence of adult stem cells. The red inhibitory bars define inhibitory effects whose intensities must be increased to maintain the quiescence of adult stem cells. See text for more details. Abbreviations: Ac, acetyl group; ACC1, acetyl-CoA carboxylase 1; ACLY, ATP citrate lyase; CAD, acyl-CoA dehydrogenase; CAT, carnitine acylcarnitine translocase; CEH, enoyl-CoA hydratase; CHAD, hydroxyacyl-CoA dehydrogenase; CKAT, ketothiolase; CPT1 and CPT2, carnitine palmitoyltransferases 1 and 2 (respectively); FACS, fatty acyl-CoA synthase; FASN, fatty acid synthase; MIG12, midline-1-interacting G12-like protein; PGC-1α, peroxisome proliferator-activated receptor-gamma coactivator 1α; PML, promyelocytic leukaemia protein; PPARδ, peroxisome proliferator-activating receptor type δ; SPOT14, the 14th spot of proteins; THRSP, thyroid hormone-inducible hepatic protein.

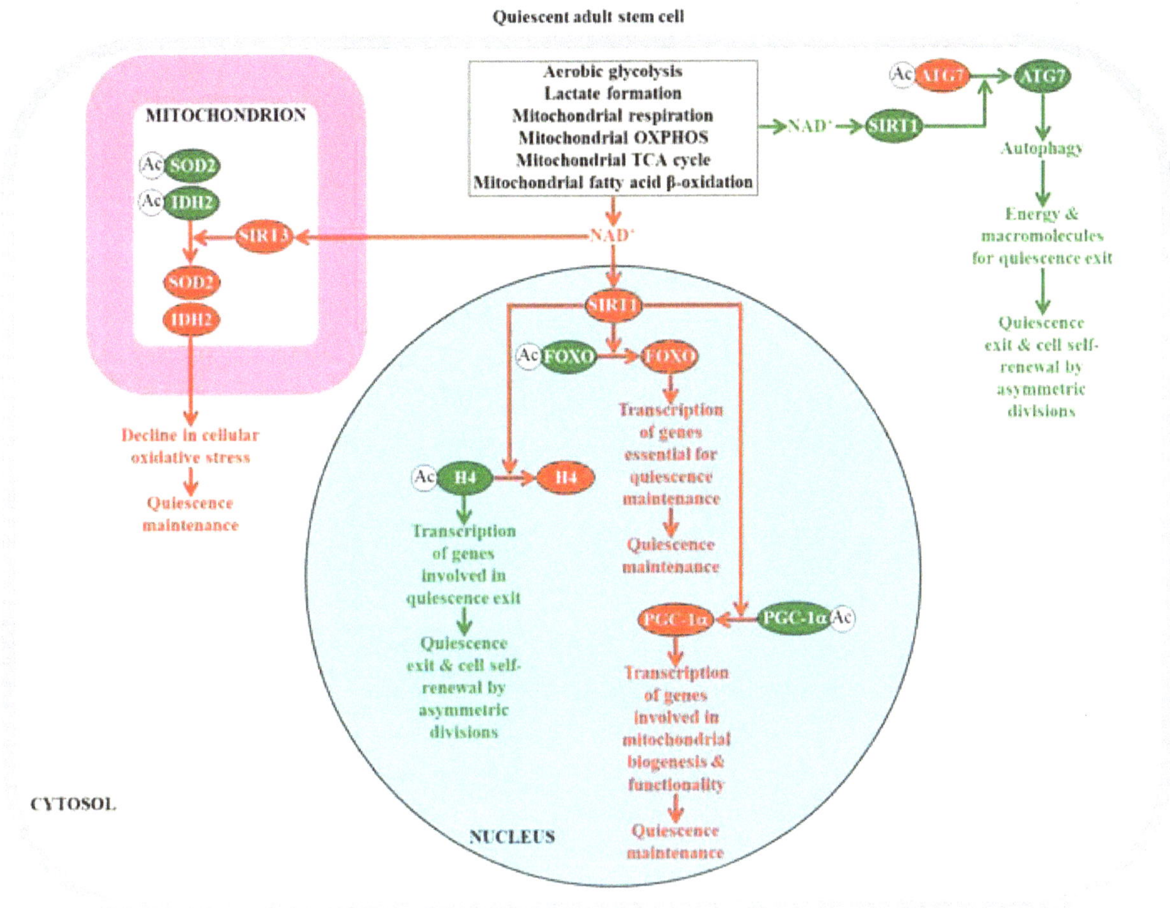

Figure 3. NAD^+ concentration within adult stem cells defines how efficiently these cells can maintain quiescence or self-renew by undergoing asymmetric divisions. The NAD^+-activated sirtuin SIRT1 in the nucleus is required for the maintenance of quiescence in adult stem cells, because this SIRT1 deacetylates histone H4 and the transcriptional factors FOXO and PGC-1α. The NAD^+-activated sirtuin SIRT3 in mitochondria is essential for quiescence maintenance by adult stem cells, because this SIRT3 deacetylates and activates superoxide dismutase SOD2 and isocitrate dehydrogenase IDH2, both of which weaken cellular oxidative stress. The NAD^+-activated sirtuin SIRT1 in the cytosol is required for the transition from quiescence to self-renewal by asymmetric divisions, because this SIRT1 deacetylates and activates the autophagy-related protein ATG7 to promote autophagy, which provides the energy and macromolecules required for such transitions. Proteins, metabolites, and processes whose activities, concentrations, and rates must be increased to maintain the quiescence of adult stem cells are displayed in red. Proteins, metabolites, and processes whose activities, concentrations, and rates must be increased to promote the self-renewal of adult stem cells by asymmetric divisions are displayed in green. The red arrows define processes whose intensities must be increased to maintain the quiescence of adult stem cells. The green arrows define processes whose intensities must be decreased to maintain the quiescence of adult stem cells. See text for more details. Abbreviations: Ac, acetyl group; ATG7, the autophagy-related protein 7; FOXO, transcriptional factors of the Forkhead family; H4, histone H4; IDH2, mitochondrial isocitrate dehydrogenase 2; OXPHOS, oxidative phosphorylation; PGC-1α, peroxisome proliferator-activated receptor-gamma coactivator 1α; SIRT1 and SIRT3, NAD^+-dependent protein deacetylases sirtuin 1 and sirtuin 3 (respectively); SOD2, mitochondrial manganese superoxide dismutase.

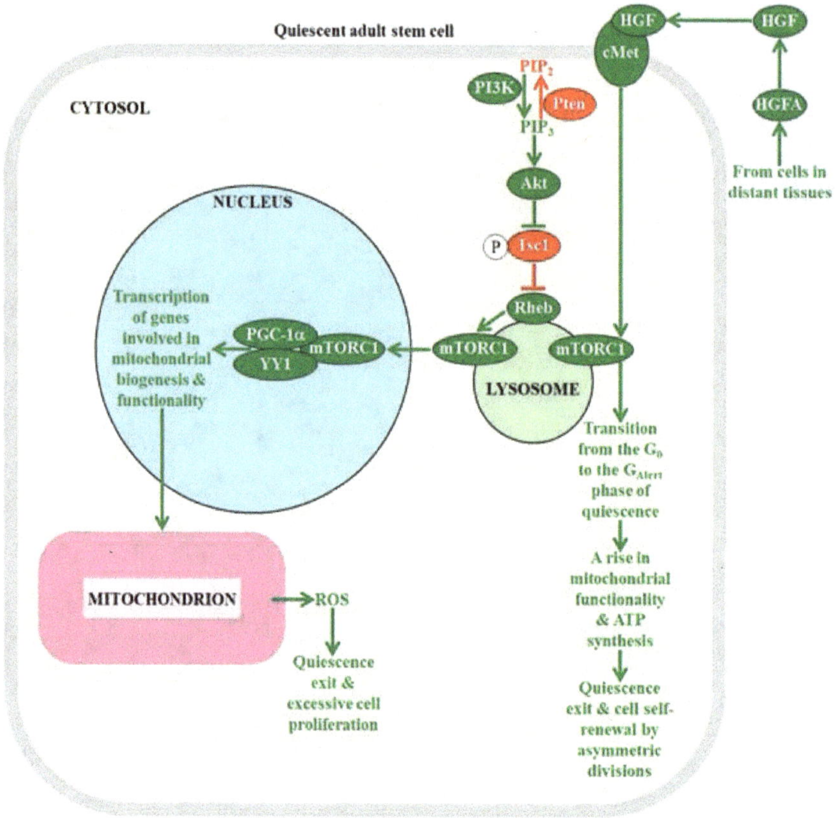

Figure 4. The intensity of information flow through the mTORC1-signaling pathway defines the fate of quiescent adult stem cells. A low intensity of mTORC1 signaling in adult stem cells decreases the extent of mitochondrial ROS production and release, thereby preventing the exit of these cells from the quiescent state and their excessive proliferation. An activation of mTORC1 signaling in response to hepatocyte growth factor, a cell-extrinsic pro-mitogenic signal, commits quiescent adult stem cells to cell cycle entry, proliferation, and differentiation. Proteins, metabolites, and processes whose activities, concentrations, and rates must be increased to maintain the quiescence of adult stem cells are displayed in red. Proteins, metabolites, and processes whose activities, concentrations, and rates need to be increased to promote the exit of adult stem cells from the state of quiescence are displayed in green. The red arrow defines the chemical reaction whose rate must be increased to maintain the quiescence of adult stem cells. The red inhibitory bar defines the inhibitory effect whose intensity must be increased to maintain the quiescence of adult stem cells. The green arrows define chemical reactions or processes whose rates or intensities must be increased to promote the exit of adult stem cells from the state of quiescence. See the text for more details. Abbreviations: Akt1, RAC-alpha serine/threonine protein kinase 1 or v-akt murine thymoma viral oncogene homolog 1; cMet, mesenchymal–epithelial transition factor; G_{Alert}, the "alert" phase of quiescence; HGF, hepatocyte growth factor; HGFA, hepatocyte growth factor activator; mTORC1, the mammalian (or mechanistic) target of rapamycin complex 1; PGC-1α, peroxisome proliferator-activated receptor-gamma coactivator 1α; PIP_2, phosphatidylinositol 4,5-bisphosphate; PIP_3, phosphatidylinositol (3,4,5)-trisphosphate; PI3K, phosphoinositide 3-kinase; Pten, phosphatase and tensin homologue; Rheb, Ras homolog enriched in brain; ROS, reactive oxygen species; Tsc1, tuberous sclerosis 1; YY1, yin-yang 1 transcription factor.

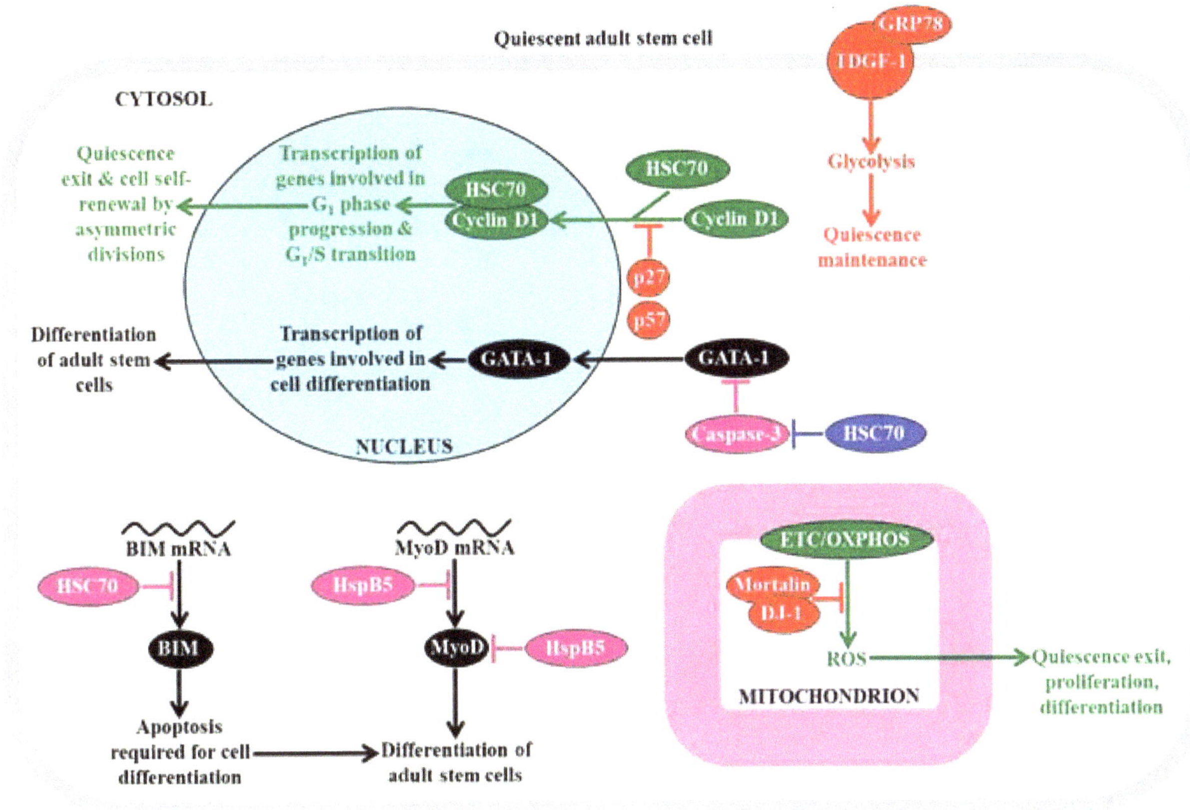

Figure 5. Several heat shock proteins (HSPs) play essential roles in preserving the quiescence, affecting the proliferation, and influencing the differentiation of adult stem cells. These HSPs control the nuclear import and degradation of some transcription factors, as well as the translation and stability of certain proteins that promote cell differentiation, glycolysis, and concentrations of mitochondrially-generated reactive oxygen species (ROS). Proteins, metabolites, and processes whose activities, concentrations, and rates must be increased to maintain the quiescence of adult stem cells are displayed in red. Proteins, metabolites, and processes whose activities, concentrations, and rates must be increased to promote the exit of adult stem cells from the state of quiescence are displayed in green. Proteins and processes whose activities and rates must be increased to promote the differentiation of adult stem cells are displayed in black. Proteins whose activities must be increased to suppress the differentiation of adult stem cells are displayed in pink. See text for more details. Abbreviations: BIM, Bcl-2-like protein 11; GATA-1, GATA-binding factor 1; GRP78, immunoglobulin heavy chain-binding protein homolog; HSC70, heat shock cognate 71 kDa protein; HspB5, alpha-crystallin B chain; MyoD, myoblast determination protein D; TDGF-1, teratocarcinoma-derived growth factor 1.

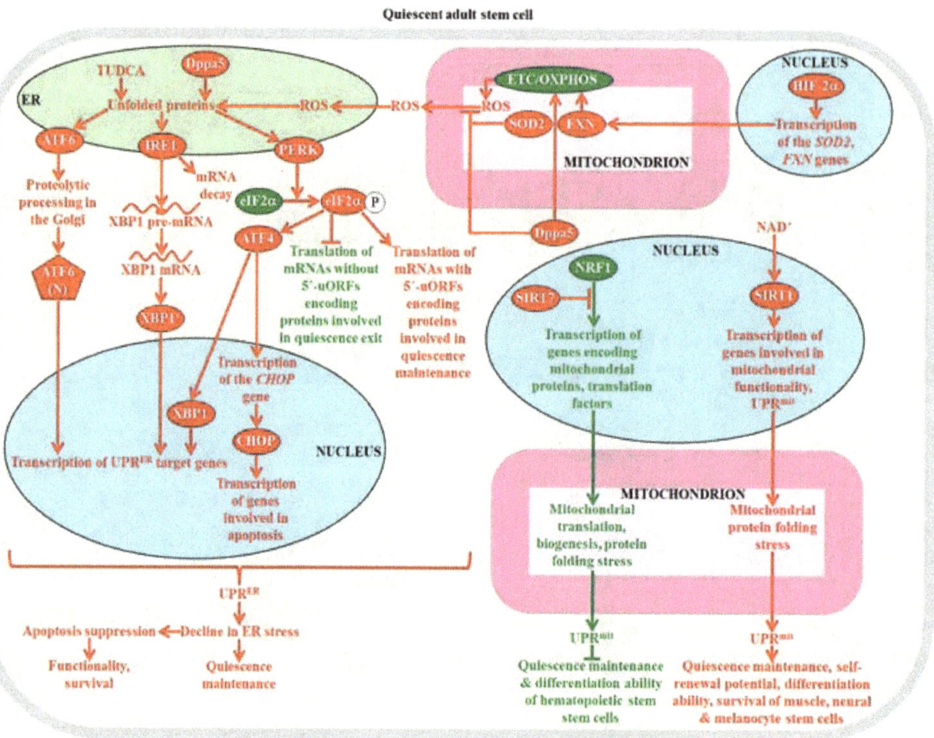

Figure 6. The unfolded protein response (UPR^{ER}) and (UPR^{mit}) systems of proteostasis restoration in adult stem cells are required for the maintenance of their quiescence, self-renewal proficiency, proliferation potential, differentiation competence, functionality, and viability. A stimulation of the ATF6 (activating transcription factor 6), IRE1 (inositol requiring enzyme 1), and PERK (PKR-like endoplasmic reticulum kinase) branches of the UPR^{ER} system is essential for the maintenance, self-renewal, functionality, and survival of adult stem cells. A SIRT7-dependent inhibition of the UPR^{mit} system is indispensable for sustaining the quiescence and differentiation capability of hematopoietic stem cells. A NAD^+/SIRT1-dependent stimulation of the UPR^{mit} system is required for the maintenance of the quiescence, self-renewal potential, differentiation ability, and viability of muscle stem cells, neural stem cells, and melanocyte stem cells. Proteins, metabolites, and processes whose activities, concentrations, and rates must be increased to maintain the quiescence of adult stem cells are displayed in red. Proteins, metabolites, and processes whose activities, concentrations, and rates need to be increased to promote the exit of adult stem cells from the state of quiescence are displayed in green. See text for more details. Abbreviations: ATF4, activating transcription factor 4; ATF6(N), N-terminal cytosolic fragment; CHOP, C/EBP homologous protein; Dppa5, developmental pluripotency-associated 5 protein; eIF2α, eukaryotic translation initiation factor 2α; ER, the endoplasmic reticulum; ETC, electron transport chain; FXN, frataxin; HIF-2α, hypoxia-inducible factor 2α; NRF1, nuclear respiratory factor 1; OXPHOS, oxidative phosphorylation; ROS, reactive oxygen species; SIRT1 and SIRT7, sirtuin 1 and sirtuin 7 (respectively); SOD2, mitochondrial manganese superoxide dismutase; TUDCA, tauroursodeoxycholic acid; uORFs, upstream open reading frames; XBP1, X-box binding protein 1; $XBP1^S$, X-box binding protein 1 translated as a protein product the spliced mRNA for XBP1.

Mechanisms through which the augmented glycolytic flow in adult stem cells can contribute to the maintenance of the quiescent state and number of these cells by regulating some downstream cellular processes require further investigation. One possibility is that such flow allows the glycolytic intermediate glucose-6-phosphate to enter the pentose phosphate pathway (PPP), which generates nicotinamide adenine dinucleotide phosphate (NADPH) (Figure 1) [123]. NADPH is not only the source of cellular reducing equivalents required for the synthesis of nucleic acids and lipids; it is also the electron donor that is essential for sustaining cellular redox homeostasis via the glutathione reductase system [123]. Since this system protects cellular macromolecules from oxidative damage inflicted by ROS, the intensified glycolytic flow in adult stem cells can defend macromolecules in these cells against ROS-dependent oxidative damage (Figure 1) [96,124–126]. The decline in mitochondrial OXPHOS, which is also characteristic of adult stem cells and generates the bulk of ROS, can contribute to the maintenance of the quiescent state and number of these cells through the two mechanisms described in Section 2.3.

2.2. Fatty Acid Oxidation and Synthesis Define the Fate of Quiescent Adult Stem Cells

Since mitochondrial transport and the oxidation of pyruvate are actively suppressed in adult stem cells (see above), the transport of fatty acid to mitochondria and the β-oxidation of fatty acids in mitochondria define the rate of mitochondrial respiration in these quiescent cells [43,97].

The efficiencies of mitochondrial fatty acid transport and β-oxidation regulate the self-renewal potential and proliferation capacity of adult stem cells [28,95,97]. A promyelocytic leukaemia protein (PML)/peroxisome proliferator-activated receptor-gamma coactivator 1α (PGC-1α)/peroxisome proliferator-activating receptor type δ (PPARδ)-dependent activation of transcription of nuclear genes involved in mitochondrial fatty acid transport and β-oxidation within hematopoietic stem cells is essential for the self-renewal of these cells by asymmetric divisions, in favor of symmetric differentiating divisions [127–129]; this is likely because such activation promotes the mitophagic degradation of damaged and dysfunctional mitochondria (Figure 2) [130].

The self-renewal of neural stem cells by asymmetric divisions also requires the efficiency of mitochondrial fatty acid β-oxidation to reach a certain threshold; it remains unknown why and how such optimal efficiency of mitochondrial fatty acid β-oxidation can fuel asymmetric divisions of neural stem cells but not their symmetric differentiating divisions [95,131,132].

Moreover, an optimal efficiency of mitochondrial fatty acid β-oxidation is needed for the self-renewal of quiescent skeletal muscle stem cells; however, the functionality and viability of these cells are impaired if such efficiency exceeds a certain, oxidative damage-inducing level [95,133,134].

Taken together, these findings indicate that there is a certain optimal efficiency of mitochondrial fatty acid β-oxidation at which this metabolic pathway actively supports the self-renewal potential and proliferation capacity of adult stem cells [95]. Mechanisms underlying this effect of mitochondrial fatty acid β-oxidation are presently unknown. One possible mechanism may involve the demonstrated ability of mitochondrial fatty acid β-oxidation to generate the bulk of NADPH [28,135], which is essential for sustaining cellular redox homeostasis via the glutathione reductase system in adult stem cells (see Section 2.1).

The self-renewal potential and proliferation capacity of adult stem cells can be controlled not only by the efficiencies of mitochondrial fatty acid transport and β-oxidation, but also by the efficiency with which fatty acids are synthesized in the cytosol. Specifically, the acetyl-CoA carboxylase (ACC) and fatty acid synthase (FASN)-dependent synthesis of fatty acids in the cytosol must be inhibited by thyroid hormone-inducible hepatic protein (THRSP; also known as the 14th spot of proteins [SPOT14] protein) to sustain the quiescent state of adult neural stem cells (Figure 2) [136]. This is most likely because certain concentrations of endogenous fatty acids can stimulate the exit of these cells from the quiescent state and their subsequent proliferation and differentiation [28,136]. However, some exogenously added acids and a high-fat diet rich in fatty acids exhibit the opposite effect on the quiescence and proliferation of a different kind of adult stem cell, specifically of intestinal stem cells [137]. In fact, endogenous fatty acids promote the quiescent state of these stem cells, and suppress their proliferation and differentiation [137].

In sum, these findings support the notion that a balance between the mitochondrial β-oxidation of fatty acids and their synthesis in the cytosol defines the fate of adult stem cells, because this balance controls the concentration of fatty acids within these cells. A regulated change of this balance can increase or decrease the intracellular concentration of fatty acids, thereby altering the efficiency with which these cells can sustain quiescence, self-renew by asymmetric divisions, or differentiate. It is also conceivable that different kinds of adult stem cells may differ in the threshold level of fatty acid concentrations that are capable of regulating the fate of these cells.

2.3. A Dual Role of ROS in Defining the Homeostasis and Functionality of Quiescent Adult Stem Cells

Since mitochondrial respiration is the major source of ROS within mammalian cells [138], the suppression of mitochondrial respiration and OXPHOS observed in adult stem cells elicits a significant decline in ROS within these cells [96,139,140].

The low concentration of ROS is a hallmark of adult stem cells, and it plays a dual essential role in sustaining the homeostasis, functionality, and long-term survival of these cells [2,71,95–97,124–126,141–145].

One role of such regulated decline in ROS is to protect the molecules of proteins, lipids, and nucleic acids within adult stem cells (including hematopoietic stems cells, neural stem cells, spermatogonial stem cells, and tracheal stem cells) against oxidative damage inflicted by ROS concentrations exceeding a toxic threshold [71,96,105,146–150]. If ROS concentrations within adult stem cells exceed such a toxic threshold, the DNA and other macromolecules in these cells are oxidatively damaged; this causes cell death, a decline in the number of adult stem cells, and ultimately leads to the exhaustion of the pool of these cells [71,151,152]. The protection of cellular macromolecules against ROS-dependent oxidative damage within adult stem cells is further enhanced by the high efficiencies of the antioxidant defense and DNA repair systems that are characteristic of these cells [96,124–126,153–155]. The antioxidant defense and DNA repair systems within adult stem cells include the following: (1) the NADPH-dependent glutathione reductase system for sustaining cellular redox homeostasis, which is fueled by the intensified glycolytic flow within these cells, as described in Section 2.1 (Figure 1); (2) the antioxidant system driven by the transcriptional activator FoxO3 of the forkhead family, which is activated by the NAD^+-dependent protein deacetylase sirtuin 1 (SIRT1); this system includes peroxisomal and mitochondrial CAT, mitochondrial SOD2, and mitochondrial thioredoxin-dependent peroxide reductase (PRDX3) [156–162]; (3) the antioxidant system orchestrated by the nuclear respiratory factor 2 (NRF2); this system includes enzymes involved in the synthesis of reduced glutathione and thioredoxin, NADPH-generating enzymes of the TCA cycle and pentose phosphate pathway, several forms of PRDX, and cytosolic thioredoxin reductase 1 (TXNRD1) [163,164]; and 4) the non-homologous end-joining (NHEJ) pathway for repairing DNA double-strand breaks [2,165]. In sum, the intensity of oxidative stress in adult stem cells is low. Such intensity is known to be defined by a balance between the efficiencies of cellular ROS production, ROS-inflicted oxidative damage, ROS detoxification, and oxidative damage repair [166–169]. Thus, the low concentration of ROS within adult stem cells, their high antioxidant capacity, and their enhanced ability to repair oxidatively damaged DNA protect these cells from excessive oxidative stress and damage.

It needs to be emphasized that the FoxO3-dependent and NRF2-dependent antioxidant defense systems, as well as the NHEJ pathway of DNA repair, are indispensable for the quiescence and/or long-term survival of adult stem cells. In fact, the FoxO3-dependent antioxidant defense system is essential for the self-renewal of neural stem cells by asymmetric divisions that allow maintaining a pool of these cells in a quiescent state [157,159,170,171]. Furthermore, the NRF2-dependent antioxidant defense system is required to preserve a pool of intestinal stem cells in the state of quiescence [163,164,172,173]. Moreover, the NHEJ pathway of DNA repair is needed for assuring the long-term survival of adult stem cells [2,174].

Another role of the regulated decline in ROS within quiescent adult stem cells is to suppress their symmetric differentiating divisions. These divisions: 1) are stimulated by ROS concentrations that exceed a certain threshold but remain non-toxic; and 2) cause proliferation and then the terminal differentiation of the cells, thereby exhausting the pool of quiescent adult stem cells [71,96,99,139,140,147,148,150,175–178]. Such stem cell proliferation-based and differentiation-based exhaustion of the pool of quiescent adult stem cells in response to a rise in ROS concentrations to a level below the toxic threshold has been reported for hematopoietic stems cells, intestinal stem cells, and skeletal muscle stem cells [71,157,159,163,164,170,171,175,179–182].

The downstream targets of ROS concentrations that elicit the cell proliferation-based and differentiation-based exhaustion of the pool of quiescent adult stem cells remain to be characterized. One of these targets of ROS in hematopoietic stems cells can be the p38α mitogen-activated protein kinase signaling pathway [183,184]. In response to increased ROS concentrations, this pathway stimulates the transcription factor Mitf (microphthalmia-associated transcription factor) that then activates the transcription of a gene for a rate-limiting enzyme of purine metabolism [184–186]. The resulting remodeling of purine metabolism alters the levels of amino acids and purine nucleotides, thus promoting cell cycle progression and cell proliferation in response to increased ROS concentrations [184–186].

2.4. Some Mitochondrial TCA Cycle Intermediates Contribute to Quiescence Maintenance by Adult Stem Cells

Recent findings suggest that the suppression of mitochondrial respiration and OXPHOS is not the only mitochondria-related factor involved in sustaining the homeostasis and functionality of adult stem cells. Specifically, it has been shown that some intermediates of the mitochondrial TCA cycle play essential roles in determining the fate of these cells; these intermediates include acetyl CoA, oxaloacetate, citrate, and α-ketoglutarate [31,77,94,187–191].

The essential roles of these TCA cycle intermediates in the fate of adult stem cells is due to their abilities to be cofactors or substrates for chromatin-modifying enzymes that catalyze some epigenetic modifications in the nucleus, such as histone acetylation/deacetylation and histone methylation, as well as DNA methylation and hypermethylation [2,31,71,77,94,187–196]. Some of these mitochondrial metabolism-driven modifications of histones and DNA have been observed only in neural stem cells, skeletal muscle stem cells, adipose-derived mesenchymal stem cells, muscle-derived mesenchymal stem cells, and bone marrow-derived mesenchymal stem cells, but not in their fully differentiated progeny; such stem cell-specific epigenetic modifications in the nucleus play essential roles in maintaining quiescence, regulating self-renewal and proliferation, and/or suppressing the differentiation of these adult stem cells [2,31,77,133,197–212].

Many of these stem cell-specific epigenetic modifications in the nucleus are known to activate or repress the transcription of genes implicated in different aspects of fate programming in adult stem cells, including the maintenance of their quiescence and self-renewal ability as well as their regulated proliferation and differentiation [2,31,77,188,189,197–203,206,207,210]. Nuclear genes whose transcription is activated in quiescent neural stem cells, muscle stem cells, hair follicle stem cells, umbilical cord-derived mesenchymal stem cells, and bone marrow-derived mesenchymal stem cells include genes that encode proteins that are involved in the G1/S cell cycle transition, epigenetic modifications in the nucleus, transcription of genes implicated in stem cell fate decisions, stemness, and microRNA formation [2,189,213–216]. Nuclear genes whose transcription is repressed in quiescent neural stem cells, muscle stem cells, hair follicle stem cells, adipose-derived mesenchymal stem cells, muscle-derived mesenchymal stem cells, and bone marrow-derived mesenchymal stem cells include genes that encode proteins implicated in DNA replication, chromosome segregation, cell cycle delay at several checkpoints, cell cycle progression, lineage specificity, and mitochondrial functionality [2,188,213–216].

Taken together, these findings suggest that certain mitochondrial metabolism-driven modifications of the epigenetic landscape within the nucleus of adult stem cells can alter the efficiencies with which some transcription factors activate or repress the expression of nuclear genes that are involved in the quiescent state maintenance by adult stem cells and/or in their response to environmental cues, proliferation, and differentiation [2,31,77,78,94,96].

Further investigation is required on the mechanisms through which the TCA cycle intermediates acetyl CoA, oxaloacetate, citrate, and α-ketoglutarate can maintain the homeostasis and functionality of adult stem cells by promoting epigenetic modifications of nuclear genes and altering the epigenetic landscape of these cells. In hematopoietic stems cells, skeletal muscle stem cells, and hair follicle stem cells, the histone 3 methyltransferases EZH1 and EZH2 (enhancer of zeste proteins 1 and 2, respectively) are essential components of such mechanisms; in fact, the downregulation of both proteins leads to a depletion of the pool of these quiescent adult stem cells, whereas the upregulation of EZH2 decelerates the exhaustion of hematopoietic stems cells [217–220].

2.5. NAD$^+$ Concentration within Adult Stem Cells Defines Their Fate

Relative rates of aerobic glycolysis, lactate formation, mitochondrial respiration, OXPHOS, mitochondrial TCA cycle, and mitochondrial fatty acid β-oxidation control the cellular concentrations of the oxidized and reduced forms of nicotinamide dinucleotide (NAD$^+$ and NADH, respectively) and, thus, the NAD$^+$/NADH ratio in adult stem cells [94,96,221]. The NAD$^+$/NADH ratio plays an essential role in defining the fate of adult stem cells not only because NAD$^+$ is a cofactor of all these metabolic processes, but also because NAD$^+$ is an activator of SIRT1 in the cytosol and SIRT3 in mitochondria [222–224].

A body of evidence supports the essential role of NAD$^+$-activated SIRT1 in defining the fate of adult neural stem cells. However, there are two conflicting views on how exactly NAD$^+$-activated SIRT1 can influence the fate of these cells. On the one hand, some studies suggest that NAD$^+$-activated SIRT1 promotes the quiescence of adult neural stem cells and suppresses their proliferation and differentiation. These studies have shown that (1) the genetic inactivation or pharmacological inhibition of SIRT1 in adult neural stem cells promotes their exit from quiescence and stimulates their proliferation and differentiation [225–229], and (2) SIRT1 overexpression or its resveratrol-driven activation preserves the quiescence of adult neural stem cells and suppresses their proliferation and differentiation [226,229]. On the other hand, other studies have suggested that NAD$^+$-activated SIRT1 suppresses the quiescence of adult neural stem cells and promotes their proliferation and differentiation. These other studies have demonstrated that (1) SIRT1 genetic downregulation or pharmacological inhibition promotes the quiescence of these cells and suppresses their proliferation and differentiation; and (2) SIRT1 overexpression stimulates the quiescence exit of these cells and accelerates their proliferation and differentiation in a mechanism that involves a transient translocation of SIRT1 from the cytosol into the nucleus [230–232]. In sum, the exact role of NAD$^+$-activated SIRT1 in defining the fate of adult neural stem cells remains controversial and requires further investigation.

The essential role of NAD$^+$ concentration and SIRT1 activity in defining the fate of adult stem cells is underscored by the finding that a decline in NAD$^+$ concentration within skeletal muscle stem cells lowers SIRT1 activity; this causes an increase in the extent of histone H4 acetylation and ultimately activates the transcription of nuclear genes involved in the transition from quiescence to the proliferation and differentiation of these stem cells [133,233]. Thus, one role of the NAD$^+$-dependent protein deacetylase SIRT1 in maintaining the quiescence of adult skeletal muscle stem cells is linked to its known ability to suppress the transcription of certain genes by specifically remodeling their epigenetic landscape through histone H4 deacetylation (Figure 3) [234–236].

Another mechanism through which NAD$^+$-activated SIRT1 contributes to quiescence maintenance in adult neural stem cells and adult skeletal muscle stem cells consists of the SIRT1-dependent deacetylation and activation of PGC-1α (a transcriptional activator of mitochondrial biogenesis) to promote mitochondrial functionality (Figure 3) [75,237–239].

It needs to be emphasized that the exact role of NAD$^+$-activated SIRT1 in the quiescence of adult skeletal muscle stem cells requires further investigation. Specifically, it has been demonstrated that when SIRT1 is activated by NAD$^+$ in these stem cells, it promotes autophagy by deacetylating and stimulating the autophagy-related protein 7 (ATG7) to provide the energy and macromolecules required for the transition from quiescence to proliferation followed by differentiation (Figure 3) [240,241]. This finding suggests that under certain conditions, NAD$^+$-activated SIRT1 can act via an autophagy-based mechanism that stimulates the exit from quiescence and promotes the proliferation and differentiation of adult skeletal muscle stem cells.

Of note, it has been proposed that NAD^+-activated SIRT1 in hematopoietic stem cells and neural stem cells may help to sustain their quiescent state by deacetylating another quiescence-related target of SIRT1, namely the DNA-binding forkhead box O (FOXO) transcription factors [48]. The SIRT1-dependent deacetylation of the FOXO transcriptional factors is known to enhance their ability to activate the transcription of many genes that are essential for preserving the quiescence of hematopoietic stem cells and neural stem cells, preventing their premature differentiation and maintaining their viability (Figure 3) [48,157,159,170,171,242,243].

SIRT3, a mitochondrial form of the NAD^+-dependent sirtuins, is essential for the maintenance of quiescence in adult hematopoietic stem cells [46,244,245]. Since NAD^+-stimulated SIRT3 deacetylates and activates some mitochondrial proteins involved in oxidative stress protection, it contributes to the quiescence maintenance of these cells by diminishing oxidative stress inside and outside of their mitochondria [46,244,245]. Specifically, when activated by NAD^+, SIRT3 deacetylates and activates SOD2, which is a major mitochondrial antioxidant enzyme; this reduces mitochondrial superoxide and weakens cellular oxidative stress (Figure 3) [245–247]. NAD^+-stimulated SIRT3 also deacetylates and activates isocitrate dehydrogenase 2 (IDH2) [244,248]. Mitochondrial IDH2 catalyzes a reaction that yields NADPH, the electron donor that is essential for sustaining cellular redox homeostasis via the glutathione reductase and thioredoxin reductase systems [123]. Thus, the SIRT3-driven deacetylation and activation of IDH2 also lessens cellular oxidative stress (Figure 3) [244,248].

2.6. A Low-Energy Status of Adult Stem Cells Helps Sustain Their Quiescence

As noted above, low efficiencies of OXPHOS and ATP synthesis in mitochondria are characteristic features of the metabolic signature of quiescent adult stem cells [94,96,97]. This causes a rise in the intracellular concentrations of adenosine monophosphate (AMP) and adenosine diphosphate (ADP), thereby creating a low-energy stress and activating the liver kinase B1 (LKB1; a master energy-sensing protein kinase) and the AMP-activated protein kinase (AMPK; a downstream phosphorylation target of LKB1) [249–252].

LKB1 is essential for the quiescence maintenance, functionality, and survival of hematopoietic stem cells in mice. In fact, a depletion of LKB has the following two temporally separated effects on hematopoietic stem cells and on the multipotent progenitors formed from these adult stem cells: (1) an initial loss of stem cell quiescence and the resulting rise in the number of cells comprising each of these two cell populations; and (2) a subsequent decline in the number, and the ultimate depletion, of both cell populations [253–255]. The hematopoietic stem cells of mice depleted of LKB1 lost the ability to regenerate the hematopoietic system of control mice, and this decline in the functionality of LKB1-depleted hematopoietic stem cells is followed by their apoptotic death [253–255]. A downstream target of LKB1 in hematopoietic stem cells is mitochondrial functionality, as LKB1 depletion in these cells decreases the expression of the transcriptional activators of mitochondrial biogenesis PGC-1α and PGC-1β, lowers mitochondrial ATP synthesis, and impairs mitochondrial integrity by decreasing mitochondrial membrane potential [253–255]. The decline in the integrity of mitochondria observed within LKB1-depleted hematopoietic stem cells is likely to be responsible for their accelerated apoptotic death [254]. These cells also undergo an induction of autophagy, which plays an essential protective role in the survival of LKB1-depleted hematopoietic stem cells [254]. It is conceivable that the ability of LKB1 to sustain the functionality and integrity of mitochondria, thereby decelerating apoptotic cell death, is linked to the essential role of this master energy-sensing protein kinase in preserving the quiescence, functionality, and survival of hematopoietic stem cells [253–256]. The involvement of LKB1 in preserving the quiescence of hematopoietic stem cells is complemented by the essential role of autophagy—a degradative elimination of dysfunctional macromolecules and organelles—in sustaining the quiescent state of these adult stem cells [257]. Although AMPK—the downstream phosphorylation and activation target of LKB1—is known to promote autophagy because it phosphorylates the autophagy-initiating protein kinase ULK1 [252]—a mechanism through which autophagic degradation is actively stimulated and sustained in hematopoietic stem cells to preserve their quiescence—it also requires further investigation.

The essential role of LKB1 in sustaining the quiescence, functionality, and survival of hematopoietic stem cells is not due to its activating effect on AMPK in these cells [253–255]. AMPK is a sensor of energetic stress and mitochondrial dysfunction that does not influence the fate of hematopoietic stem cells, neither before nor after being phosphorylated and activated by LKB1 [253–255,258]. Phosphorylated and activated AMPK is known to suppress the mammalian (or mechanistic) target of rapamycin complex 1 (mTORC1) signaling pathway [48,252], whose genetic enhancement elicits a depletion of hematopoietic stem cells [259–264] (see Section 2.7 for more details). Despite such an essential role of a low-intensity mTORC1 signaling in maintaining hematopoietic stem cell quiescence, the indispensable role of LKB1 in sustaining the quiescence, functionality, and survival of hematopoietic stem cells is not caused by the LKB1-driven and AMPK-dependent activation of the mTORC1 signaling pathway [253–255,258].

Although LKB1 controls the fates of hematopoietic stem cells and the multipotent progenitors formed from these cells, it does not affect the abundance or functionality of the fully differentiated progeny of such cells [253–255]. In contrast, LKB1 is not required for sustaining the quiescence, functionality, and survival of a different type of adult stem cells, namely intestinal stem cells [265]. However, LKB1 is essential for the normal differentiation and maturation of intestinal stem cells; mechanisms underlying such effects of LKB1 are presently unknown [265–267]. Thus, LKB1 can differently influence the self-renewal, proliferation, and differentiation of different types of adult stem cells.

2.7. The Maintenance of mTORC1 Signaling at Low Intensity in Adult Stem Cells Is Essential for Sustaining Their Quiescence, Self-Renewal, and Functionality

The mTORC1 signaling pathway is a key signaling hub that—in response to changes in extracellular and intracellular nutrients, pro-mitogenic stimuli, and stresses—alters the efficiencies of many anabolic and catabolic cellular processes to ensure a proper adaptation of the cell to such changes [268,269]. The anabolic processes controlled by mTORC1 include glycolysis and the pentose phosphate pathway, lipid and nucleotide synthesis, and protein synthesis [268,269]. Among the catabolic processes controlled by mTORC1 are autophagy and lysosome biogenesis, and the ubiquitin-dependent proteasomal degradation of proteins [268,269]. mTORC1 also controls cellular energy homeostasis by activating the YY1 (yin-yang 1)/PGC-1α-dependent transcription of nuclear genes involved in mitochondrial biogenesis and functionality [270–272].

Since some of the cellular processes regulated by mTORC1 can be involved in creating the metabolic signature of adult stem cells that is essential for their quiescence (see Sections 2.1–2.6), and because some of the processes creating such signatures are known to control mTORC1 via feedback regulation mechanisms [28,270–272], it is conceivable that mTORC1 may play an essential role in defining the fate of quiescent adult stem cells. In fact, an overactivation of the mTORC1 pathway by a mutation that depletes the protein inhibitor Pten (phosphatase and tensin homologue) of this pathway causes an exit of hematopoietic stem cells from quiescence, leads to a decline in functionality of these cells, decreases their self-renewal potential, alters their differentiation pattern, and eventually results in an exhaustion of the hematopoietic stem cell population pool in a cell-autonomous, mTORC1-dependent fashion (Figure 4) [259,260]. Furthermore, an enhancement of the mTORC1 pathway by a constitutive expression of the upstream protein activator Akt1 (RAC-alpha serine/threonine protein kinase 1 or v-akt murine thymoma viral oncogene homolog 1) of mTORC1 transiently increases the abundance of hematopoietic stem cells; then, it causes their excessive proliferation, and ultimately elicits the apoptotic death of hematopoietic stem cells and the resulting depletion of their pool in an mTORC1-dependent manner (Figure 4) [263,264]. Moreover, an overstimulation of the information flow through the mTORC1 pathway by a mutation that conditionally deletes the upstream protein inhibitor Tsc1 (tuberous sclerosis

1) of mTORC1 promotes an exit of hematopoietic stem cells from the quiescent state, impairs their functionality and self-renewal ability, promotes their apoptotic death, and eventually depletes the pool of hematopoietic stem cells in an mTORC1-dependent fashion (Figure 4) [261,262]. These effects of Tsc1 deletion on the fate of hematopoietic stem cells (1) coincide with a rise in the abundance of mitochondria and a rise in cellular ROS; and (2) can be reversed with the help of the antioxidant *N*-acetylcysteine, a ROS antagonist [261]. Thus, the maintenance of mTORC1 signaling at low intensity in hematopoietic stem cells is essential for sustaining their quiescence, because it allows the suppression of the YY1/PGC-1α-dependent transcription of nuclear genes involved in mitochondrial biogenesis and functionality [270]. Such suppression prevents a rise of mitochondrially-produced cellular ROS above a threshold level that is capable of inducing the quiescence exit and proliferation of these adult stem cells (Figure 4) [261].

The intensity of information flow through the mTORC1 signaling pathway also defines the fate of a different type of quiescent adult stem cells, namely neural stem cells, as well as the neural progenitor cells that are formed from them. In fact, a mutation that conditionally deletes Tsc1 to enhance this pathway impairs the migration patterns of both neural stem cells and neural progenitor cells in the subventricular zone of the brain [273]. Moreover, a downregulation of the mTORC1 signaling pathway by caloric restriction in Paneth cells of the intestinal stem cell niche triggers a cell non-autonomous mechanism that promotes the self-renewal of intestinal stem cells and improves their functionality [274]. Thus, the fate of intestinal stem cells also depends on the intensity of information flow through the mTORC1 signaling pathway. Downstream cellular processes whose regulation by mTORC1 controls quiescence maintenance, self-renewal, and functionality of neural stem cells and intestinal stem cells are presently unknown.

The nature of the intracellular pro-mitogenic and/or anti-mitogenic signals whose ability to control mTORC1 in a cell-autonomous manner defines the fate of quiescent adult stem cells requires further investigation. Recent studies uncovered a cell-nonautonomous mechanism of such mTORC1 control in muscle stem cells. Specifically, it was demonstrated that the abilities of muscle stem cells to respond to injury-induced systemic signals from distant tissues by retaining a pool of quiescent stem cells and by creating a population of differentiated cells for distant tissue repair are under tight control of the mTORC1 signaling within these adult stem cells [20,275,276]. Tissue injury stimulates the circulating protease hepatocyte growth factor activator (HGFA); then, HGFA relays a signal to muscle stem cells in tissues distant to the zone of injury by proteolytically activating HGF to stimulate the HGF receptor cMet (mesenchymal–epithelial transition factor) and promote mTORC1 signaling in these stem cells via a presently unknown mechanism (Figure 4) [20,275,276]. Once promoted, mTORC1 orchestrates a transition of adult stem cells from the G_0 phase to the "alert" (G_{Alert}) phase of quiescence; this increases the cell size, mitochondrial activity, and ATP concentration and, ultimately commits these stem cells to cell cycle entry, proliferation, and differentiation (Figure 4) [20,275,276].

2.8. Several Mechanisms of Proteostasis Maintenance in Quiescent Adult Stem Cells Define Their Fate

As discussed in Section 2.3, an essential role of ROS in defining the homeostasis and functionality of quiescent adult stem cells consists in the ability of ROS concentrations that exceed a toxic threshold to inflict oxidative damage to cellular proteins. Several mechanisms for maintaining protein homeostasis (proteostasis) within these cells are known to play essential roles in preserving the quiescence, self-renewal, proliferation capacity, differentiation potential, and long-term survival of adult stem cells. Some of these mechanisms prevent a collapse of cellular proteostasis by regulating protein synthesis and folding, whereas other mechanisms are involved in the proteasomal or autophagic degradation of damaged and dysfunctional proteins and organelles [29,277–280]. These mechanisms are integrated into a proteostatic network orchestrated by several signaling pathways and transcriptional factors that define the fate of adult stem cells [29,278,279]. The common traits of the proteostatic network operating in adult stem cells include the following: (1) a suppression of protein synthesis on free ribosomes in the cytosol; (2) a rise in the concentrations of heat shock proteins (HSPs) that act as chaperones or co-chaperones to assist the proper folding and stability of newly synthesized proteins; (3) an activation of the unfolded protein response (UPR) systems in the endoplasmic reticulum (ER) and mitochondria (UPR^{ER} and UPR^{mit}, respectively); (4) an enhancement of the ubiquitin system for the ubiquitin/proteasome-dependent proteolytic clearance of improperly folded proteins, cell-cycle regulators, and transcriptional factors, as well as for the proteasome-independent regulation of surface protein receptors, histones, ribosome assembly factors, and vesicle transport proteins; and (5) a stimulation of autophagy, a quality control mechanism for the regulated lysosomal degradation of dysfunctional or excessive proteins and organelles, in some types of adult stem cells or its maintenance at a basal level in other types of such cells (Figures 5 and 6) [29,79,277–284]. The involvement of each of these proteostatic mechanisms in the homeostasis and functionality of adult stem cells is outlined below in this section.

2.8.1. Protein Synthesis on Free Ribosomes in the Cytosol

The rate of protein synthesis in hematopoietic stem cells is significantly lower than that in differentiating progenitor cells formed from them, which is likely because the repressor 4EBP1 (eukaryotic translation initiation factor 4E-binding protein 1) of cap-dependent translation is less phosphorylated and more active in these adult stem cells [285]. The protein synthesis rate that is maintained in hematopoietic stem cells is optimal for sustaining their quiescence and self-renewal potential. In support of this notion, it was shown that (1) a mutation that increases such a rate within hematopoietic stem cells in an mTORC1-dependent manner depletes their pool; (2) a mutation that decreases the protein synthesis rate within hematopoietic stem cells weakens their self-renewal ability; and (3) a combination of these two mutations restores the "optimal" protein synthesis rate within hematopoietic stem cells and salvages the above effects of both mutations on stem cell quiescence and self-renewal [259,285]. Therefore, the 4EBP1-dependent decline in protein synthesis rate observed in hematopoietic stem cells is required for the maintenance of their homeostasis and functionality. The efficiency of ribosome assembly in hematopoietic stem cells is an essential contributing factor to such an indispensable role of the "optimal" protein synthesis rate in defining the fate of these adult stem cells. In fact, a mutation in the ribosome protein Rpl22l impairs the emergence of hematopoietic stem cells [286]. Furthermore, a depletion of the transcription factor Runx1 in hematopoietic stem cells weakens ribosome biogenesis, decelerates protein synthesis, decreases cell susceptibility to apoptotic death, and makes these adult stem cells more resistant to genotoxic and ER stresses [287]. Moreover, a mutation that impairs the maturation and nuclear export of the pre-60S ribosomal subunit in hematopoietic stem cells causes an exhaustion of the pools of quiescent cells and the multipotent progenitors formed from them, but not of the pool of mature hematopoietic cells [288]. In addition, a decline in ribosome abundance within hematopoietic stem cells suppresses the translation of a specific set of mRNAs that are essential for erythroid lineage commitment after these stem cells exit the quiescent state [289].

Akin to hematopoietic stem cell quiescence, self-renewal, and differentiation, the fate of neural stem cells also depends on the rate of mTORC1-regulated protein synthesis. Specifically, the constitutive activation of 4EBP1 (which represses cap-dependent translation) in neural stem cells with hyperactive mTORC1 and protein synthesis exceeding the optimal rate has been shown to restore the optimal rate of protein synthesis, increase self-renewal potential, and slow down the accelerated differentiation of these adult stem cells [290].

Protein synthesis on free ribosomes in the cytosol also defines the homeostasis and functionality of epidermal stem cells, as a mutation that impairs the recycling and rescue of ribosomes stalled before protein synthesis completion has been demonstrated to increase the synthesis rates of all the cellular proteins in an mTORC1-dependent manner, cause the excessive proliferation of these adult stem cells, and alter their normal differentiation pattern [291]. Since a suppression of mTORC1 signaling by rapamycin in epidermal stem cells carrying this mutation decreases the global protein synthesis rate and salvages the above effects of the mutation of the fate of epidermal stem cells, the maintenance of a protein synthesis rate below a certain threshold is essential for sustaining the homeostasis and functionality of these adult stem cells [291].

The fate of skeletal muscle stem cells depends on the synthesis rates of myogenic factor 5 (Myf5) and myoblast determination protein (MyoD) that are translated from a distinct set of mRNA templates. In quiescent skeletal muscle stem cells, the translation of these mRNAs is selectively suppressed either by a protein kinase R (PKR)-like endoplasmic reticulum kinase (PERK)-dependent phosphorylation of translation initiation factor eIF2α [292] or by their association with certain microRNAs [293,294]. This causes an accumulation of such mRNAs in cytoplasmic mRNP (messenger ribonucleoprotein) granules, thus silencing their translation [292–294]. Such silencing is essential for the maintenance of a reversible quiescent state by skeletal muscle stem cells [292–294]. Furthermore, the dissociation of the cytoplasmic mRNP granules caused either by an eIF2α dephosphorylation or by a downregulation of the microRNAs allows the translation of these mRNAs in skeletal muscle stem cells, and is required for both their exit from quiescence and their entry into a differentiation program [292–294].

2.8.2. HSP Concentrations

Many HSPs are chaperones or co-chaperones that assist the proper folding and stability of newly synthesized proteins [295,296]. The concentrations of some HSPs in various types of quiescent adult stem cells exceed those in the fully differentiated progeny of such cells [279,297]. Specifically, the abundance of HSP70 protein 5 (HSPA5), HSP70 protein 8 (HSPA8), and HOP (an HSP70-HSP90 organizing protein) in neural stem cells and mesenchymal stem cells is higher than in their differentiated progeny [298]. Adipose-derived stem cells exhibit higher concentrations of HSP27 (HSPB1), αB-crystallin (HSPB5), HSP20 (HSPB6), and HSP60 than the fully differentiated progeny of such cells [299].

Some of these HSPs play essential roles in preserving the quiescence, abundance, survival, proliferation capacity, and differentiation potential of adult stem cells, as outlined below.

Mechanisms underlying such effects of some HSPs have begun to emerge. HSC70 (HSPA8) is essential for the cytokine-mediated survival of hematopoietic stem cells and prevents their differentiation; this is because this HSP decreases the stability of mRNA encoding BIM, which is a BH3-only pro-apoptotic factor that compromises stem cell viability but is required for apoptosis during hematopoiesis and leukemogenesis (Figure 5) [300]. HSC70 (HSPA8) also interacts with cyclin D1 and cyclin-dependent kinase inhibitors p27 and p57 in the cytosol of hematopoietic stem cells [301]. Both p27 and p57 prevent the nuclear import of the HSC70/cyclin D1 complex, thereby allowing the maintenance of quiescence of hematopoietic stem cells (Figure 5) [301]. The GRP78 member of the HSP70 protein family binds to teratocarcinoma-derived growth factor 1 (TDGF-1) on the surface of hematopoietic stem cells, and this binding allows maintaining the quiescent state of these adult cells via the TDGF-1-dependent induction of glycolysis (Figure 5) [302]. HSP70 (HSPA5) indirectly stimulates the erythroid differentiation of hematopoietic stem cells because it prevents the caspase-3-mediated proteolysis of GATA sequence protein 1 (GATA-1), which is a transcriptional factor that is essential for the terminal differentiation of erythroid progenitors formed from these adult stem cells (Figure 5) [303]. The HSP mortalin in the mitochondria of hematopoietic stem cells interacts with the antioxidant deglycase protein 1(DJ-1), which is implicated in Parkinson's disease, and the mortalin/DJ-1 complex allows sustaining hematopoietic stem cell quiescence, abundance, and self-renewal capacity, because it protects the mitochondria of these cells from ROS accumulation and oxidative macromolecular damage (Figure 5) [304].

An overexpression of αB-crystallin (HspB5), a small HSP that is essential for muscle development and homeostasis [305,306], slows down the differentiation of skeletal muscle stem cells; this effect of αB-crystallin (HspB5) is due to its ability to decelerate synthesis and accelerate the degradation of MyoD, which is a master protein regulator of such differentiation (Figure 5) [307]. Moreover, HSP70 (HSPA5) is indispensable for the osteogenic and chondrogenic differentiation of human mesenchymal stem cells, perhaps because it enhances the expression of the bone morphogenetic protein 2 member of the transforming growth factor β(TGF-β) superfamily of secreted polypeptide factors [308,309].

2.8.3. The UPR^{ER} and UPR^{mit} Systems

If the HSPs-assisted folding of newly synthesized proteins is not enough to sustain their proper conformations, the build-up of misfolded and unfolded proteins in the ER and mitochondria activates the UPR^{ER} and UPR^{mit} systems (respectively) to refold or degrade these proteins and restore cellular proteostasis [310–313].

When activated, the UPR^{ER} system allows restoring proteostasis in the ER, because it decelerates protein synthesis to decrease protein flow to the ER, promotes a refolding of some improperly folded proteins accumulated in this organelle, and directs other improperly folded proteins amassed in the ER for degradation by ER-associated degradation (ERAD) or autophagy [310,311,314]. If these protective processes that are integrated into the UPR^{ER} system are unable to reinstate proteostasis in the ER, a coordinated action of the ER and mitochondria triggers the mitochondria-controlled apoptotic death of the entire cell [315].

When the UPR^{mit} system is activated, it enables proteostasis reinstatement in mitochondria because it stimulates the refolding of some improperly folded proteins that accumulated in these organelles with the help of mitochondrial chaperone systems and because it also promotes the proteolytic degradation of other improperly folded proteins with the help of proteolytic systems in mitochondria [312,313,316,317].

As outlined below, both the UPR^{ER} and UPR^{mit} systems of proteostasis restoration are indispensable for maintaining the quiescence, self-renewal, proliferation capacity, differentiation potential, and functionality of adult stem cells.

The RNA binding protein Dppa5 (developmental pluripotency-associated 5 protein), the tauroursodeoxycholic bile acid, and hypoxia-inducible factor 2α (HIF-2α) stimulate the UPR^{ER} system to elicit a decline in ER stress within hematopoietic stem cells and protect these cells from apoptotic death caused by excessive ER stress [318–320]. Such stimulation of the UPR^{ER} system is required for the maintenance, self-renewal, functionality, and survival of hematopoietic stem cells (Figure 6) [318–320]. If ER stress in the quiescent hematopoietic stem cells of humans exceeds a certain threshold and cannot be resolved by the UPR^{ER} system, these cells commit suicide by undergoing apoptotic death [321]. This prevents the propagation of dysfunctional quiescent hematopoietic stem cells that amass improperly folded and aggregated proteins in the ER [321]. Progenitor cell populations that are formed from these human quiescent hematopoietic stem cells following their activation can avoid an ER stress-induced apoptotic death, because they undergo an adaptive enhancement of the UPR^{ER} system and can resolve ER stress [321]. The UPR^{ER} system is also indispensable for the lymphopoietic and erythropoietic differentiation programs of primed mouse hematopoietic stem cells; however, mechanisms underlying such effects of the UPR^{ER} system require further investigation [322–324].

Of note, the UPR^{ER} system does not always define the fate of hematopoietic stem cells, because under certain conditions, ER stress can be resolved with the help of chemical compounds assisting in maintaining proteostasis within the ER. Specifically, bile acids secreted from maternal and fetal liver act as chemical chaperones that prevent the accumulation of improperly folded and aggregated proteins in the ER, thereby decreasing ER stress and allowing the expansion of a population of hematopoietic stem cells during hematopoiesis in the fetal liver of mice [325].

The protein kinase PERK of the UPR^{ER} phosphorylates the eukaryotic translation initiation factor 2α (eIF2α) in mouse skeletal muscle stem cells, thus suppressing the translation of many mRNAs that lack upstream open reading frames (uORFs) in their 5′ untranslated regions [292]. mRNAs whose translation is suppressed by eIF2α phosphorylation in these adult stem cells encode the proteins that are needed for quiescence exit followed by proliferation and myogenic differentiation, whereas mRNAs with uORFs whose translation is not suppressed by such phosphorylation encode proteins involved in quiescence maintenance (Figure 6) [292]. Mutations that prevent the PERK-dependent eIF2α phosphorylation impair the abilities of skeletal muscle stem cells to maintain quiescence and self-renew, while an inhibitor of eIF2a dephosphorylation increases the self-renewal potential of these cells and improves their functionality [292]. Thus, the PERK arm of the UPR^{ER} system controls the quiescence, self-renewal, differentiation, and functionality of skeletal muscle stem cells in mice. The activation of this arm of the UPR^{ER} system following muscle injury in mice is also essential for the survival of progenitor cells formed from primed skeletal muscle stem cells and for the differentiation of these progenitor cells during regenerative myogenesis and muscle formation [326].

In the nucleus of mouse quiescent hematopoietic stem cells, the histone deacetylase SIRT7 is very abundant and interacts with the transcription factor nuclear respiratory factor 1 (NRF1), which in its free form activates the transcription of genes encoding mitochondrial ribosomal proteins and translation factors [327]. The interaction between NRF1 and SIRT7 impairs the ability of NRF1 to activate the transcription of these genes, thus inhibiting mitochondrial translation and biogenesis, lowering mitochondrial protein stress, and suppressing the UPR^{mit} system (Figure 6) [327]. Such SIRT7-driven suppression of the UPR^{mit} system is essential for maintaining the quiescence and differentiation potential of hematopoietic stem cells [327].

Pharmacological interventions that rise the intracellular concentration of NAD^+ in mice have been shown to stimulate the protein deacetylase SIRT1, which then increases mitochondrial functionality and activates the UPR^{mit} system by increasing the abundance of two members of the prohibitin protein family of mitochondrial stress sensors and effectors (Figure 6) [75,239]. Such NAD^+/SIRT1-dependent activation of the UPR^{mit} system (including prohibitins) is indispensable for the quiescence, self-renewal, differentiation, and viability of muscle stem cells, neural stem cells, and melanocyte stem cells in mice (Figure 6) [75,239].

2.8.4. The Ubiquitin System

The enhancement of the ubiquitin system characteristic of quiescent adult stem cells is sometimes considered only as a mechanism for the ubiquitin/proteasome-dependent proteolytic clearance of improperly folded proteins whose proper conformations in these stem cells cannot be restored by their HSPs-assisted folding and/or by their UPR^{ER} and UPR^{mit}-dependent refolding or degradation [29,278,279]. However, the ubiquitin system is known to play essential proteolysis-related and proteolysis-unrelated roles in preserving the quiescence, self-renewal, proliferation capacity, and differentiation potential of adult stem cells, not because it helps to clear improperly folded proteins, but mainly because it regulates the stability, conformation, activity, localization, protein-binding specificity, or vesicular trafficking of properly folded cell-cycle regulators, surface protein receptors, transcription factors, histones, ribosome assembly factors, and vesicle transport proteins that define the fate of these stem cells [281,283,284].

The specificity with which ubiquitin is covalently attached to certain lysine residues of the proteins that define the fate of adult stem cells depends on many E3 ubiquitin ligases, each ubiquitinating a distinct set of protein targets [284,328]. The ubiquitin E3 ligases c-Cbl, Itch, Fbw7, Skp2, and Huwe1 are indispensable for sustaining quiescence and preventing the excessive self-renewal and overproliferation of hematopoietic stem cells, thus precluding a depletion of this adult stem cell population and impeding an exhaustion of hematopoiesis [29,281,283,284,329–346]. This is because these ubiquitin E3 ligases ubiquitinate and prime for proteasome degradation a distinct group of proteins that are essential for maintaining hematopoietic stem cell homeostasis by regulating signal transduction, the transcription of many nuclear genes, cell growth and proliferation, cell cycle progression, and mitochondria-controlled apoptosis; among these proteins are Notch1, c-Kit, STAT5, c-Myc, n-Myc, cyclin E, p27, and Mcl-1 [29,281,283,284,329–346]. A depletion of the ubiquitin E3 ligases c-Cbl, Itch, Fbw7, Skp2 and Huwe1 in hematopoietic stem cells elicits their loss of quiescence, enhances their self-renewal, increases their abundance, prompts their overproliferation, decelerates their differentiation, and eventually causes a depletion of the hematopoietic stem cell population [29,281,283,284,340,343,347–351].

When hematopoietic stem cells move out from their hypoxic niche in the low-oxygen environment of the bone marrow to enter the differentiation program, the ubiquitin E3 ligase VHL (von Hippel–Lindau) ubiquitinates the hypoxia-inducible transcription factor HIF-1α, thus promoting its proteasomal degradation [116,352]. HIF-1α is a master controller of the transcription program for sustaining the quiescence, functionality, and survival of the hematopoietic stem cells sustained within the low-tension oxygen niche [117,120,353]. The VHL-driven proteasomal degradation of HIF-1α in the hematopoietic stem cell niche is required for the migration of these cells from the niche and for the ensuing exit of these cells from quiescence and entry into differentiation [116]. In fact, VHL depletion increases the stability of HIF-1α, promotes the quiescence of hematopoietic stem cells and their early progenitors, and impairs the proliferation and differentiation of these cells during hematopoiesis [116].

In adult neural stem cells, the ubiquitin E3 ligase APC/C (anaphase-promoting complex) controls a balance between the cell quiescence maintenance program and the programs for cell quiescence exit, proliferation, and differentiation, because it primes for proteasome degradation or non-proteolytically activates certain cell-cycle regulation proteins, transcription factors, translation factors, and cell surface receptor proteins [284,354–359]. HUWE1 (HECT, UBA and WWE domain containing protein 1), another ubiquitin E3 ligase in adult neural stem cells, stimulates a re-entry of early neural progenitor cells into the quiescent state, because it ubiquitinates and primes some transcription factors for proteasome degradation, cell-cycle regulation proteins, and apoptotic death regulators [284,360–364].

In sum, the above findings indicate that the ability of ubiquitin E3 ligases to prime for proteasome degradation (or, in some cases, to activate in a non-proteolytic manner) a distinct set of proteins in different types of adult stem cells is essential for controlling a balance between the processes of cell quiescence maintenance, exit, and re-entry. As it has been reviewed elsewhere, the ubiquitin E3 ligases-dependent proteasome degradation is also indispensable for regulated self-renewal, which is a response to signals emerging from the niche, proliferation, differentiation, functionality and survival of various adult stem cells [281,283,284].

2.8.5. Autophagy

Autophagy, a quality control mechanism for regulated lysosomal degradation of damaged or dysfunctional proteins and organelles, is required for sustaining the quiescent state, self-renewal ability, proliferation capacity, differentiation potential, fitness, functionality, and/or long-term survival of quiescent adult stem cells [29,78,79,278,279,282,365,366].

In different types of adult stem cells, the activity of autophagy is either higher or lower than that in the differentiating progenitor cells formed from them [29,78,79,278,279,282,365,367].

Autophagy activity in hematopoietic, dermal, epidermal, and mesenchymal stem cells exceeds that in progenitor cells derived from these adult stem cells [368,369]. Such a rise in autophagic activity within adult hematopoietic stem cells is due to the induced expression of many pro-autophagy genes, which is driven by the forkhead transcription factor FoxO3 [369–371]. The increase of autophagic activity within hematopoietic stem cells is essential for sustaining their quiescent state, self-renewal ability, differentiation potential, high resistance to stresses, fitness, functionality, and viability [257,368,369,371–375]. In fact, mutations eliminating several key protein components of autophagic machinery impair these essential features of hematopoietic stem cells [257,368,369,371–375]. These mutations increase the abundance of mitochondria, stimulate mitochondrial ROS production, enhance ROS-inflicted oxidative damage to cellular components, and accelerate mitochondria-controlled apoptotic cell death [257,371–375]. Therefore, it is believed that the FoxO3-induced autophagy is essential for the quiescence, self-renewal, differentiation, stress resistance, fitness, functionality, and viability of hematopoietic stem cells, because it selectively eliminates functional and dysfunctional mitochondria to suppress the excessive formation of ROS in these organelles, lower oxidative cellular damage, and prevent mitochondria-controlled cell death [257,371–375].

Autophagy activity in neural stem cells and cardiac stem cells is lower than that in the progenitor cells formed from these adult stem cells; such activity further rises during the differentiation of both types of progenitor cells [376–378]. Mutations eliminating the Atg5 and Ambra1 protein components of autophagic machinery in neural stem cells and the pharmacological interventions that suppress autophagy in both these types of adult stem cells impair early steps of stem and progenitor cell differentiation [376–378]. In contrast, pharmacological interventions that stimulate autophagy in cardiac stem cells promote the differentiation of these stem cells and their early progenitors [377,378]. It is conceivable that autophagy activation in progenitor cells formed from neural stem cells and cardiac stem cells is required to fulfill the high-energy demands of the differentiation process [376–378]. Of note, akin to Atg5 and Ambra1 depletions, a depletion of the autophagy-inducing protein FIP200 impairs the differentiation of early progenitors of neural stem cells [379]. Since such an FIP200-dependent impairment of neural stem cell progenitors can be salvaged with the help of an anti-oxidant chemical compound, autophagy activation in these progenitor cells may not only provide energy to fuel the differentiation process, but may also suppress excessive oxidative damage to cellular components during differentiation [379]. FIP200 depletion also causes a progressive depletion of the pool of neural stem cells because it triggers their apoptotic death [379]. Thus, the basal level of autophagy activity observed in these adult stem cells plays an essential role in protecting them from the apoptotic death caused by excessive cellular stress.

Similar to the autophagy activity in neural stem cells and cardiac stem cells, such activity in the muscle stem cells of young mice is lower than the autophagy activity in the progenitor cells that are derived from them [365,367]. The basal level of autophagy activity in these muscle stem cells is essential for the establishment and maintenance of their quiescence state, as a depletion of the Atg7 protein component of autophagic machinery in these cells impairs the reversible G_0 state of quiescence, decreases stem cell number and functionality, and promotes entry into the irreversible G_0 state of senescence [365,367]. The entry of autophagy-deficient muscle stem cells into the irreversible senescent state is caused by a build-up of dysfunctional mitochondria, an accumulation of ROS in excessive concentrations, a rise in oxidative damage to cellular components, and a resulting decline of proteostasis in these cells [365,367]. The accumulation of excessive ROS in autophagy-deficient muscle stem cells is responsible for their entry into the irreversible senescent state; in fact, an anti-oxidant chemical compound that decreases cellular ROS has been shown to prevent such senescence entry and restore the self-renewal of autophagy-deficient muscle stem cells [365,367].

In addition to the essential role of autophagy in establishing and maintaining the quiescence of muscle stem cells, autophagy is also indispensable for the exit of muscle stem cells from the quiescent state, the activation of their myogenic differentiation, and the progression through several stages of such differentiation and muscle regeneration. Specifically, during the transition of muscle stem cells from the quiescent state to the activation state, autophagy activity rises in a SIRT1-dependent manner to provide the nutrients and ATP needed for the energy-demanding process of entry into myogenic differentiation [240]. Furthermore, in response to muscle injury, autophagy is stimulated in early progenitors of muscle stem cells, and the extent of such autophagy stimulation defines the efficiency of muscle regeneration via a presently unknown mechanism [380]. Moreover, autophagy is also involved in myotube formation during muscle regeneration, but the mechanism of such involvement remains to be investigated [381].

2.9. Cell Cycle Regulatory Proteins Are Essential for Sustaining the Quiescence, Self-Renewal, Functionality, and Differentiation Potential of Adult Stem Cells

Several cell cycle regulatory proteins are integrated into a network of cell-intrinsic mechanisms that define the fate of quiescent adult stem cells [2,4,382–387].

One of these proteins is the tumor suppressor protein p53, which is a transcription factor that can arrest the cell cycle at the G_1/S checkpoint because in response to DNA damage, it activates the expression of the cyclin-dependent kinase Cdk2 inhibitor p21 [388–390]. A depletion of p53 in hematopoietic stem cells, which promotes quiescence exit and cell cycle entry, enhances self-renewal and raises the number of fully functional hematopoietic stem cells [391–394]. Thus, p53 is essential for sustaining the quiescent state of hematopoietic stem cells and inhibiting their proliferation and self-renewal. The essential role of p53 in sustaining the pool of hematopoietic stem cells at a certain level is independent of p21 [394] but requires Necdin, which is a growth-suppressing protein whose expression is activated by p53 at the transcriptional level [395]. The ability of p53 to fully sustain the functional hematopoietic stem cells by promoting the apoptotic death of those of them that build-up excessive DNA damage is under the control of Aspp1, which is a member of the family of apoptosis-stimulating proteins of p53 [396].

p53 also suppresses the proliferation and self-renewal of neural stem cells and promotes the apoptotic death of those of them that are dysfunctional (likely because they amass DNA damage). In fact, p53 depletion in neural stem cells stimulates their proliferation and mitigates their apoptotic death [397]. The mechanisms underlying these effects of p53 in neural stem cells are presently unknown.

Three members of the retinoblastoma protein family (pRBs) are tumor suppressor proteins that, in their hypophosphorylated forms, can arrest the cell cycle at the G_1/S checkpoint, because they are transcriptional repressors of genes that are essential for G_1/S transition [398,399]. If pRBs are hyperphosphorylated by different cyclin/cyclin-dependent kinase complexes in response to certain pro-mitogenic stimuli, they unable to suppress cell cycle entry at the G_1/S checkpoint [399,400]. As outlined below, similar to p53, pRBs also define the fate of different types of quiescent adult stem cells.

A simultaneous depletion of all the pRBs in adult hematopoietic stem cells elicits the exit of these stem cells from quiescence, impairs the reconstitution ability of these stem cells in a transplantation assay, causes an excessive proliferation of both stem cells and their early hematopoietic progenitors, and promotes apoptosis in lymphoid (but not in myeloid) progenitor populations [401]. Hence, a collective action of pRBs is essential for sustaining the quiescence of hematopoietic stem cells, preventing their unbalanced proliferation, maintaining their transplantation functionality, and retaining an unbiased differentiation of the lymphoid and myeloid cell lineages in the hematopoietic system.

A depletion of a single member of the pRBs family in muscle stem cells causes their permanent exit from the quiescent state, accelerates cell cycle re-entry in both stem cells and their progenitor myoblast cells (thus substantially expanding these two cell populations), and significantly decelerates terminal differentiation into myotubes; these effects of the depletion of a single pRB member deteriorate muscle fiber formation, slow muscle growth, and delay muscle repair [402]. Thus, even a partial decline in the abundance of pRBs alters the fate of muscle stem cells.

Among the cell cycle regulatory proteins that define the fate of quiescent adult stem cells are several cyclin-dependent kinase inhibitors. Their essential roles in maintaining the functionality of adult stem cells are discussed below.

As mentioned in Section 2.8.2, the interaction of cyclin-dependent kinase inhibitors p27 and p57 with the HSC70/cyclin D1 complex in the cytosol of hematopoietic stem cells prevents the nuclear import of this protein complex [301]. A depletion of both p27 and p57 in mice permits the nuclear import of the HSC70/cyclin D1 complex, thereby stimulating pRB hyperphosphorylation by the complex formed between cyclin D1 and cyclin-dependent kinases Cdk4/6 in the nucleus and impairing the ability of pRB to arrest the cell cycle of hematopoietic stem cells at the G_1/S checkpoint [301]. Due to these effects, mouse hematopoietic stem cells depleted of both p27 and p57 fail to maintain quiescence, are decreased in number, have low self-renewal activity, and exhibit a loss of the reconstitution ability in a transplantation assay [301]. Thus, a collective action of p27 and p57 is essential for sustaining the quiescence, self-renewal, and functionality of hematopoietic stem cells.

A depletion of the cyclin-dependent kinase 2 (Cdk2) inhibitor p21 in mice impairs the abilities of hematopoietic stem cells and neural stem cells to sustain quiescence, lowers their self-renewal potentials, reduces their reconstitution abilities in a transplantation assay, decreases their numbers, and ultimately causes an exhaustion of their pools [403,404]. Hence, p21 is indispensable for the maintenance of the quiescence, self-renewal ability, and fitness in both hematopoietic stem cells and neural stem cells.

3. Conclusions

In this review, we compared many metabolic, signal transduction, gene expression, epigenetic, stress survival, cell cycle regulation, and other traits of different types of mammalian and human adult stem cells. Our comparison indicates that adult stem cells have evolved an intricate network of cell-intrinsic mechanisms that control the establishment and preservation of these traits. These mechanisms regulate quiescence entry, maintenance, and exit in response to certain extrinsic pro-mitogenic and anti-mitogenic cues from the microenvironment of adult stem cells. One important challenge is to understand how the numerous cell-intrinsic mechanisms of quiescence entry, maintenance, and exit are integrated in space and time within mammalian and human adult stem cells. The other challenge is to decipher the hierarchical order and relative contributions of the different traits of adult stem cells in the ability of these cells to enter, sustain, and exit quiescence in response to specific cell-extrinsic factors within different tissue-specific microenvironments. Future work will also aim at understanding how the history of spatial and temporal changes in cell growth and division conditions is translated into the pattern of quiescence entry, maintenance, and exit in different types of adult stem cells. Since the impairment of a balance between the quiescence, proliferation, and differentiation of adult stem cells has been implicated in the pathophysiology of many diseases of old age, addressing these challenges in the future will increase our understanding of how this balance can be controlled to delay cellular and organismal aging and postpone the onset of aging-associated diseases.

Author Contributions: K.M., P.D., Y.M., D.M. and V.I.T. wrote the text. V.I.T. prepared the figures.

Acknowledgments: We are grateful to current and former members of the Titorenko laboratory for discussions.

References

1. Gray, J.V.; Petsko, G.A.; Johnston, G.C.; Ringe, D.; Singer, R.A.; Werner-Washburne, M. "Sleeping beauty": Quiescence in *Saccharomyces cerevisiae*. *Microbiol. Mol. Biol. Rev.* **2004**, *68*, 187–206. [CrossRef] [PubMed]
2. Cheung, T.H.; Rando, T.A. Molecular regulation of stem cell quiescence. *Nat. Rev. Mol. Cell. Biol.* **2013**, *14*, 329–340. [CrossRef] [PubMed]
3. Dhawan, J.; Laxman, S. Decoding the stem cell quiescence cycle—Lessons from yeast for regenerative biology. *J. Cell Sci.* **2015**, *128*, 4467–4474. [CrossRef] [PubMed]
4. Rumman, M.; Dhawan, J.; Kassem, M. Concise Review: Quiescence in Adult Stem Cells: Biological Significance and Relevance to Tissue Regeneration. *Stem Cells* **2015**, *33*, 2903–2912. [CrossRef]
5. Pardee, A.B. A restriction point for control of normal animal cell proliferation. *Proc. Natl. Acad. Sci. USA* **1974**, *71*, 1286–1290. [CrossRef] [PubMed]
6. Foster, D.A.; Yellen, P.; Xu, L.; Saqcena, M. Regulation of G1 Cell Cycle Progression: Distinguishing the Restriction Point from a Nutrient-Sensing Cell Growth Checkpoint(s). *Genes Cancer* **2010**, *1*, 1124–1131. [CrossRef]
7. Hartwell, L.H.; Culotti, J.; Pringle, J.R.; Reid, B.J. Genetic control of the cell division cycle in yeast. *Science* **1974**, *183*, 46–51. [CrossRef]
8. De Virgilio, C. The essence of yeast quiescence. *FEMS Microbiol. Rev.* **2012**, *36*, 306–339. [CrossRef]
9. Cameron, I.L.; Bols, N.C. Effect of cell population density on G_2 arrest in *Tetrahymena*. *J. Cell Biol.* **1975**, *67*, 518–522. [CrossRef]
10. Drewinko, B.; Yang, L.Y.; Barlogie, B.; Trujillo, J.M. Cultured human tumour cells may be arrested in all stages of the cycle during stationary phase: Demonstration of quiescent cells in G_1, S and G_2 phase. *Cell Tissue Kinet.* **1984**, *17*, 453–463. [CrossRef]
11. Costello, G.; Rodgers, L.; Beach, D. Fission yeast enters the stationary phase G_0 state from either mitotic G_1 or G_2. *Curr. Genet.* **1986**, *11*, 119–125. [CrossRef]

12. Baisch, H. Different quiescence states of three culture cell lines detected by acridine orange staining of cellular RNA. *Cytometry* **1988**, *9*, 325–331. [CrossRef] [PubMed]
13. Wei, W.; Nurse, P.; Broek, D. Yeast cells can enter a quiescent state through G_1, S, G_2, or M phase of the cell cycle. *Cancer Res.* **1993**, *53*, 1867–1870.
14. Takeo, K.; Tanaka, R.; Miyaji, M.; Nishimura, K. Unbudded G_2 as well as G_1 arrest in the stationary phase of the basidiomycetous yeast *Cryptococcus neoformans*. *FEMS Microbiol. Lett.* **1995**, *29*, 231–235.
15. Cooper, S. Reappraisal of serum starvation, the restriction point, G_0, and G_1 phase arrest points. *FASEB J.* **2003**, *17*, 333–340. [CrossRef]
16. Klosinska, M.M.; Crutchfield, C.A.; Bradley, P.H.; Rabinowitz, J.D.; Broach, J.R. Yeast cells can access distinct quiescent states. *Genes Dev.* **2011**, *25*, 336–349. [CrossRef]
17. Daignan-Fornier, B.; Sagot, I. Proliferation/quiescence: The controversial "aller-retour". *Cell Div.* **2011**, *6*, 10. [CrossRef] [PubMed]
18. Laporte, D.; Lebaudy, A.; Sahin, A.; Pinson, B.; Ceschin, J.; Daignan-Fornier, B.; Sagot, I. Metabolic status rather than cell cycle signals control quiescence entry and exit. *J. Cell Biol.* **2011**, *192*, 949–957. [CrossRef]
19. Roche, B.; Arcangioli, B.; Martienssen, R. Transcriptional reprogramming in cellular quiescence. *RNA Biol.* **2017**, *14*, 843–853. [CrossRef]
20. Rodgers, J.T.; King, K.Y.; Brett, J.O.; Cromie, M.J.; Charville, G.W.; Maguire, K.K.; Brunson, C.; Mastey, N.; Liu, L.; Tsai, C.R.; et al. mTORC1 controls the adaptive transition of quiescent stem cells from G_0 to G_{Alert}. *Nature* **2014**, *510*, 393–396. [CrossRef]
21. McGann, C.J.; Odelberg, S.J.; Keating, M.T. Mammalian myotube dedifferentiation induced by newt regeneration extract. *Proc. Natl. Acad. Sci. USA* **2001**, *98*, 13699–13704. [CrossRef]
22. Beauséjour, C.M.; Krtolica, A.; Galimi, F.; Narita, M.; Lowe, S.W.; Yaswen, P.; Campisi, J. Reversal of human cellular senescence: Roles of the p53 and p16 pathways. *EMBO J.* **2003**, *22*, 4212–4222. [CrossRef]
23. Fausto, N. Liver regeneration and repair: Hepatocytes, progenitor cells, and stem cells. *Hepatology* **2004**, *39*, 1477–1487. [CrossRef]
24. Pajcini, K.V.; Corbel, S.Y.; Sage, J.; Pomerantz, J.H.; Blau, H.M. Transient inactivation of Rb and ARF yields regenerative cells from postmitotic mammalian muscle. *Cell Stem Cell* **2010**, *7*, 198–213. [CrossRef]
25. Clevers, H. Stem cells. What is an adult stem cell? *Science* **2015**, *350*, 1319–1320. [CrossRef]
26. Coller, H.A.; Sang, L.; Roberts, J.M. A new description of cellular quiescence. *PLoS Biol.* **2006**, *4*, e83. [CrossRef]
27. Ochocki, J.D.; Simon, M.C. Nutrient-sensing pathways and metabolic regulation in stem cells. *J. Cell Biol.* **2013**, *203*, 23–33. [CrossRef] [PubMed]
28. Ito, K.; Suda, T. Metabolic requirements for the maintenance of self-renewing stem cells. *Nat. Rev. Mol. Cell Biol.* **2014**, *15*, 243–256. [CrossRef] [PubMed]
29. García-Prat, L.; Sousa-Victor, P.; Muñoz-Cánoves, P. Proteostatic and Metabolic Control of Stemness. *Cell Stem Cell* **2017**, *20*, 593–608. [CrossRef]
30. Kwon, J.S.; Everetts, N.J.; Wang, X.; Wang, W.; Della Croce, K.; Xing, J.; Yao, G. Controlling Depth of Cellular Quiescence by an Rb-E2F Network Switch. *Cell Rep.* **2017**, *20*, 3223–3235. [CrossRef] [PubMed]
31. Ren, R.; Ocampo, A.; Liu, G.H.; Izpisua Belmonte, J.C. Regulation of Stem Cell Aging by Metabolism and Epigenetics. *Cell Metab.* **2017**, *26*, 460–474. [CrossRef] [PubMed]
32. Bi, S.; Wang, H.; Kuang, W. Stem cell rejuvenation and the role of autophagy in age retardation by caloric restriction: An update. *Mech. Ageing Dev.* **2018**, *175*, 46–54. [CrossRef]
33. Lewis, D.B.; Gattie, G.T. The ecology of quiescent microbes. *ASM News* **1991**, *57*, 27–32.
34. Finkel, S.E. Long-term survival during stationary phase: Evolution and the GASP phenotype. *Nat. Rev. Microbiol.* **2006**, *4*, 113–120. [CrossRef] [PubMed]
35. Werner-Washburne, M.; Roy, S.; Davidson, G.S. Aging and the survival of quiescent and non-quiescent cells in yeast stationary-phase cultures. *Subcell. Biochem.* **2012**, *57*, 123–143. [PubMed]
36. Rittershaus, E.S.; Baek, S.H.; Sassetti, C.M. The normalcy of dormancy: Common themes in microbial quiescence. *Cell Host Microbe* **2013**, *13*, 643–651. [CrossRef] [PubMed]
37. Scheres, B. Stem-cell niches: Nursery rhymes across kingdoms. *Nat. Rev. Mol. Cell Biol.* **2007**, *8*, 345–354. [CrossRef] [PubMed]
38. Shim, J.; Mukherjee, T.; Banerjee, U. Direct sensing of systemic and nutritional signals by haematopoietic progenitors in *Drosophila*. *Nat. Cell Biol.* **2012**, *14*, 394–400. [CrossRef]

39. Heyman, J.; Kumpf, R.P.; De Veylder, L. A quiescent path to plant longevity. *Trends Cell Biol.* **2014**, *24*, 443–448. [CrossRef]
40. Seidel, H.S.; Kimble, J. Cell-cycle quiescence maintains *Caenorhabditis elegans* germline stem cells independent of GLP-1/Notch. *eLife* **2015**, *4*, e10832. [CrossRef]
41. Narbonne, P.; Gerhold, A.R.; Maddox, P.S.; Labbé, J.C. The C. *elegans* GSCs: A Powerful Model for In Vivo Study of Adult Stem Cell Regulation. *Int. J. Stem Cell Res. Ther.* **2016**, *3*, 044. [CrossRef]
42. Rovere, F.D.; Fattorini, L.; Ronzan, M.; Falasca, G.; Altamura, M.M. The quiescent center and the stem cell niche in the adventitious roots of *Arabidopsis thaliana*. *Plant Signal. Behav.* **2016**, *11*, e1176660. [CrossRef] [PubMed]
43. Schell, J.C.; Wisidagama, D.R.; Bensard, C.; Zhao, H.; Wei, P.; Tanner, J.; Flores, A.; Mohlman, J.; Sorensen, L.K.; Earl, C.S.; et al. Control of intestinal stem cell function and proliferation by mitochondrial pyruvate metabolism. *Nat. Cell Biol.* **2017**, *19*, 1027–1036. [CrossRef]
44. Velappan, Y.; Signorelli, S.; Considine, M.J. Cell cycle arrest in plants: What distinguishes quiescence, dormancy and differentiated G_1? *Ann. Bot.* **2017**, *120*, 495–509. [CrossRef] [PubMed]
45. Macedo, J.C.; Vaz, S.; Logarinho, E. Mitotic Dysfunction Associated with Aging Hallmarks. *Adv. Exp. Med. Biol.* **2017**, *1002*, 153–188.
46. Ahlqvist, K.J.; Suomalainen, A.; Hämäläinen, R.H. Stem cells, mitochondria and aging. *Biochim. Biophys. Acta* **2015**, *1847*, 1380–1386. [CrossRef] [PubMed]
47. Eridani, S.; Sgaramella, V.; Cova, L. Stem cells: From embryology to cellular therapy? An appraisal of the present state of art. *Cytotechnology* **2004**, *44*, 125–141. [CrossRef]
48. Mihaylova, M.M.; Sabatini, D.M.; Yilmaz, Ö.H. Dietary and metabolic control of stem cell function in physiology and cancer. *Cell Stem Cell* **2014**, *14*, 292–305. [CrossRef]
49. Ito, K.; Ito, K. Metabolism and the Control of Cell Fate Decisions and Stem Cell Renewal. *Annu. Rev. Cell Dev. Biol.* **2016**, *32*, 399–409. [CrossRef]
50. Santoro, A.; Vlachou, T.; Carminati, M.; Pelicci, P.G.; Mapelli, M. Molecular mechanisms of asymmetric divisions in mammary stem cells. *EMBO Rep.* **2016**, *17*, 1700–1720. [CrossRef]
51. Moore, D.L.; Jessberger, S. Creating Age Asymmetry: Consequences of Inheriting Damaged Goods in Mammalian Cells. *Trends Cell Biol.* **2017**, *27*, 82–92. [CrossRef] [PubMed]
52. Shen, Q.; Goderie, S.K.; Jin, L.; Karanth, N.; Sun, Y.; Abramova, N.; Vincent, P.; Pumiglia, K.; Temple, S. Endothelial cells stimulate self-renewal and expand neurogenesis of neural stem cells. *Science* **2004**, *304*, 1338–1340. [CrossRef]
53. Morrison, S.J.; Kimble, J. Asymmetric and symmetric stem-cell divisions in development and cancer. *Nature* **2006**, *441*, 1068–1074. [CrossRef]
54. Clayton, E.; Doupé, D.P.; Klein, A.M.; Winton, D.J.; Simons, B.D.; Jones, P.H. A single type of progenitor cell maintains normal epidermis. *Nature* **2007**, *446*, 185–189. [CrossRef]
55. Cicalese, A.; Bonizzi, G.; Pasi, C.E.; Faretta, M.; Ronzoni, S.; Giulini, B.; Brisken, C.; Minucci, S.; Di Fiore, P.P.; Pelicci, P.G. The tumor suppressor p53 regulates polarity of self-renewing divisions in mammary stem cells. *Cell* **2009**, *138*, 1083–1095. [CrossRef]
56. Zhang, Y.V.; Cheong, J.; Ciapurin, N.; McDermitt, D.J.; Tumbar, T. Distinct self-renewal and differentiation phases in the niche of infrequently dividing hair follicle stem cells. *Cell Stem Cell* **2009**, *5*, 267–278. [CrossRef]
57. Snippert, H.J.; van der Flier, L.G.; Sato, T.; van Es, J.H.; van den Born, M.; Kroon-Veenboer, C.; Barker, N.; Klein, A.M.; van Rheenen, J.; Simons, B.D.; et al. Intestinal crypt homeostasis results from neutral competition between symmetrically dividing Lgr5 stem cells. *Cell* **2010**, *143*, 134–144. [CrossRef]
58. O'Brien, L.E.; Soliman, S.S.; Li, X.; Bilder, D. Altered modes of stem cell division drive adaptive intestinal growth. *Cell* **2011**, *147*, 603–614. [CrossRef]
59. Shahriyari, L.; Komarova, N.L. Symmetric vs. asymmetric stem cell divisions: An adaptation against cancer? *PLoS ONE* **2013**, *8*, e76195. [CrossRef]
60. Katajisto, P.; Döhla, J.; Chaffer, C.L.; Pentinmikko, N.; Marjanovic, N.; Iqbal, S.; Zoncu, R.; Chen, W.; Weinberg, R.A.; Sabatini, D.M. Stem cells. Asymmetric apportioning of aged mitochondria between daughter cells is required for stemness. *Science* **2015**, *348*, 340–343. [CrossRef]
61. Ocampo, A.; Reddy, P.; Martinez-Redondo, P.; Platero-Luengo, A.; Hatanaka, F.; Hishida, T.; Li, M.; Lam, D.; Kurita, M.; Beyret, E.; et al. In vivo amelioration of age-associated hallmarks by partial reprogramming. *Cell* **2016**, *167*, 1719–1733. [CrossRef] [PubMed]

62. Wu, J.; Izpisua Belmonte, J.C. Stem Cells: A Renaissance in Human Biology Research. *Cell* **2016**, *165*, 1572–1585. [CrossRef] [PubMed]
63. Wu, J.; Ocampo, A.; Izpisua Belmonte, J.C. Cellular metabolism and induced pluripotency. *Cell* **2016**, *166*, 1371–1385. [CrossRef]
64. Ahmed, A.S.; Sheng, M.H.; Wasnik, S.; Baylink, D.J.; Lau, K.W. Effect of aging on stem cells. *World, J. Exp. Med.* **2017**, *7*, 1–10. [CrossRef] [PubMed]
65. García-Prat, L.; Sousa-Victor, P.; Muñoz-Cánoves, P. Functional dysregulation of stem cells during aging: A focus on skeletal muscle stem cells. *FEBS J.* **2013**, *280*, 4051–4062. [CrossRef]
66. Li, M.; Izpisua Belmonte, J.C. Genetic rejuvenation of old muscle. *Nature* **2014**, *506*, 304–305. [CrossRef]
67. Sousa-Victor, P.; Gutarra, S.; García-Prat, L.; Rodriguez-Ubreva, J.; Ortet, L.; Ruiz-Bonilla, V.; Jardí, M.; Ballestar, E.; González, S.; Serrano, A.L.; et al. Geriatric muscle stem cells switch reversible quiescence into senescence. *Nature* **2014**, *506*, 316–321. [CrossRef]
68. Goodell, M.A.; Rando, T.A. Stem cells and healthy aging. *Science* **2015**, *350*, 1199–1204. [CrossRef]
69. Akunuru, S.; Geiger, H. Aging, Clonality, and Rejuvenation of Hematopoietic Stem Cells. *Trends Mol. Med.* **2016**, *22*, 701–712. [CrossRef]
70. Almada, A.E.; Wagers, A.J. Molecular circuitry of stem cell fate in skeletal muscle regeneration, ageing and disease. *Nat. Rev. Mol. Cell Biol.* **2016**, *17*, 267–279. [CrossRef]
71. Chandel, N.S.; Jasper, H.; Ho, T.T.; Passegué, E. Metabolic regulation of stem cell function in tissue homeostasis and organismal ageing. *Nat. Cell Biol.* **2016**, *18*, 823–832. [CrossRef] [PubMed]
72. Ocampo, A.; Reddy, P.; Izpisua Belmonte, J.C. Anti-Aging Strategies Based on Cellular Reprogramming. *Trends Mol. Med.* **2016**, *22*, 725–738. [CrossRef] [PubMed]
73. Schultz, M.B.; Sinclair, D.A. When stem cells grow old: Phenotypes and mechanisms of stem cell aging. *Development* **2016**, *143*, 3–14. [CrossRef]
74. Soria-Valles, C.; López-Otín, C. iPSCs: On the Road to Reprogramming Aging. *Trends Mol. Med.* **2016**, *22*, 713–724. [CrossRef] [PubMed]
75. Zhang, H.; Ryu, D.; Wu, Y.; Gariani, K.; Wang, X.; Luan, P.; D'Amico, D.; Ropelle, E.R.; Lutolf, M.P.; Aebersold, R.; et al. NAD^+ repletion improves mitochondrial and stem cell function and enhances life span in mice. *Science* **2016**, *352*, 1436–1443. [CrossRef]
76. Artoni, F.; Kreipke, R.E.; Palmeira, O.; Dixon, C.; Goldberg, Z.; Ruohola-Baker, H. Loss of *foxo* rescues stem cell aging in *Drosophila* germ line. *eLife* **2017**, *6*, e27842. [CrossRef
77. Brunet, A.; Rando, T.A. Interaction between epigenetic and metabolism in aging stem cells. *Curr. Opin. Cell Biol.* **2017**, *45*, 1–7. [CrossRef]
78. García-Prat, L.; Muñoz-Cánoves, P. Aging, metabolism and stem cells: Spotlight on muscle stem cells. *Mol. Cell Endocrinol.* **2017**, *445*, 109–117. [CrossRef]
79. Revuelta, M.; Matheu, A. Autophagy in stem cell aging. *Aging Cell* **2017**, *16*, 912–915. [CrossRef] [PubMed]
80. Solanas, G.; Peixoto, F.O.; Perdiguero, E.; Jardí, M.; Ruiz-Bonilla, V.; Datta, D.; Symeonidi, A.; Castellanos, A.; Welz, P.S.; Caballero, J.M.; et al. Aged Stem Cells Reprogram Their Daily Rhythmic Functions to Adapt to Stress. *Cell* **2017**, *170*, 678–692. [CrossRef]
81. Keyes, B.E.; Fuchs, E. Stem cells: Aging and transcriptional fingerprints. *J. Cell Biol.* **2018**, *217*, 79–92. [CrossRef] [PubMed]
82. Mahmoudi, S.; Brunet, A. Bursts of Reprogramming: A Path to Extend Lifespan? *Cell* **2016**, *167*, 1672–1674. [CrossRef]
83. Meyer, K.; Yankner, B.A. Slowing Down Aging. *Cell Metab.* **2017**, *26*, 592–593. [CrossRef] [PubMed]
84. Zhang, Y.; Kim, M.S.; Jia, B.; Yan, J.; Zuniga-Hertz, J.P.; Han, C.; Cai, D. Hypothalamic stem cells control ageing speed partly through exosomal miRNAs. *Nature* **2017**, *548*, 52–57. [CrossRef]
85. Brack, A.S.; Conboy, M.J.; Roy, S.; Lee, M.; Kuo, C.J.; Keller, C.; Rando, T.A. Increased Wnt signaling during aging alters muscle stem cell fate and increases fibrosis. *Science* **2007**, *317*, 807–810. [CrossRef]
86. Chakkalakal, J.V.; Jones, K.M.; Basson, M.A.; Brack, A.S. The aged niche disrupts muscle stem cell quiescence. *Nature* **2012**, *490*, 355–360. [CrossRef]
87. Conboy, I.M.; Rando, T.A. Heterochronic parabiosis for the study of the effects of aging on stem cells and their niches. *Cell Cycle* **2012**, *11*, 2260–2267. [CrossRef]
88. Doles, J.; Storer, M.; Cozzuto, L.; Roma, G.; Keyes, W.M. Age-associated inflammation inhibits epidermal stem cell function. *Genes Dev.* **2012**, *26*, 2144–2153. [CrossRef] [PubMed]

89. Keyes, B.E.; Segal, J.P.; Heller, E.; Lien, W.H.; Chang, C.Y.; Guo, X.; Oristian, D.S.; Zheng, D.; Fuchs, E. Nfatc1 orchestrates aging in hair follicle stem cells. *Proc. Natl. Acad. Sci. USA* **2013**, *110*, E4950–E4959. [CrossRef] [PubMed]
90. Chen, C.C.; Murray, P.J.; Jiang, T.X.; Plikus, M.V.; Chang, Y.T.; Lee, O.K.; Widelitz, R.B.; Chuong, C.M. Regenerative hair waves in aging mice and extra-follicular modulators follistatin, dkk1, and sfrp4. *J. Investig. Dermatol.* **2014**, *134*, 2086–2096. [CrossRef] [PubMed]
91. So, W.K.; Cheung, T.H. Molecular Regulation of Cellular Quiescence: A Perspective from Adult Stem Cells and Its Niches. *Methods Mol. Biol.* **2018**, *1686*, 1–25. [PubMed]
92. Hsu, Y.C.; Fuchs, E. A family business: Stem cell progeny join the niche to regulate homeostasis. *Nat. Rev. Mol. Cell Biol.* **2012**, *13*, 103–114. [CrossRef] [PubMed]
93. Scadden, D.T. Nice neighborhood: Emerging concepts of the stem cell niche. *Cell* **2014**, *157*, 41–50. [CrossRef] [PubMed]
94. Khacho, M.; Slack, R.S. Mitochondrial activity in the regulation of stem cell self-renewal and differentiation. *Curr Opin Cell Biol.* **2017**, *49*, 1–8. [CrossRef] [PubMed]
95. Shyh-Chang, N.; Ng, H.H. The metabolic programming of stem cells. *Genes Dev.* **2017**, *31*, 336–346. [CrossRef]
96. Lisowski, P.; Kannan, P.; Mlody, B.; Prigione, A. Mitochondria and the dynamic control of stem cell homeostasis. *EMBO Rep.* **2018**, *19*, e45432. [CrossRef]
97. Wei, P.; Dove, K.K.; Bensard, C.; Schell, J.C.; Rutter, J. The Force Is Strong with This One: Metabolism (Over)powers Stem Cell Fate. *Trends Cell Biol.* **2018**, *28*, 551–559. [CrossRef]
98. Zhang, J.; Nuebel, E.; Daley, G.Q.; Koehler, C.M.; Teitell, M.A. Metabolic regulation in pluripotent stem cells during reprogramming and self-renewal. *Cell Stem Cell* **2012**, *11*, 589–595. [CrossRef]
99. Shyh-Chang, N.; Daley, G.Q.; Cantley, L.C. Stem cell metabolism in tissue development and aging. *Development* **2013**, *140*, 2535–2547. [CrossRef]
100. Folmes, C.D.; Nelson, T.J.; Martinez-Fernandez, A.; Arrell, D.K.; Lindor, J.Z.; Dzeja, P.P.; Ikeda, Y.; Perez-Terzic, C.; Terzic, A. Somatic oxidative bioenergetics transitions into pluripotency-dependent glycolysis to facilitate nuclear reprogramming. *Cell Metab.* **2011**, *14*, 264–271. [CrossRef] [PubMed]
101. Varum, S.; Rodrigues, A.S.; Moura, M.B.; Momcilovic, O.; Easley, C.A.; Ramalho-Santos, J.; Van Houten, B.; Schatten, G. Energy metabolism in human pluripotent stem cells and their differentiated counterparts. *PLoS ONE* **2011**, *6*, e20914. [CrossRef]
102. Stringari, C.; Edwards, R.A.; Pate, K.T.; Waterman, M.L.; Donovan, P.J.; Gratton, E. Metabolic trajectory of cellular differentiation in small intestine by Phasor Fluorescence Lifetime Microscopy of NADH. *Sci. Rep.* **2012**, *2*, 568. [CrossRef] [PubMed]
103. Flores, A.; Schell, J.; Krall, A.S.; Jelinek, D.; Miranda, M.; Grigorian, M.; Braas, D.; White, A.C.; Zhou, J.L.; Graham, N.A.; et al. Lactate dehydrogenase activity drives hair follicle stem cell activation. *Nat. Cell Biol.* **2017**, *19*, 1017–1026. [CrossRef]
104. St John, J.C.; Ramalho-Santos, J.; Gray, H.L.; Petrosko, P.; Rawe, V.Y.; Navara, C.S.; Simerly, C.R.; Schatten, G.P. The expression of mitochondrial DNA transcription factors during early cardiomyocyte in vitro differentiation from human embryonic stem cells. *Cloning Stem Cells* **2005**, *7*, 141–153. [CrossRef] [PubMed]
105. Prigione, A.; Fauler, B.; Lurz, R.; Lehrach, H.; Adjaye, J. The senescence-related mitochondrial/oxidative stress pathway is repressed in human induced pluripotent stem cells. *Stem Cells* **2010**, *28*, 721–733. [CrossRef]
106. Zhang, J.; Khvorostov, I.; Hong, J.S.; Oktay, Y.; Vergnes, L.; Nuebel, E.; Wahjudi, P.N.; Setoguchi, K.; Wang, G.; Do, A.; et al. UCP2 regulates energy metabolism and differentiation potential of human pluripotent stem cells. *EMBO J.* **2011**, *30*, 4860–4873. [CrossRef]
107. Schuijers, J.; Clevers, H. Adult mammalian stem cells: The role of Wnt, Lgr5 and R-spondins. *EMBO J.* **2012**, *31*, 2685–2696. [CrossRef] [PubMed]
108. Sánchez-Aragó, M.; García-Bermúdez, J.; Martínez-Reyes, I.; Santacatterina, F.; Cuezva, J.M. Degradation of IF1 controls energy metabolism during osteogenic differentiation of stem cells. *EMBO Rep.* **2013**, *14*, 638–644. [CrossRef] [PubMed]
109. Takubo, K.; Nagamatsu, G.; Kobayashi, C.I.; Nakamura-Ishizu, A.; Kobayashi, H.; Ikeda, E.; Goda, N.; Rahimi, Y.; Johnson, R.S.; Soga, T.; et al. Regulation of glycolysis by Pdk functions as a metabolic checkpoint for cell cycle quiescence in hematopoietic stem cells. *Cell Stem Cell* **2013**, *12*, 49–61. [CrossRef] [PubMed]

110. Maryanovich, M.; Zaltsman, Y.; Ruggiero, A.; Goldman, A.; Shachnai, L.; Zaidman, S.L.; Porat, Z.; Golan, K.; Lapidot, T.; Gross, A. An MTCH2 pathway repressing mitochondria metabolism regulates haematopoietic stem cell fate. *Nat. Commun.* **2015**, *6*, 7901. [CrossRef]
111. Wanet, A.; Arnould, T.; Najimi, M.; Renard, P. Connecting Mitochondria, Metabolism, and Stem Cell Fate. *Stem Cells Dev.* **2015**, *24*, 1957–1971. [CrossRef]
112. Prieto, J.; León, M.; Ponsoda, X.; Sendra, R.; Bort, R.; Ferrer-Lorente, R.; Raya, A.; López-García, C.; Torres, J. Early ERK1/2 activation promotes DRP1-dependent mitochondrial fission necessary for cell reprogramming. *Nat. Commun.* **2016**, *7*, 11124. [CrossRef]
113. Schell, J.C.; Rutter, J. Mitochondria link metabolism and epigenetics in haematopoiesis. *Nat. Cell Biol.* **2017**, *19*, 589–591. [CrossRef]
114. Eliasson, P.; Rehn, M.; Hammar, P.; Larsson, P.; Sirenko, O.; Flippin, L.A.; Cammenga, J.; Jönsson, J.I. Hypoxia mediates low cell-cycle activity and increases the proportion of long-term-reconstituting hematopoietic stem cells during in vitro culture. *Exp. Hematol.* **2010**, *38*, 301–310. [CrossRef]
115. Simsek, T.; Kocabas, F.; Zheng, J.; Deberardinis, R.J.; Mahmoud, A.I.; Olson, E.N.; Schneider, J.W.; Zhang, C.C.; Sadek, H.A. The distinct metabolic profile of hematopoietic stem cells reflects their location in a hypoxic niche. *Cell Stem Cell* **2010**, *7*, 380–390. [CrossRef]
116. Takubo, K.; Goda, N.; Yamada, W.; Iriuchishima, H.; Ikeda, E.; Kubota, Y.; Shima, H.; Johnson, R.S.; Hirao, A.; Suematsu, M.; et al. Regulation of the HIF-1alpha level is essential for hematopoietic stem cells. *Cell Stem Cell* **2010**, *7*, 391–402. [CrossRef]
117. Suda, T.; Takubo, K.; Semenza, G.L. Metabolic regulation of hematopoietic stem cells in the hypoxic niche. *Cell Stem Cell* **2011**, *9*, 298–310. [CrossRef]
118. Klimmeck, D.; Hansson, J.; Raffel, S.; Vakhrushev, S.Y.; Trumpp, A.; Krijgsveld, J. Proteomic cornerstones of hematopoietic stem cell differentiation: Distinct signatures of multipotent progenitors and myeloid committed cells. *Mol. Cell. Proteom.* **2012**, *11*, 286–302. [CrossRef]
119. Spencer, J.A.; Ferraro, F.; Roussakis, E.; Klein, A.; Wu, J.; Runners, J.M.; Zaher, W.; Mortensen, L.J.; Alt, C.; Turcotte, R.; et al. Direct measurement of local oxygen concentration in the bone marrow of live animals. *Nature* **2014**, *508*, 269–273. [CrossRef]
120. Zhang, C.C.; Sadek, H.A. Hypoxia and metabolic properties of hematopoietic stem cells. *Antioxid. Redox Signal.* **2014**, *20*, 1891–1901. [CrossRef]
121. Vannini, N.; Girotra, M.; Naveiras, O.; Nikitin, G.; Campos, V.; Giger, S.; Roch, A.; Auwerx, J.; Lutolf, M.P. Specification of haematopoietic stem cell fate via modulation of mitochondrial activity. *Nat. Commun.* **2016**, *7*, 13125. [CrossRef]
122. Pattappa, G.; Thorpe, S.D.; Jegard, N.C.; Heywood, H.K.; de Bruijn, J.D.; Lee, D.A. Continuous and uninterrupted oxygen tension influences the colony formation and oxidative metabolism of human mesenchymal stem cells. *Tissue Eng. Part C Methods* **2013**, *19*, 68–79. [CrossRef]
123. Stincone, A.; Prigione, A.; Cramer, T.; Wamelink, M.M.; Campbell, K.; Cheung, E.; Olin-Sandoval, V.; Grüning, N.M.; Krüger, A.; Tauqeer Alam, M.; et al. The return of metabolism: Biochemistry and physiology of the pentose phosphate pathway. *Biol. Rev. Camb. Philos. Soc.* **2015**, *90*, 927–963. [CrossRef]
124. Tsatmali, M.; Walcott, E.C.; Crossin, K.L. Newborn neurons acquire high levels of reactive oxygen species and increased mitochondrial proteins upon differentiation from progenitors. *Brain Res.* **2005**, *1040*, 137–150. [CrossRef] [PubMed]
125. Jang, Y.Y.; Sharkis, S.J. A low level of reactive oxygen species selects for primitive hematopoietic stem cells that may reside in the low-oxygenic niche. *Blood* **2007**, *110*, 3056–3063. [CrossRef]
126. Atashi, F.; Modarressi, A.; Pepper, M.S. The role of reactive oxygen species in mesenchymal stem cell adipogenic and osteogenic differentiation: A review. *Stem Cells Dev.* **2015**, *24*, 1150–1163. [CrossRef]
127. Ito, K.; Bernardi, R.; Morotti, A.; Matsuoka, S.; Saglio, G.; Ikeda, Y.; Rosenblatt, J.; Avigan, D.E.; Teruya-Feldstein, J.; Pandolfi, P.P. PML targeting eradicates quiescent leukaemia-initiating cells. *Nature* **2008**, *453*, 1072–1078. [CrossRef] [PubMed]
128. Ito, K.; Carracedo, A.; Weiss, D.; Arai, F.; Ala, U.; Avigan, D.E.; Schafer, Z.T.; Evans, R.M.; Suda, T.; Lee, C.H.; et al. A PML–PPAR-δ pathway for fatty acid oxidation regulates hematopoietic stem cell maintenance. *Nat. Med.* **2012**, *18*, 1350–1358. [CrossRef] [PubMed]
129. Ito, K.; Ito, K. Newly Identified Roles of PML in Stem Cell Biology. *Front. Oncol.* **2013**, *3*, 50. [CrossRef]

130. Ito, K.; Turcotte, R.; Cui, J.; Zimmerman, S.E.; Pinho, S.; Mizoguchi, T.; Arai, F.; Runnels, J.M.; Alt, C.; Teruya-Feldstein, J.; et al. Self-renewal of a purified Tie2^{+} hematopoietic stem cell population relies on mitochondrial clearance. *Science* **2016**, *354*, 1156–1160. [CrossRef] [PubMed]
131. Stoll, E.A.; Makin, R.; Sweet, I.R.; Trevelyan, A.J.; Miwa, S.; Horner, P.J.; Turnbull, D.M. Neural Stem Cells in the Adult Subventricular Zone Oxidize Fatty Acids to Produce Energy and Support Neurogenic Activity. *Stem Cells* **2015**, *33*, 2306–2319. [CrossRef]
132. Xie, Z.; Jones, A.; Deeney, J.T.; Hur, S.K.; Bankaitis, V.A. Inborn Errors of Long-Chain Fatty Acid β-Oxidation Link Neural Stem Cell Self-Renewal to Autism. *Cell Rep.* **2016**, *14*, 991–999. [CrossRef] [PubMed]
133. Ryall, J.G.; Dell'Orso, S.; Derfoul, A.; Juan, A.; Zare, H.; Feng, X.; Clermont, D.; Koulnis, M.; Gutierrez-Cruz, G.; Fulco, M.; et al. The NAD^{+}-dependent SIRT1 deacetylase translates a metabolic switch into regulatory epigenetics in skeletal muscle stem cells. *Cell Stem Cell* **2015**, *16*, 171–183. [CrossRef]
134. Fukawa, T.; Yan-Jiang, B.C.; Min-Wen, J.C.; Jun-Hao, E.T.; Huang, D.; Qian, C.N.; Ong, P.; Li, Z.; Chen, S.; Mak, S.Y.; et al. Excessive fatty acid oxidation induces muscle atrophy in cancer cachexia. *Nat. Med.* **2016**, *22*, 666–671. [CrossRef]
135. Carracedo, A.; Cantley, L.C.; Pandolfi, P.P. Cancer metabolism: Fatty acid oxidation in the limelight. *Nat. Rev. Cancer* **2013**, *13*, 227–232. [CrossRef] [PubMed]
136. Knobloch, M.; Braun, S.M.; Zurkirchen, L.; von Schoultz, C.; Zamboni, N.; Araúzo-Bravo, M.J.; Kovacs, W.J.; Karalay, O.; Suter, U.; Machado, R.A.; et al. Metabolic control of adult neural stem cell activity by Fasn-dependent lipogenesis. *Nature* **2013**, *493*, 226–230. [CrossRef] [PubMed]
137. Beyaz, S.; Mana, M.D.; Roper, J.; Kedrin, D.; Saadatpour, A.; Hong, S.J.; Bauer-Rowe, K.E.; Xifaras, M.E.; Akkad, A.; Arias, E.; et al. High-fat diet enhances stemness and tumorigenicity of intestinal progenitors. *Nature* **2016**, *531*, 53–58. [CrossRef] [PubMed]
138. Murphy, M.P. How mitochondria produce reactive oxygen species. *Biochem. J.* **2009**, *417*, 1–13. [CrossRef]
139. Bigarella, C.L.; Liang, R.; Ghaffari, S. Stem cells and the impact of ROS signaling. *Development* **2014**, *141*, 4206–4218. [CrossRef]
140. Liang, R.; Ghaffari, S. Stem cells, redox signaling, and stem cell aging. *Antioxid. Redox Signal.* **2014**, *20*, 1902–1916. [CrossRef]
141. Cervantes, R.B.; Stringer, J.R.; Shao, C.; Tischfield, J.A.; Stambrook, P.J. Embryonic stem cells and somatic cells differ in mutation frequency and type. *Proc. Natl. Acad. Sci. USA* **2002**, *99*, 3586–3590. [CrossRef]
142. Kirby, D.M.; Rennie, K.J.; Smulders-Srinivasan, T.K.; Acin-Perez, R.; Whittington, M.; Enriquez, J.A.; Trevelyan, A.J.; Turnbull, D.M.; Lightowlers, R.N. Transmitochondrial embryonic stem cells containing pathogenic mtDNA mutations are compromised in neuronal differentiation. *Cell Prolif.* **2009**, *42*, 413–424. [CrossRef] [PubMed]
143. Ahlqvist, K.J.; Hämäläinen, R.H.; Yatsuga, S.; Uutela, M.; Terzioglu, M.; Götz, A.; Forsström, S.; Salven, P.; Angers-Loustau, A.; Kopra, O.H.; et al. Somatic progenitor cell vulnerability to mitochondrial DNA mutagenesis underlies progeroid phenotypes in Polg mutator mice. *Cell Metab.* **2012**, *15*, 100–109. [CrossRef] [PubMed]
144. Wahlestedt, M.; Ameur, A.; Moraghebi, R.; Norddahl, G.L.; Sten, G.; Woods, N.B.; Bryder, D. Somatic cells with a heavy mitochondrial DNA mutational load render induced pluripotent stem cells with distinct differentiation defects. *Stem Cells* **2014**, *32*, 1173–1182. [CrossRef]
145. Ma, H.; Folmes, C.D.; Wu, J.; Morey, R.; Mora-Castilla, S.; Ocampo, A.; Ma, L.; Poulton, J.; Wang, X.; Ahmed, R.; et al. Metabolic rescue in pluripotent cells from patients with mtDNA disease. *Nature* **2015**, *524*, 234–238. [CrossRef] [PubMed]
146. Armstrong, L.; Tilgner, K.; Saretzki, G.; Atkinson, S.P.; Stojkovic, M.; Moreno, R.; Przyborski, S.; Lako, M. Human induced pluripotent stem cell lines show stress defense mechanisms and mitochondrial regulation similar to those of human embryonic stem cells. *Stem Cells* **2010**, *28*, 661–673. [CrossRef] [PubMed]
147. Le Belle, J.E.; Orozco, N.M.; Paucar, A.A.; Saxe, J.P.; Mottahedeh, J.; Pyle, A.D.; Wu, H.; Kornblum, H.I. Proliferative neural stem cells have high endogenous ROS levels that regulate self-renewal and neurogenesis in a PI3K/Akt-dependant manner. *Cell Stem Cell* **2011**, *8*, 59–71. [CrossRef]
148. Morimoto, H.; Iwata, K.; Ogonuki, N.; Inoue, K.; Atsuo, O.; Kanatsu-Shinohara, M.; Morimoto, T.; Yabe-Nishimura, C.; Shinohara, T. ROS are required for mouse spermatogonial stem cell self-renewal. *Cell Stem Cell* **2013**, *12*, 774–786. [CrossRef]

149. Kohli, L.; Passed, E. Surviving changes: The metabolic journey of hematopoietic stem cells. *Trends Cell Biol.* **2014**, *24*, 479–487. [CrossRef] [PubMed]
150. Paul, M.K.; Bisht, B.; Darmawan, D.O.; Chiou, R.; Ha, V.L.; Wallace, W.D.; Chon, A.T.; Hegab, A.E.; Grogan, T.; Elashoff, D.A.; et al. Dynamic changes in intracellular ROS levels regulate airway basal stem cell homeostasis through Nrf2-dependent Notch signaling. *Cell Stem Cell* **2014**, *15*, 199–214. [CrossRef] [PubMed]
151. Bakker, S.T.; Passegué, E. Resilient and resourceful: Genome maintenance strategies in hematopoietic stem cells. *Exp. Hematol.* **2013**, *41*, 915–923. [CrossRef]
152. Adams, P.D.; Jasper, H.; Rudolph, K.L. Aging-Induced Stem Cell Mutations as Drivers for Disease and Cancer. *Cell Stem Cell* **2015**, *16*, 601–612. [CrossRef]
153. Maynard, S.; Swistowska, A.M.; Lee, J.W.; Liu, Y.; Liu, S.T.; Da Cruz, A.B.; Rao, M.; de Souza-Pinto, N.C.; Zeng, X.; Bohr, V.A. Human embryonic stem cells have enhanced repair of multiple forms of DNA damage. *Stem Cells* **2008**, *26*, 2266–2274. [CrossRef]
154. Saretzki, G.; Walter, T.; Atkinson, S.; Passos, J.F.; Bareth, B.; Keith, W.N.; Stewart, R.; Hoare, S.; Stojkovic, M.; Armstrong, L.; et al. Downregulation of multiple stress defense mechanisms during differentiation of human embryonic stem cells. *Stem Cells* **2008**, *26*, 455–464. [CrossRef]
155. Dannenmann, B.; Lehle, S.; Hildebrand, D.G.; Kübler, A.; Grondona, P.; Schmid, V.; Holzer, K.; Fröschl, M.; Essmann, F.; Rothfuss, O.; et al. High glutathione and glutathione peroxidase-2 levels mediate cell-type-specific DNA damage protection in human induced pluripotent stem cells. *Stem Cell Rep.* **2015**, *4*, 886–898. [CrossRef]
156. Miyamoto, K.; Miyamoto, T.; Kato, R.; Yoshimura, A.; Motoyama, N.; Suda, T. FoxO3a regulates hematopoietic homeostasis through a negative feedback pathway in conditions of stress or aging. *Blood* **2008**, *112*, 4485–4493. [CrossRef]
157. Renault, V.M.; Rafalski, V.A.; Morgan, A.A.; Salih, D.A.; Brett, J.O.; Webb, A.E.; Villeda, S.A.; Thekkat, P.U.; Guillerey, C.; Denko, N.C.; et al. FoxO3 regulates neural stem cell homeostasis. *Cell Stem Cell* **2009**, *5*, 527–539. [CrossRef]
158. Matsui, K.; Ezoe, S.; Oritani, K.; Shibata, M.; Tokunaga, M.; Fujita, N.; Tanimura, A.; Sudo, T.; Tanaka, H.; McBurney, M.W.; et al. NAD-dependent histone deacetylase, SIRT1, plays essential roles in the maintenance of hematopoietic stem cells. *Biochem. Biophys. Res. Commun.* **2012**, *418*, 811–817. [CrossRef]
159. Webb, A.E.; Pollina, E.A.; Vierbuchen, T.; Urbán, N.; Ucar, D.; Leeman, D.S.; Martynoga, B.; Sewak, M.; Rando, T.A.; Guillemot, F.; et al. FOXO3 shares common targets with ASCL1 genome-wide and inhibits ASCL1-dependent neurogenesis. *Cell Rep.* **2013**, *4*, 477–491. [CrossRef]
160. Rimmelé, P.; Bigarella, C.L.; Liang, R.; Izac, B.; Dieguez-Gonzalez, R.; Barbet, G.; Donovan, M.; Brugnara, C.; Blander, J.M.; Sinclair, D.A.; et al. Aging-like phenotype and defective lineage specification in SIRT1-deleted hematopoietic stem and progenitor cells. *Stem Cell Rep.* **2014**, *3*, 44–59. [CrossRef]
161. Mehta, A.; Zhao, J.L.; Sinha, N.; Marinov, G.K.; Mann, M.; Kowalczyk, M.S.; Galimidi, R.P.; Du, X.; Erikci, E.; Regev, A.; et al. The MicroRNA-132 and MicroRNA-212 Cluster Regulates Hematopoietic Stem Cell Maintenance and Survival with Age by Buffering FOXO3 Expression. *Immunity* **2015**, *42*, 1021–1032. [CrossRef]
162. Rimmelé, P.; Liang, R.; Bigarella, C.L.; Kocabas, F.; Xie, J.; Serasinghe, M.N.; Chipuk, J.; Sadek, H.; Zhang, C.C.; Ghaffari, S. Mitochondrial metabolism in hematopoietic stem cells requires functional FOXO3. *EMBO Rep.* **2015**, *16*, 1164–1176. [CrossRef] [PubMed]
163. Wakabayashi, N.; Itoh, K.; Wakabayashi, J.; Motohashi, H.; Noda, S.; Takahashi, S.; Imakado, S.; Kotsuji, T.; Otsuka, F.; Roop, D.R.; et al. Keap1-null mutation leads to postnatal lethality due to constitutive Nrf2 activation. *Nat. Genet.* **2003**, *35*, 238–245. [CrossRef] [PubMed]
164. Hochmuth, C.E.; Biteau, B.; Bohmann, D.; Jasper, H. Redox regulation by Keap1 and Nrf2 controls intestinal stem cell proliferation in Drosophila. *Cell Stem Cell* **2011**, *8*, 188–199. [CrossRef] [PubMed]
165. Mohrin, M.; Bourke, E.; Alexander, D.; Warr, M.R.; Barry-Holson, K.; Le Beau, M.M.; Morrison, C.G.; Passegué, E. Hematopoietic stem cell quiescence promotes error-prone DNA repair and mutagenesis. *Cell Stem Cell* **2010**, *7*, 174–185. [CrossRef] [PubMed]
166. Finkel, T.; Holbrook, N.J. Oxidants, oxidative stress and the biology of ageing. *Nature* **2000**, *408*, 239–247. [CrossRef] [PubMed]
167. D'Autréaux, B.; Toledano, M.B. ROS as signalling molecules: Mechanisms that generate specificity in ROS homeostasis. *Nat. Rev. Mol. Cell Biol.* **2007**, *8*, 813–824. [CrossRef]

168. Giorgio, M.; Trinei, M.; Migliaccio, E.; Pelicci, P.G. Hydrogen peroxide: A metabolic by-product or a common mediator of ageing signals? *Nat. Rev. Mol. Cell Biol.* **2007**, *8*, 722–728. [CrossRef] [PubMed]
169. Schieber, M.; Chandel, N.S. ROS function in redox signaling and oxidative stress. *Curr. Biol.* **2014**, *24*, R453–R462. [CrossRef]
170. Miyamoto, K.; Araki, K.Y.; Naka, K.; Arai, F.; Takubo, K.; Yamazaki, S.; Matsuoka, S.; Miyamoto, T.; Ito, K.; Ohmura, M.; et al. Foxo3a is essential for maintenance of the hematopoietic stem cell pool. *Cell Stem Cell* **2007**, *1*, 101–112. [CrossRef]
171. Tothova, Z.; Kollipara, R.; Huntly, B.J.; Lee, B.H.; Castrillon, D.H.; Cullen, D.E.; McDowell, E.P.; Lazo-Kallanian, S.; Williams, I.R.; Sears, C.; et al. FoxOs are critical mediators of hematopoietic stem cell resistance to physiologic oxidative stress. *Cell* **2007**, *128*, 325–339. [CrossRef] [PubMed]
172. Sykiotis, G.P.; Bohmann, D. Keap1/Nrf2 signaling regulates oxidative stress tolerance and lifespan in Drosophila. *Dev. Cell* **2008**, *14*, 76–85. [CrossRef]
173. Blanpain, C.; Mohrin, M.; Sotiropoulou, P.A.; Passegué, E. DNA-damage response in tissue-specific and cancer stem cells. *Cell Stem Cell* **2011**, *8*, 16–29. [CrossRef]
174. Lombard, D.B.; Chua, K.F.; Mostoslavsky, R.; Franco, S.; Gostissa, M.; Alt, F.W. DNA repair, genome stability, and aging. *Cell* **2005**, *120*, 497–512. [CrossRef]
175. Owusu-Ansah, E.; Banerjee, U. Reactive oxygen species prime Drosophila haematopoietic progenitors for differentiation. *Nature* **2009**, *461*, 537–541. [CrossRef]
176. Tormos, K.V.; Anso, E.; Hamanaka, R.B.; Eisenbart, J.; Joseph, J.; Kalyanaraman, B.; Chandel, N.S. Mitochondrial complex III ROS regulate adipocyte differentiation. *Cell Metab.* **2011**, *14*, 537–544. [CrossRef] [PubMed]
177. Lyublinskaya, O.G.; Borisov, Y.G.; Pugovkina, N.A.; Smirnova, I.S.; Obidina, J.V.; Ivanova, J.S.; Zenin, V.V.; Shatrova, A.N.; Borodkina, A.V.; Aksenov, N.D.; et al. Reactive Oxygen Species Are Required for Human Mesenchymal Stem Cells to Initiate Proliferation after the Quiescence Exit. *Oxid. Med. Cell. Longev.* **2015**, *2015*, 502105. [CrossRef]
178. Khacho, M.; Clark, A.; Svoboda, D.S.; Azzi, J.; MacLaurin, J.G.; Meghaizel, C.; Sesaki, H.; Lagace, D.C.; Germain, M.; Harper, M.E.; et al. Mitochondrial Dynamics Impacts Stem Cell Identity and Fate Decisions by Regulating a Nuclear Transcriptional Program. *Cell Stem Cell* **2016**, *19*, 232–247. [CrossRef] [PubMed]
179. Juntilla, M.M.; Patil, V.D.; Calamito, M.; Joshi, R.P.; Birnbaum, M.J.; Koretzky, G.A. AKT1 and AKT2 maintain hematopoietic stem cell function by regulating reactive oxygen species. *Blood* **2010**, *115*, 4030–4038. [CrossRef]
180. Biteau, B.; Jasper, H. EGF signaling regulates the proliferation of intestinal stem cells in Drosophila. *Development* **2011**, *138*, 1045–1055. [CrossRef]
181. Malinska, D.; Kudin, A.P.; Bejtka, M.; Kunz, W.S. Changes in mitochondrial reactive oxygen species synthesis during differentiation of skeletal muscle cells. *Mitochondrion* **2012**, *12*, 144–148. [CrossRef]
182. Ueda, T.; Nagamachi, A.; Takubo, K.; Yamasaki, N.; Matsui, H.; Kanai, A.; Nakata, Y.; Ikeda, K.; Konuma, T.; Oda, H.; et al. Fbxl10 overexpression in murine hematopoietic stem cells induces leukemia involving metabolic activation and upregulation of Nsg2. *Blood* **2015**, *125*, 3437–3446. [CrossRef]
183. Ito, K.; Hirao, A.; Arai, F.; Takubo, K.; Matsuoka, S.; Miyamoto, K.; Ohmura, M.; Naka, K.; Hosokawa, K.; Ikeda, Y.; et al. Reactive oxygen species act through p38 MAPK to limit the lifespan of hematopoietic stem cells. *Nat. Med.* **2006**, *12*, 446–451. [CrossRef]
184. Karigane, D.; Kobayashi, H.; Morikawa, T.; Ootomo, Y.; Sakai, M.; Nagamatsu, G.; Kubota, Y.; Goda, N.; Matsumoto, M.; Nishimura, E.K.; et al. p38α Activates Purine Metabolism to Initiate Hematopoietic Stem/Progenitor Cell Cycling in Response to Stress. *Cell Stem Cell* **2016**, *19*, 192–204. [CrossRef]
185. Kwon, B. p38α-mediated purine metabolism is linked to exit from quiescence of hematopoietic stem cells. *Stem Cell Investig.* **2016**, *3*, 69. [CrossRef]
186. Essers, M.A.G. Stressed-Out HSCs Turn Up p38α and Purine to Proliferate. *Cell Stem Cell* **2016**, *19*, 143–144. [CrossRef]
187. Wellen, K.E.; Hatzivassiliou, G.; Sachdeva, U.M.; Bui, T.V.; Cross, J.R.; Thompson, C.B. ATP-citrate lyase links cellular metabolism to histone acetylation. *Science* **2009**, *324*, 1076–1080. [CrossRef]
188. Sørensen, A.L.; Timoskainen, S.; West, F.D.; Vekterud, K.; Boquest, A.C.; Ahrlund-Richter, L.; Stice, S.L.; Collas, P. Lineage-specific promoter DNA methylation patterns segregate adult progenitor cell types. *Stem Cells Dev.* **2010**, *19*, 1257–1266. [CrossRef]

189. Yannarelli, G.; Pacienza, N.; Cuniberti, L.; Medin, J.; Davies, J.; Keating, A. Brief report: The potential role of epigenetics on multipotent cell differentiation capacity of mesenchymal stromal cells. *Stem Cells* **2013**, *31*, 215–220. [CrossRef]
190. Kaelin, W.G.; McKnight, S.L. Influence of metabolism on epigenetics and disease. *Cell* **2013**, *153*, 56–69. [CrossRef]
191. Hwang, I.Y.; Kwak, S.; Lee, S.; Kim, H.; Lee, S.E.; Kim, J.H.; Kim, Y.A.; Jeon, Y.K.; Chung, D.H.; Jin, X.; et al. Psat1-Dependent Fluctuations in α-Ketoglutarate Affect the Timing of ESC Differentiation. *Cell Metab.* **2016**, *24*, 494–501. [CrossRef] [PubMed]
192. Carey, B.W.; Finley, L.W.; Cross, J.R.; Allis, C.D.; Thompson, C.B. Intracellular α-ketoglutarate maintains the pluripotency of embryonic stem cells. *Nature* **2015**, *518*, 413–416. [CrossRef] [PubMed]
193. Moussaieff, A.; Rouleau, M.; Kitsberg, D.; Cohen, M.; Levy, G.; Barasch, D.; Nemirovski, A.; Shen-Orr, S.; Laevsky, I.; Amit, M.; et al. Glycolysis-mediated changes in acetyl-CoA and histone acetylation control the early differentiation of embryonic stem cells. *Cell Metab.* **2015**, *21*, 392–402. [CrossRef] [PubMed]
194. Ryall, J.G.; Cliff, T.; Dalton, S.; Sartorelli, V. Metabolic Reprogramming of Stem Cell Epigenetics. *Cell Stem Cell* **2015**, *17*, 651–662. [CrossRef] [PubMed]
195. TeSlaa, T.; Chaikovsky, A.C.; Lipchina, I.; Escobar, S.L.; Hochedlinger, K.; Huang, J.; Graeber, T.G.; Braas, D.; Teitell, M.A. α-Ketoglutarate Accelerates the Initial Differentiation of Primed Human Pluripotent Stem Cells. *Cell Metab.* **2016**, *24*, 485–493. [CrossRef] [PubMed]
196. Zhu, C.; Gao, Y.; Guo, H.; Xia, B.; Song, J.; Wu, X.; Zeng, H.; Kee, K.; Tang, F.; Yi, C. Single-Cell 5-Formylcytosine Landscapes of Mammalian Early Embryos and ESCs at Single-Base Resolution. *Cell Stem Cell* **2017**, *20*, 720–731. [CrossRef]
197. Chambers, S.M.; Shaw, C.A.; Gatza, C.; Fisk, C.J.; Donehower, L.A.; Goodell, M.A. Aging hematopoietic stem cells decline in function and exhibit epigenetic dysregulation. *PLoS Biol.* **2007**, *5*, e201. [CrossRef]
198. Noer, A.; Lindeman, L.C.; Collas, P. Histone H3 modifications associated with differentiation and long-term culture of mesenchymal adipose stem cells. *Stem Cells Dev.* **2009**, *18*, 725–736. [CrossRef]
199. Weishaupt, H.; Sigvardsson, M.; Attema, J.L. Epigenetic chromatin states uniquely define the developmental plasticity of murine hematopoietic stem cells. *Blood* **2010**, *115*, 247–256. [CrossRef]
200. Florian, M.C.; Dörr, K.; Niebel, A.; Daria, D.; Schrezenmeier, H.; Rojewski, M.; Filippi, M.D.; Hasenberg, A.; Gunzer, M.; Scharffetter-Kochanek, K.; et al. Cdc42 activity regulates hematopoietic stem cell aging and rejuvenation. *Cell Stem Cell* **2012**, *10*, 520–530. [CrossRef] [PubMed]
201. Beerman, I.; Bock, C.; Garrison, B.S.; Smith, Z.D.; Gu, H.; Meissner, A.; Rossi, D.J. Proliferation-dependent alterations of the DNA methylation landscape underlie hematopoietic stem cell aging. *Cell Stem Cell* **2013**, *12*, 413–425. [CrossRef]
202. Geiger, H.; de Haan, G.; Florian, M.C. The ageing haematopoietic stem cell compartment. *Nat. Rev. Immunol.* **2013**, *13*, 376–389.
203. Liu, L.; Cheung, T.H.; Charville, G.W.; Hurgo, B.M.; Leavitt, T.; Shih, J.; Brunet, A.; Rando, T.A. Chromatin modifications as determinants of muscle stem cell quiescence and chronological aging. *Cell Rep.* **2013**, *4*, 189–204. [CrossRef]
204. Benayoun, B.A.; Pollina, E.A.; Ucar, D.; Mahmoudi, S.; Karra, K.; Wong, E.D.; Devarajan, K.; Daugherty, A.C.; Kundaje, A.B.; Mancini, E.; et al. H3K4me3 breadth is linked to cell identity and transcriptional consistency. *Cell* **2014**, *158*, 673–688. [CrossRef]
205. Challen, G.A.; Sun, D.; Mayle, A.; Jeong, M.; Luo, M.; Rodriguez, B.; Mallaney, C.; Celik, H.; Yang, L.; Xia, Z.; et al. Dnmt3a and Dnmt3b have overlapping and distinct functions in hematopoietic stem cells. *Cell Stem Cell* **2014**, *15*, 350–364. [CrossRef]
206. Sun, D.; Luo, M.; Jeong, M.; Rodriguez, B.; Xia, Z.; Hannah, R.; Wang, H.; Le, T.; Faull, K.F.; Chen, R.; et al. Epigenomic profiling of young and aged HSCs reveals concerted changes during aging that reinforce self-renewal. *Cell Stem Cell* **2014**, *14*, 673–688. [CrossRef]
207. Beerman, I.; Rossi, D.J. Epigenetic Control of Stem Cell Potential during Homeostasis, Aging, and Disease. *Cell Stem Cell* **2015**, *16*, 613–625. [CrossRef]
208. Mayle, A.; Yang, L.; Rodriguez, B.; Zhou, T.; Chang, E.; Curry, C.V.; Challen, G.A.; Li, W.; Wheeler, D.; Rebel, V.I.; et al. Dnmt3a loss predisposes murine hematopoietic stem cells to malignant transformation. *Blood* **2015**, *125*, 629–638. [CrossRef]

209. Ugarte, F.; Sousae, R.; Cinquin, B.; Martin, E.W.; Krietsch, J.; Sanchez, G.; Inman, M.; Tsang, H.; Warr, M.; Passegué, E.; et al. Progressive Chromatin Condensation and H3K9 Methylation Regulate the Differentiation of Embryonic and Hematopoietic Stem Cells. *Stem Cell Rep.* **2015**, *5*, 728–740. [CrossRef]
210. Zhang, W.; Li, J.; Suzuki, K.; Qu, J.; Wang, P.; Zhou, J.; Liu, X.; Ren, R.; Xu, X.; Ocampo, A.; et al. Aging stem cells. A Werner syndrome stem cell model unveils heterochromatin alterations as a driver of human aging. *Science* **2015**, *348*, 1160–1163. [CrossRef]
211. Boonsanay, V.; Zhang, T.; Georgieva, A.; Kostin, S.; Qi, H.; Yuan, X.; Zhou, Y.; Braun, T. Regulation of Skeletal Muscle Stem Cell Quiescence by Suv4-20h1-Dependent Facultative Heterochromatin Formation. *Cell Stem Cell* **2016**, *18*, 229–242. [CrossRef] [PubMed]
212. Faralli, H.; Wang, C.; Nakka, K.; Benyoucef, A.; Sebastian, S.; Zhuang, L.; Chu, A.; Palii, C.G.; Liu, C.; Camellato, B.; et al. UTX demethylase activity is required for satellite cell-mediated muscle regeneration. *J. Clin. Investig.* **2016**, *126*, 1555–1565. [CrossRef] [PubMed]
213. Pagano, M.; Pepperkok, R.; Verde, F.; Ansorge, W.; Draetta, G. Cyclin A is required at two points in the human cell cycle. *EMBO J.* **1992**, *11*, 961–971. [CrossRef]
214. Blanpain, C.; Lowry, W.E.; Geoghegan, A.; Polak, L.; Fuchs, E. Self-renewal, multipotency, and the existence of two cell populations within an epithelial stem cell niche. *Cell* **2004**, *118*, 635–648. [CrossRef]
215. Fukada, S.; Uezumi, A.; Ikemoto, M.; Masuda, S.; Segawa, M.; Tanimura, N.; Yamamoto, H.; Miyagoe-Suzuki, Y.; Takeda, S. Molecular signature of quiescent satellite cells in adult skeletal muscle. *Stem Cells* **2007**, *25*, 2448–2459. [CrossRef]
216. Forsberg, E.C.; Passegué, E.; Prohaska, S.S.; Wagers, A.J.; Koeva, M.; Stuart, J.M.; Weissman, I.L. Molecular signatures of quiescent, mobilized and leukemia-initiating hematopoietic stem cells. *PLoS ONE* **2010**, *5*, e8785. [CrossRef]
217. Kamminga, L.M.; Bystrykh, L.V.; de Boer, A.; Houwer, S.; Douma, J.; Weersing, E.; Dontje, B.; de Haan, G. The Polycomb group gene Ezh2 prevents hematopoietic stem cell exhaustion. *Blood* **2006**, *107*, 2170–2179. [CrossRef] [PubMed]
218. Ezhkova, E.; Lien, W.H.; Stokes, N.; Pasolli, H.A.; Silva, J.M.; Fuchs, E. EZH1 and EZH2 cogovern histone H3K27 trimethylation and are essential for hair follicle homeostasis and wound repair. *Genes Dev.* **2011**, *25*, 485–498. [CrossRef]
219. Juan, A.H.; Derfoul, A.; Feng, X.; Ryall, J.G.; Dell'Orso, S.; Pasut, A.; Zare, H.; Simone, J.M.; Rudnicki, M.A.; Sartorelli, V. Polycomb EZH2 controls self-renewal and safeguards the transcriptional identity of skeletal muscle stem cells. *Genes Dev.* **2011**, *25*, 789–794. [CrossRef]
220. Hidalgo, I.; Herrera-Merchan, A.; Ligos, J.M.; Carramolino, L.; Nuñez, J.; Martinez, F.; Dominguez, O.; Torres, M.; Gonzalez, S. Ezh1 is required for hematopoietic stem cell maintenance and prevents senescence-like cell cycle arrest. *Cell Stem Cell* **2012**, *11*, 649–662. [CrossRef] [PubMed]
221. Locasale, J.W.; Cantley, L.C. Metabolic flux and the regulation of mammalian cell growth. *Cell Metab.* **2011**, *14*, 443–451. [CrossRef] [PubMed]
222. Libert, S.; Guarente, L. Metabolic and neuropsychiatric effects of calorie restriction and sirtuins. *Annu. Rev. Physiol.* **2013**, *75*, 669–684. [CrossRef] [PubMed]
223. Imai, S.; Guarente, L. NAD^+ and sirtuins in aging and disease. *Trends Cell Biol.* **2014**, *24*, 464–471. [CrossRef]
224. Yu, A.; Dang, W. Regulation of stem cell aging by SIRT1—Linking metabolic signaling to epigenetic modifications. *Mol. Cell. Endocrinol.* **2017**, *455*, 75–82. [CrossRef] [PubMed]
225. Rafalski, V.A.; Ho, P.P.; Brett, J.O.; Ucar, D.; Dugas, J.C.; Pollina, E.A.; Chow, L.M.; Ibrahim, A.; Baker, S.J.; Barres, B.A.; et al. Expansion of oligodendrocyte progenitor cells following SIRT1 inactivation in the adult brain. *Nat. Cell Biol.* **2013**, *15*, 614–624. [CrossRef]
226. Saharan, S.; Jhaveri, D.J.; Bartlett, P.F. SIRT1 regulates the neurogenic potential of neural precursors in the adult subventricular zone and hippocampus. *J. Neurosci. Res.* **2013**, *91*, 642–659. [CrossRef] [PubMed]
227. Zuccaro, E.; Arlotta, P. The quest for myelin in the adult brain. *Nat. Cell Biol.* **2013**, *15*, 572–575. [CrossRef] [PubMed]
228. Hu, B.; Guo, Y.; Chen, C.; Li, Q.; Niu, X.; Guo, S.; Zhang, A.; Wang, Y.; Deng, Z. Repression of SIRT1 promotes the differentiation of mouse induced pluripotent stem cells into neural stem cells. *Cell Mol. Neurobiol.* **2014**, *34*, 905–912. [CrossRef]
229. Fujita, Y.; Yamashita, T. Sirtuins in Neuroendocrine Regulation and Neurological Diseases. *Front. Neurosci.* **2018**, *12*, 778. [CrossRef]

230. Hisahara, S.; Chiba, S.; Matsumoto, H.; Tanno, M.; Yagi, H.; Shimohama, S.; Sato, M.; Horio, Y. Histone deacetylase SIRT1 modulates neuronal differentiation by its nuclear translocation. *Proc. Natl. Acad. Sci. USA* **2008**, *105*, 15599–15604. [CrossRef]
231. Ma, C.Y.; Yao, M.J.; Zhai, Q.W.; Jiao, J.W.; Yuan, X.B.; Poo, M.M. SIRT1 suppresses self-renewal of adult hippocampal neural stem cells. *Development* **2014**, *141*, 4697–4709. [CrossRef] [PubMed]
232. Fawal, M.A.; Davy, A. Impact of Metabolic Pathways and Epigenetics on Neural Stem Cells. *Epigenet. Insights* **2018**, *11*, 2516865718820946. [CrossRef]
233. Diaz-Ruiz, A.; Gonzalez-Freire, M.; Ferrucci, L.; Bernier, M.; Cabo, R. SIRT1 synchs satellite cell metabolism with stem cell fate. *Cell Stem Cell* **2015**, *16*, 103–104. [CrossRef]
234. Yun, J.; Johnson, J.L.; Hanigan, C.L.; Locasale, J.W. Interactions between epigenetics and metabolism in cancers. *Front. Oncol.* **2012**, *2*, 163. [CrossRef] [PubMed]
235. Gut, P.; Verdin, E. The nexus of chromatin regulation and intermediary metabolism. *Nature* **2013**, *502*, 489–498. [CrossRef] [PubMed]
236. Sharma, A.; Diecke, S.; Zhang, W.Y.; Lan, F.; He, C.; Mordwinkin, N.M.; Chua, K.F.; Wu, J.C. The role of SIRT6 protein in aging and reprogramming of human induced pluripotent stem cells. *J. Biol. Chem.* **2013**, *288*, 18439–18447. [CrossRef] [PubMed]
237. Rodgers, J.T.; Lerin, C.; Haas, W.; Gygi, S.P.; Spiegelman, B.M.; Puigserver, P. Nutrient control of glucose homeostasis through a complex of PGC-1α and SIRT1. *Nature* **2005**, *434*, 113–118. [CrossRef]
238. O'Brien, L.C.; Keeney, P.M.; Bennett, J.P. Differentiation of Human Neural Stem Cells into Motor Neurons Stimulates Mitochondrial Biogenesis and Decreases Glycolytic Flux. *Stem Cells Dev.* **2015**, *24*, 1984–1994. [CrossRef] [PubMed]
239. Guarente, L. The resurgence of NAD^+. *Science* **2016**, *352*, 1396–1397. [CrossRef] [PubMed]
240. Tang, A.H.; Rando, T.A. Induction of autophagy supports the bioenergetic demands of quiescent muscle stem cell activation. *EMBO J.* **2014**, *33*, 2782–2797. [CrossRef] [PubMed]
241. Wagers, A.J. How stem cells get "turned on". *EMBO J.* **2014**, *33*, 2743–2744. [CrossRef]
242. Brunet, A.; Sweeney, L.B.; Sturgill, J.F.; Chua, K.F.; Greer, P.L.; Lin, Y.; Tran, H.; Ross, S.E.; Mostoslavsky, R.; Cohen, H.Y.; et al. Stress-dependent regulation of FOXO transcription factors by the SIRT1 deacetylase. *Science* **2004**, *303*, 2011–2015. [CrossRef]
243. Kobayashi, Y.; Furukawa-Hibi, Y.; Chen, C.; Horio, Y.; Isobe, K.; Ikeda, K.; Motoyama, N. SIRT1 is critical regulator of FOXO-mediated transcription in response to oxidative stress. *Int. J. Mol. Med.* **2005**, *16*, 237–243. [CrossRef]
244. Yu, W.; Dittenhafer-Reed, K.E.; Denu, J.M. SIRT3 protein deacetylates isocitrate dehydrogenase 2 (IDH2) and regulates mitochondrial redox status. *J. Biol. Chem.* **2012**, *287*, 14078–14086. [CrossRef] [PubMed]
245. Brown, K.; Xie, S.; Qiu, X.; Mohrin, M.; Shin, J.; Liu, Y.; Zhang, D.; Scadden, D.T.; Chen, D. SIRT3 reverses aging-associated degeneration. *Cell Rep.* **2013**, *3*, 319–327. [CrossRef] [PubMed]
246. Qiu, X.; Brown, K.; Hirschey, M.D.; Verdin, E.; Chen, D. Calorie restriction reduces oxidative stress by SIRT3-mediated SOD2 activation. *Cell Metab.* **2010**, *12*, 662–667. [CrossRef] [PubMed]
247. Tao, R.; Coleman, M.C.; Pennington, J.D.; Ozden, O.; Park, S.H.; Jiang, H.; Kim, H.S.; Flynn, C.R.; Hill, S.; McDonald, W.H.; et al. Sirt3-mediated deacetylation of evolutionarily conserved lysine 122 regulates MnSOD activity in response to stress. *Mol. Cell* **2010**, *40*, 893–904. [CrossRef]
248. Someya, S.; Yu, W.; Hallows, W.C.; Xu, J.; Vann, J.M.; Leeuwenburgh, C.; Tanokura, M.; Denu, J.M.; Prolla, T.A. Sirt3 mediates reduction of oxidative damage and prevention of age-related hearing loss under caloric restriction. *Cell* **2010**, *143*, 802–812. [CrossRef]
249. Shackelford, D.B.; Shaw, R.J. The LKB1-AMPK pathway: Metabolism and growth control in tumour suppression. *Nat. Rev. Cancer* **2009**, *9*, 563–575. [PubMed]
250. Mihaylova, M.M.; Shaw, R.J. The AMPK signalling pathway coordinates cell growth, autophagy and metabolism. *Nat. Cell Biol.* **2011**, *13*, 1016–1023. [CrossRef]
251. Hardie, D.G.; Alessi, D.R. LKB1 and AMPK and the cancer-metabolism link—Ten years after. *BMC Biol.* **2013**, *11*, 36. [CrossRef]
252. Herzig, S.; Shaw, R.J. AMPK: Guardian of metabolism and mitochondrial homeostasis. *Nat. Rev. Mol. Cell Biol.* **2018**, *19*, 121–135. [CrossRef]

253. Gan, B.; Hu, J.; Jiang, S.; Liu, Y.; Sahin, E.; Zhuang, L.; Fletcher-Sananikone, E.; Colla, S.; Wang, Y.A.; Chin, L.; et al. Lkb1 regulates quiescence and metabolic homeostasis of haematopoietic stem cells. *Nature* **2010**, *468*, 701–704. [CrossRef]
254. Gurumurthy, S.; Xie, S.Z.; Alagesan, B.; Kim, J.; Yusuf, R.Z.; Saez, B.; Tzatsos, A.; Ozsolak, F.; Milos, P.; Ferrari, F.; et al. The Lkb1 metabolic sensor maintains haematopoietic stem cell survival. *Nature* **2010**, *468*, 659–663. [CrossRef]
255. Nakada, D.; Saunders, T.L.; Morrison, S.J. Lkb1 regulates cell cycle and energy metabolism in haematopoietic stem cells. *Nature* **2010**, *468*, 653–658. [CrossRef]
256. Durand, E.M.; Zon, L.I. Stem cells: The blood balance. *Nature* **2010**, *468*, 644–645. [CrossRef]
257. Mortensen, M.; Soilleux, E.J.; Djordjevic, G.; Tripp, R.; Lutteropp, M.; Sadighi-Akha, E.; Stranks, A.J.; Glanville, J.; Knight, S.; Jacobsen, S.E.; et al. The autophagy protein Atg7 is essential for hematopoietic stem cell maintenance. *J. Exp. Med.* **2011**, *208*, 455–467. [CrossRef] [PubMed]
258. Krock, B.; Skuli, N.; Simon, M.C. The tumor suppressor LKB1 emerges as a critical factor in hematopoietic stem cell biology. *Cell Metab.* **2011**, *13*, 8–10. [CrossRef]
259. Yilmaz, O.H.; Valdez, R.; Theisen, B.K.; Guo, W.; Ferguson, D.O.; Wu, H.; Morrison, S.J. Pten dependence distinguishes haematopoietic stem cells from leukaemia-initiating cells. *Nature* **2006**, *441*, 475–482. [CrossRef]
260. Zhang, J.; Grindley, J.C.; Yin, T.; Jayasinghe, S.; He, X.C.; Ross, J.T.; Haug, J.S.; Rupp, D.; Porter-Westpfahl, K.S.; Wiedemann, L.M.; et al. PTEN maintains haematopoietic stem cells and acts in lineage choice and leukaemia prevention. *Nature* **2006**, *441*, 518–522. [CrossRef]
261. Chen, C.; Liu, Y.; Liu, R.; Ikenoue, T.; Guan, K.L.; Liu, Y.; Zheng, P. TSC-mTOR maintains quiescence and function of hematopoietic stem cells by repressing mitochondrial biogenesis and reactive oxygen species. *J. Exp. Med.* **2008**, *205*, 2397–2408. [CrossRef]
262. Gan, B.; Sahin, E.; Jiang, S.; Sanchez-Aguilera, A.; Scott, K.L.; Chin, L.; Williams, D.A.; Kwiatkowski, D.J.; DePinho, R.A. mTORC1-dependent and -independent regulation of stem cell renewal, differentiation, and mobilization. *Proc. Natl. Acad. Sci. USA* **2008**, *105*, 19384–19389. [CrossRef] [PubMed]
263. Kharas, M.G.; Gritsman, K. Akt: A double-edged sword for hematopoietic stem cells. *Cell Cycle* **2010**, *9*, 1223–1224. [CrossRef]
264. Kharas, M.G.; Okabe, R.; Ganis, J.J.; Gozo, M.; Khandan, T.; Paktinat, M.; Gilliland, D.G.; Gritsman, K. Constitutively active AKT depletes hematopoietic stem cells and induces leukemia in mice. *Blood* **2010**, *115*, 1406–1415. [CrossRef]
265. Shorning, B.Y.; Zabkiewicz, J.; McCarthy, A.; Pearson, H.B.; Winton, D.J.; Sansom, O.J.; Ashworth, A.; Clarke, A.R. Lkb1 deficiency alters goblet and paneth cell differentiation in the small intestine. *PLoS ONE* **2009**, *4*, e4264. [CrossRef]
266. Yeung, T.M.; Chia, L.A.; Kosinski, C.M.; Kuo, C.J. Regulation of self-renewal and differentiation by the intestinal stem cell niche. *Cell. Mol. Life Sci.* **2011**, *68*, 2513–2523. [CrossRef] [PubMed]
267. Richmond, C.A.; Shah, M.S.; Carlone, D.L.; Breault, D.T. Factors regulating quiescent stem cells: Insights from the intestine and other self-renewing tissues. *J. Physiol.* **2016**, *594*, 4805–4813. [CrossRef]
268. Saxton, R.A.; Sabatini, D.M. mTOR Signaling in Growth, Metabolism, and Disease. *Cell* **2017**, *168*, 960–976. [CrossRef] [PubMed]
269. Kim, J.; Guan, K.L. mTOR as a central hub of nutrient signalling and cell growth. *Nat. Cell Biol.* **2019**, *21*, 63–71. [CrossRef] [PubMed]
270. Cunningham, J.T.; Rodgers, J.T.; Arlow, D.H.; Vazquez, F.; Mootha, V.K.; Puigserver, P. mTOR controls mitochondrial oxidative function through a YY1-PGC-1α transcriptional complex. *Nature* **2007**, *450*, 736–740. [CrossRef]
271. Morita, M.; Gravel, S.P.; Chénard, V.; Sikström, K.; Zheng, L.; Alain, T.; Gandin, V.; Avizonis, D.; Arguello, M.; Zakaria, C.; et al. mTORC1 controls mitochondrial activity and biogenesis through 4E-BP-dependent translational regulation. *Cell Metab.* **2013**, *18*, 698–711. [CrossRef]
272. Rosario, F.J.; Gupta, M.B.; Myatt, L.; Powell, T.L.; Glenn, J.P.; Cox, L.; Jansson, T. Mechanistic Target of Rapamycin Complex 1 Promotes the Expression of Genes Encoding Electron Transport Chain Proteins and Stimulates Oxidative Phosphorylation in Primary Human Trophoblast Cells by Regulating Mitochondrial Biogenesis. *Sci. Rep.* **2019**, *9*, 246. [CrossRef]

273. Zhou, J.; Shrikhande, G.; Xu, J.; McKay, R.M.; Burns, D.K.; Johnson, J.E.; Parada, L.F. Tsc1 mutant neural stem/progenitor cells exhibit migration deficits and give rise to subependymal lesions in the lateral ventricle. *Genes Dev.* **2011**, *25*, 1595–1600. [CrossRef]
274. Yilmaz, Ö.H.; Katajisto, P.; Lamming, D.W.; Gültekin, Y.; Bauer-Rowe, K.E.; Sengupta, S.; Birsoy, K.; Dursun, A.; Yilmaz, V.O.; Selig, M.; et al. mTORC1 in the Paneth cell niche couples intestinal stem-cell function to calorie intake. *Nature* **2012**, *486*, 490–495. [CrossRef]
275. Malam, Z.; Cohn, R.D. Stem cells on alert: Priming quiescent stem cells after remote injury. *Cell Stem Cell* **2014**, *15*, 7–8. [CrossRef]
276. Rodgers, J.T.; Schroeder, M.D.; Ma, C.; Rando, T.A. HGFA Is an Injury-Regulated Systemic Factor that Induces the Transition of Stem Cells into G(Alert). *Cell Rep.* **2017**, *19*, 479–486. [CrossRef] [PubMed]
277. Buszczak, M.; Signer, R.A.; Morrison, S.J. Cellular differences in protein synthesis regulate tissue homeostasis. *Cell* **2014**, *159*, 242–251. [CrossRef]
278. Vilchez, D.; Saez, I.; Dillin, A. The role of protein clearance mechanisms in organismal ageing and age-related diseases. *Nat. Commun.* **2014**, *5*, 5659. [CrossRef]
279. Vilchez, D.; Simic, M.S.; Dillin, A. Proteostasis and aging of stem cells. *Trends Cell Biol.* **2014**, *24*, 161–170. [CrossRef] [PubMed]
280. Brombin, A.; Joly, J.S.; Jamen, F. New tricks for an old dog: Ribosome biogenesis contributes to stem cell homeostasis. *Curr. Opin. Genet. Dev.* **2015**, *34*, 61–70. [CrossRef]
281. Moran-Crusio, K.; Reavie, L.B.; Aifantis, I. Regulation of hematopoietic stem cell fate by the ubiquitin proteasome system. *Trends Immunol.* **2012**, *33*, 357–363. [CrossRef]
282. Guan, J.L.; Simon, A.K.; Prescott, M.; Menendez, J.A.; Liu, F.; Wang, F.; Wang, C.; Wolvetang, E.; Vazquez-Martin, A.; Zhang, J. Autophagy in stem cells. *Autophagy* **2013**, *9*, 830–849. [CrossRef]
283. Strikoudis, A.; Guillamot, M.; Aifantis, I. Regulation of stem cell function by protein ubiquitylation. *EMBO Rep.* **2014**, *15*, 365–382. [CrossRef]
284. Werner, A.; Manford, A.G.; Rape, M. Ubiquitin-Dependent Regulation of Stem Cell Biology. *Trends Cell Biol.* **2017**, *27*, 568–579. [CrossRef]
285. Signer, R.A.; Magee, J.A.; Salic, A.; Morrison, S.J. Haematopoietic stem cells require a highly regulated protein synthesis rate. *Nature* **2014**, *509*, 49–54. [CrossRef]
286. Zhang, Y.; Duc, A.C.; Rao, S.; Sun, X.L.; Bilbee, A.N.; Rhodes, M.; Li, Q.; Kappes, D.J.; Rhodes, J.; Wiest, D.L. Control of hematopoietic stem cell emergence by antagonistic functions of ribosomal protein paralogs. *Dev. Cell* **2013**, *24*, 411–425. [CrossRef]
287. Cai, X.; Gao, L.; Teng, L.; Ge, J.; Oo, Z.M.; Kumar, A.R.; Gilliland, D.G.; Mason, P.J.; Tan, K.; Speck, N.A. Runx1 Deficiency Decreases Ribosome Biogenesis and Confers Stress Resistance to Hematopoietic Stem and Progenitor Cells. *Cell Stem Cell* **2015**, *17*, 165–177. [CrossRef]
288. Le Bouteiller, M.; Souilhol, C.; Beck-Cormier, S.; Stedman, A.; Burlen-Defranoux, O.; Vandormael-Pournin, S.; Bernex, F.; Cumano, A.; Cohen-Tannoudji, M. Notchless-dependent ribosome synthesis is required for the maintenance of adult hematopoietic stem cells. *J. Exp. Med.* **2013**, *210*, 2351–2369. [CrossRef]
289. Khajuria, R.K.; Munschauer, M.; Ulirsch, J.C.; Fiorini, C.; Ludwig, L.S.; McFarland, S.K.; Abdulhay, N.J.; Specht, H.; Keshishian, H.; Mani, D.R.; et al. Ribosome Levels Selectively Regulate Translation and Lineage Commitment in Human Hematopoiesis. *Cell* **2018**, *173*, 90–103. [CrossRef]
290. Hartman, N.W.; Lin, T.V.; Zhang, L.; Paquelet, G.E.; Feliciano, D.M.; Bordey, A. mTORC1 targets the translational repressor 4E-BP2, but not S6 kinase 1/2, to regulate neural stem cell self-renewal in vivo. *Cell Rep.* **2013**, *5*, 433–444. [CrossRef]
291. Liakath-Ali, K.; Mills, E.W.; Sequeira, I.; Lichtenberger, B.M.; Pisco, A.O.; Sipilä, K.H.; Mishra, A.; Yoshikawa, H.; Wu, C.C.; Ly, T.; et al. An evolutionarily conserved ribosome-rescue pathway maintains epidermal homeostasis. *Nature* **2018**, *556*, 376–380. [CrossRef] [PubMed]
292. Zismanov, V.; Chichkov, V.; Colangelo, V.; Jamet, S.; Wang, S.; Syme, A.; Koromilas, A.E.; Crist, C. Phosphorylation of eIF2α Is a Translational Control Mechanism Regulating Muscle Stem Cell Quiescence and Self-Renewal. *Cell Stem Cell* **2016**, *18*, 79–90. [CrossRef] [PubMed]
293. Cheung, T.H.; Quach, N.L.; Charville, G.W.; Liu, L.; Park, L.; Edalati, A.; Yoo, B.; Hoang, P.; Rando, T.A. Maintenance of muscle stem-cell quiescence by microRNA-489. *Nature* **2012**, *482*, 524–528. [CrossRef]

294. Crist, C.G.; Montarras, D.; Buckingham, M. Muscle satellite cells are primed for myogenesis but maintain quiescence with sequestration of Myf5 mRNA targeted by microRNA-31 in mRNP granules. *Cell Stem Cell* **2012**, *11*, 118–126. [CrossRef] [PubMed]
295. Sontag, E.M.; Samant, R.S.; Frydman, J. Mechanisms and Functions of Spatial Protein Quality Control. *Annu. Rev. Biochem.* **2017**, *86*, 97–122. [CrossRef] [PubMed]
296. Klaips, C.L.; Jayaraj, G.G.; Hartl, F.U. Pathways of cellular proteostasis in aging and disease. *J. Cell Biol.* **2018**, *217*, 51–63. [CrossRef] [PubMed]
297. Fan, G.C. Role of heat shock proteins in stem cell behavior. *Prog. Mol. Biol. Transl. Sci.* **2012**, *111*, 305–322. [PubMed]
298. Baharvand, H.; Fathi, A.; van Hoof, D.; Salekdeh, G.H. Concise review: Trends in stem cell proteomics. *Stem Cells* **2007**, *25*, 1888–1903. [CrossRef]
299. DeLany, J.P.; Floyd, Z.E.; Zvonic, S.; Smith, A.; Gravois, A.; Reiners, E.; Wu, X.; Kilroy, G.; Lefevre, M.; Gimble, J.M. Proteomic analysis of primary cultures of human adipose-derived stem cells: Modulation by adipogenesis. *Mol. Cell. Proteom.* **2005**, *4*, 731–740. [CrossRef]
300. Matsui, H.; Asou, H.; Inaba, T. Cytokines direct the regulation of Bim mRNA stability by heat-shock cognate protein 70. *Mol. Cell* **2007**, *25*, 99–112. [CrossRef]
301. Zou, P.; Yoshihara, H.; Hosokawa, K.; Tai, I.; Shinmyozu, K.; Tsukahara, F.; Maru, Y.; Nakayama, K.; Nakayama, K.I.; Suda, T. p57(Kip2) and p27(Kip1) cooperate to maintain hematopoietic stem cell quiescence through interactions with Hsc70. *Cell Stem Cell* **2011**, *9*, 247–261. [CrossRef] [PubMed]
302. Miharada, K.; Karlsson, G.; Rehn, M.; Rörby, E.; Siva, K.; Cammenga, J.; Karlsson, S. Cripto regulates hematopoietic stem cells as a hypoxic-niche-related factor through cell surface receptor GRP78. *Cell Stem Cell* **2011**, *9*, 330–344. [CrossRef]
303. Ribeil, J.A.; Zermati, Y.; Vandekerckhove, J.; Cathelin, S.; Kersual, J.; Dussiot, M.; Coulon, S.; Moura, I.C.; Zeuner, A.; Kirkegaard-Sørensen, T.; et al. Hsp70 regulates erythropoiesis by preventing caspase-3-mediated cleavage of GATA-1. *Nature* **2007**, *445*, 102–105. [CrossRef]
304. Tai-Nagara, I.; Matsuoka, S.; Ariga, H.; Suda, T. Mortalin and DJ-1 coordinately regulate hematopoietic stem cell function through the control of oxidative stress. *Blood* **2014**, *123*, 41–50. [CrossRef] [PubMed]
305. Vicart, P.; Caron, A.; Guicheney, P.; Li, Z.; Prévost, M.C.; Faure, A.; Chateau, D.; Chapon, F.; Tomé, F.; Dupret, J.M.; et al. A missense mutation in the αB-crystallin chaperone gene causes a desmin-related myopathy. *Nat. Genet.* **1998**, *20*, 92–95. [CrossRef]
306. Sanbe, A.; Osinska, H.; Saffitz, J.E.; Glabe, C.G.; Kayed, R.; Maloyan, A.; Robbins, J. Desmin-related cardiomyopathy in transgenic mice: A cardiac amyloidosis. *Proc. Natl. Acad. Sci. USA* **2004**, *101*, 10132–10136. [CrossRef] [PubMed]
307. Singh, B.N.; Rao, K.S.; Rao, C.M. Ubiquitin-proteasome-mediated degradation and synthesis of MyoD is modulated by alphaB-crystallin, a small heat shock protein, during muscle differentiation. *Biochim. Biophys. Acta* **2010**, *1803*, 288–299. [CrossRef] [PubMed]
308. Chen, J.; Shi, Z.D.; Ji, X.; Morales, J.; Zhang, J.; Kaur, N.; Wang, S. Enhanced osteogenesis of human mesenchymal stem cells by periodic heat shock in self-assembling peptide hydrogel. *Tissue Eng. Part A* **2013**, *19*, 716–728. [CrossRef] [PubMed]
309. Li, C.; Sunderic, K.; Nicoll, S.B.; Wang, S. Downregulation of Heat Shock Protein 70 Impairs Osteogenic and Chondrogenic Differentiation in Human Mesenchymal Stem Cells. *Sci. Rep.* **2018**, *8*, 553. [CrossRef] [PubMed]
310. Walter, P.; Ron, D. The unfolded protein response: From stress pathway to homeostatic regulation. *Science* **2011**, *334*, 1081–1086. [CrossRef] [PubMed]
311. Gardner, B.M.; Pincus, D.; Gotthardt, K.; Gallagher, C.M.; Walter, P. Endoplasmic reticulum stress sensing in the unfolded protein response. *Cold Spring Harb. Perspect. Biol.* **2013**, *5*, a013169. [CrossRef] [PubMed]
312. Melber, A.; Haynes, C.M. UPR^{mt} regulation and output: A stress response mediated by mitochondrial-nuclear communication. *Cell Res.* **2018**, *28*, 281–295. [CrossRef] [PubMed]
313. Shpilka, T.; Haynes, C.M. The mitochondrial UPR: Mechanisms, physiological functions and implications in ageing. *Nat. Rev. Mol. Cell Biol.* **2018**, *19*, 109–120. [CrossRef]
314. Araki, K.; Nagata, K. Protein folding and quality control in the ER. *Cold Spring Harb. Perspect. Biol.* **2011**, *3*, a007526. [CrossRef] [PubMed]

315. Malhotra, J.D.; Kaufman, R.J. ER stress and its functional link to mitochondria: Role in cell survival and death. *Cold Spring Harb. Perspect. Biol.* **2011**, *3*, a004424. [CrossRef]
316. Baker, M.J.; Tatsuta, T.; Langer, T. Quality control of mitochondrial proteostasis. *Cold Spring Harb. Perspect. Biol.* **2011**, *3*, a007559. [CrossRef] [PubMed]
317. Qureshi, M.A.; Haynes, C.M.; Pellegrino, M.W. The mitochondrial unfolded protein response: Signaling from the powerhouse. *J. Biol. Chem.* **2017**, *292*, 13500–13506. [CrossRef]
318. Rouault-Pierre, K.; Lopez-Onieva, L.; Foster, K.; Anjos-Afonso, F.; Lamrissi-Garcia, I.; Serrano-Sanchez, M.; Mitter, R.; Ivanovic, Z.; de Verneuil, H.; Gribben, J.; et al. HIF-2α protects human hematopoietic stem/progenitors and acute myeloid leukemic cells from apoptosis induced by endoplasmic reticulum stress. *Cell Stem Cell* **2013**, *13*, 549–563. [CrossRef]
319. Miharada, K.; Sigurdsson, V.; Karlsson, S. Dppa5 improves hematopoietic stem cell activity by reducing endoplasmic reticulum stress. *Cell Rep.* **2014**, *7*, 1381–1392. [CrossRef]
320. Sigurdsson, V.; Miharada, K. Regulation of unfolded protein response in hematopoietic stem cells. *Int. J. Hematol.* **2018**, *107*, 627–633. [CrossRef]
321. van Galen, P.; Kreso, A.; Mbong, N.; Kent, D.G.; Fitzmaurice, T.; Chambers, J.E.; Xie, S.; Laurenti, E.; Hermans, K.; Eppert, K.; et al. The unfolded protein response governs integrity of the haematopoietic stem-cell pool during stress. *Nature* **2014**, *510*, 268–272. [CrossRef]
322. Cui, K.; Coutts, M.; Stahl, J.; Sytkowski, A.J. Novel interaction between the transcription factor CHOP (GADD153) and the ribosomal protein FTE/S3a modulates erythropoiesis. *J. Biol. Chem.* **2000**, *275*, 7591–7596. [CrossRef]
323. Skalet, A.H.; Isler, J.A.; King, L.B.; Harding, H.P.; Ron, D.; Monroe, J.G. Rapid B cell receptor-induced unfolded protein response in non-secretory B cells correlates with pro- versus antiapoptotic cell fate. *J. Biol. Chem.* **2005**, *280*, 39762–39771. [CrossRef] [PubMed]
324. Zhang, K.; Wong, H.N.; Song, B.; Miller, C.N.; Scheuner, D.; Kaufman, R.J. The unfolded protein response sensor IRE1α is required at 2 distinct steps in B cell lymphopoiesis. *J. Clin. Investig.* **2005**, *115*, 268–281. [CrossRef]
325. Sigurdsson, V.; Takei, H.; Soboleva, S.; Radulovic, V.; Galeev, R.; Siva, K.; Leeb-Lundberg, L.M.; Iida, T.; Nittono, H.; Miharada, K. Bile Acids Protect Expanding Hematopoietic Stem Cells from Unfolded Protein Stress in Fetal Liver. *Cell Stem Cell* **2016**, *18*, 522–532. [CrossRef] [PubMed]
326. Xiong, G.; Hindi, S.M.; Mann, A.K.; Gallot, Y.S.; Bohnert, K.R.; Cavener, D.R.; Whittemore, S.R.; Kumar, A. The PERK arm of the unfolded protein response regulates satellite cell-mediated skeletal muscle regeneration. *eLife* **2017**, *6*, e22871. [CrossRef] [PubMed]
327. Mohrin, M.; Shin, J.; Liu, Y.; Brown, K.; Luo, H.; Xi, Y.; Haynes, C.M.; Chen, D. Stem cell aging. A mitochondrial UPR-mediated metabolic checkpoint regulates hematopoietic stem cell aging. *Science* **2015**, *347*, 1374–1377. [CrossRef] [PubMed]
328. Yau, R.; Rape, M. The increasing complexity of the ubiquitin code. *Nat. Cell Biol.* **2016**, *18*, 579–586. [CrossRef]
329. Gupta-Rossi, N.; Le Bail, O.; Gonen, H.; Brou, C.; Logeat, F.; Six, E.; Ciechanover, A.; Israël, A. Functional interaction between SEL-10, an F-box protein, and the nuclear form of activated Notch1 receptor. *J. Biol. Chem.* **2001**, *276*, 34371–34378. [CrossRef] [PubMed]
330. Koepp, D.M.; Schaefer, L.K.; Ye, X.; Keyomarsi, K.; Chu, C.; Harper, J.W.; Elledge, S.J. Phosphorylation-dependent ubiquitination of cyclin E by the SCFFbw7 ubiquitin ligase. *Science* **2001**, *294*, 173–177. [CrossRef] [PubMed]
331. Strohmaier, H.; Spruck, C.H.; Kaiser, P.; Won, K.A.; Sangfelt, O.; Reed, S.I. Human F-box protein hCdc4 targets cyclin E for proteolysis and is mutated in a breast cancer cell line. *Nature* **2001**, *413*, 316–322. [CrossRef]
332. Goh, E.L.; Zhu, T.; Leong, W.Y.; Lobie, P.E. c-Cbl is a negative regulator of GH-stimulated STAT5-mediated transcription. *Endocrinology* **2002**, *143*, 3590–3603. [CrossRef]
333. Jehn, B.M.; Dittert, I.; Beyer, S.; von der Mark, K.; Bielke, W. c-Cbl binding and ubiquitin-dependent lysosomal degradation of membrane-associated Notch1. *J. Biol. Chem.* **2002**, *277*, 8033–8040. [CrossRef]
334. Nakayama, K.; Nagahama, H.; Minamishima, Y.A.; Miyake, S.; Ishida, N.; Hatakeyama, S.; Kitagawa, M.; Iemura, S.; Natsume, T.; Nakayama, K.I. Skp2-mediated degradation of p27 regulates progression into mitosis. *Dev. Cell* **2004**, *6*, 661–672. [CrossRef]

335. Tsunematsu, R.; Nakayama, K.; Oike, Y.; Nishiyama, M.; Ishida, N.; Hatakeyama, S.; Bessho, Y.; Kageyama, R.; Suda, T.; Nakayama, K.I. Mouse Fbw7/Sel-10/Cdc4 is required for notch degradation during vascular development. *J. Biol. Chem.* **2004**, *279*, 9417–9423. [CrossRef]
336. Welcker, M.; Orian, A.; Jin, J.; Grim, J.E.; Harper, J.W.; Eisenman, R.N.; Clurman, B.E. The Fbw7 tumor suppressor regulates glycogen synthase kinase 3 phosphorylation-dependent c-Myc protein degradation. *Proc. Natl. Acad. Sci. USA* **2004**, *101*, 9085–9090. [CrossRef]
337. Yada, M.; Hatakeyama, S.; Kamura, T.; Nishiyama, M.; Tsunematsu, R.; Imaki, H.; Ishida, N.; Okumura, F.; Nakayama, K.; Nakayama, K.I. Phosphorylation-dependent degradation of c-Myc is mediated by the F-box protein Fbw7. *EMBO J.* **2004**, *23*, 2116–2125. [CrossRef]
338. Schmidt, M.H.H.; Dikic, I. The Cbl interactome and its functions. *Nat. Rev. Mol. Cell Biol.* **2005**, *6*, 907–918. [CrossRef]
339. Zeng, S.; Xu, Z.; Lipkowitz, S.; Longley, J.B. Regulation of stem cell factor receptor signaling by Cbl family proteins (Cbl-b/c-Cbl). *Blood* **2005**, *105*, 226–232. [CrossRef]
340. Naujokat, C.; Sarić, T. Concise review: Role and function of the ubiquitin-proteasome system in mammalian stem and progenitor cells. *Stem Cells* **2007**, *25*, 2408–2418. [CrossRef]
341. Reavie, L.; Della Gatta, G.; Crusio, K.; Aranda-Orgilles, B.; Buckley, S.M.; Thompson, B.; Lee, E.; Gao, J.; Bredemeyer, A.L.; Helmink, B.A.; et al. Regulation of hematopoietic stem cell differentiation by a single ubiquitin ligase-substrate complex. *Nat. Immunol.* **2010**, *11*, 207–215. [CrossRef] [PubMed]
342. Inuzuka, H.; Shaik, S.; Onoyama, I.; Gao, D.; Tseng, A.; Maser, R.S.; Zhai, B.; Wan, L.; Gutierrez, A.; Lau, A.W.; et al. SCF(FBW7) regulates cellular apoptosis by targeting MCL1 for ubiquitylation and destruction. *Nature* **2011**, *471*, 104–109. [CrossRef] [PubMed]
343. Rathinam, C.; Matesic, L.E.; Flavell, R.A. The E3 ligase Itch is a negative regulator of the homeostasis and function of hematopoietic stem cells. *Nat. Immunol.* **2011**, *12*, 399–407. [CrossRef] [PubMed]
344. Wertz, I.E.; Kusam, S.; Lam, C.; Okamoto, T.; Sandoval, W.; Anderson, D.J.; Helgason, E.; Ernst, J.A.; Eby, M.; Liu, J.; et al. Sensitivity to antitubulin chemotherapeutics is regulated by MCL1 and FBW7. *Nature* **2011**, *471*, 110–114. [CrossRef]
345. Takeishi, S.; Matsumoto, A.; Onoyama, I.; Naka, K.; Hirao, A.; Nakayama, K.I. Ablation of Fbxw7 eliminates leukemia-initiating cells by preventing quiescence. *Cancer Cell* **2013**, *23*, 347–361. [CrossRef] [PubMed]
346. King, B.; Boccalatte, F.; Moran-Crusio, K.; Wolf, E.; Wang, J.; Kayembe, C.; Lazaris, C.; Yu, X.; Aranda-Orgilles, B.; Lasorella, A.; et al. The ubiquitin ligase Huwel regulates the maintenance and lymphoid commitment of hematopoietic stem cells. *Nat. Immunol.* **2016**, *17*, 1312–1321. [CrossRef] [PubMed]
347. Matsuoka, S.; Oike, Y.; Onoyama, I.; Iwama, A.; Arai, F.; Takubo, K.; Mashimo, Y.; Oguro, H.; Nitta, E.; Ito, K.; et al. Fbxw7 acts as a critical fail-safe against premature loss of hematopoietic stem cells and development of T-ALL. *Genes Dev.* **2008**, *22*, 986–991. [CrossRef]
348. Rathinam, C.; Thien, C.B.; Langdon, W.Y.; Gu, H.; Flavell, R.A. The E3 ubiquitin ligase c-Cbl restricts development and functions of hematopoietic stem cells. *Genes Dev.* **2008**, *22*, 992–997. [CrossRef]
349. Thompson, B.J.; Jankovic, V.; Gao, J.; Buonamici, S.; Vest, A.; Lee, J.M.; Zavadil, J.; Nimer, S.D.; Aifantis, I. Control of hematopoietic stem cell quiescence by the E3 ubiquitin ligase Fbw7. *J. Exp. Med.* **2008**, *205*, 1395–1408. [CrossRef]
350. Rodriguez, S.; Wang, L.; Mumaw, C.; Srour, E.F.; Lo Celso, C.; Nakayama, K.; Carlesso, N. The SKP2 E3 ligase regulates basal homeostasis and stress-induced regeneration of HSCs. *Blood* **2011**, *117*, 6509–6519. [CrossRef]
351. Wang, J.; Han, F.; Wu, J.; Lee, S.W.; Chan, C.H.; Wu, C.Y.; Yang, W.L.; Gao, Y.; Zhang, X.; Jeong, Y.S.; et al. The role of Skp2 in hematopoietic stem cell quiescence, pool size, and self-renewal. *Blood* **2011**, *118*, 5429–5438. [CrossRef]
352. Simon, M.C.; Keith, B. The role of oxygen availability in embryonic development and stem cell function. *Nat. Rev. Mol. Cell Biol.* **2008**, *9*, 285–296. [CrossRef]
353. Kaelin, W.G., Jr. The von Hippel-Lindau tumour suppressor protein: O_2 sensing and cancer. *Nat. Rev. Cancer* **2008**, *8*, 865–873. [CrossRef] [PubMed]
354. Konishi, Y.; Stegmüller, J.; Matsuda, T.; Bonni, S.; Bonni, A. Cdh1-APC controls axonal growth and patterning in the mammalian brain. *Science* **2004**, *303*, 1026–1030. [CrossRef]
355. Lasorella, A.; Stegmüller, J.; Guardavaccaro, D.; Liu, G.; Carro, M.S.; Rothschild, G.; de la Torre-Ubieta, L.; Pagano, M.; Bonni, A.; Iavarone, A. Degradation of Id2 by the anaphase-promoting complex couples cell cycle exit and axonal growth. *Nature* **2006**, *442*, 471–474. [CrossRef]

356. Stegmüller, J.; Konishi, Y.; Huynh, M.A.; Yuan, Z.; Dibacco, S.; Bonni, A. Cell-intrinsic regulation of axonal morphogenesis by the Cdh1-APC target SnoN. *Neuron* **2006**, *50*, 389–400. [CrossRef]
357. Yang, Y.; Kim, A.H.; Yamada, T.; Wu, B.; Bilimoria, P.M.; Ikeuchi, Y.; de la Iglesia, N.; Shen, J.; Bonni, A. A Cdc20-APC ubiquitin signaling pathway regulates presynaptic differentiation. *Science* **2009**, *326*, 575–578. [CrossRef]
358. Huang, J.; Ikeuchi, Y.; Malumbres, M.; Bonni, A. A Cdh1-APC/FMRP Ubiquitin Signaling Link Drives mGluR-Dependent Synaptic Plasticity in the Mammalian Brain. *Neuron* **2015**, *86*, 726–739. [CrossRef] [PubMed]
359. Shao, R.; Liu, J.; Yan, G.; Zhang, J.; Han, Y.; Guo, J.; Xu, Z.; Yuan, Z.; Liu, J.; Malumbres, M.; et al. Cdh1 regulates craniofacial development via APC-dependent ubiquitination and activation of Goosecoid. *Cell Res.* **2016**, *26*, 699–712. [CrossRef]
360. Adhikary, S.; Marinoni, F.; Hock, A.; Hulleman, E.; Popov, N.; Beier, R.; Bernard, S.; Quarto, M.; Capra, M.; Goettig, S.; et al. The ubiquitin ligase HectH9 regulates transcriptional activation by Myc and is essential for tumor cell proliferation. *Cell* **2005**, *123*, 409–421. [CrossRef]
361. Zhong, Q.; Gao, W.; Du, F.; Wang, X. Mule/ARF-BP1, a BH3-only E3 ubiquitin ligase, catalyzes the polyubiquitination of Mcl-1 and regulates apoptosis. *Cell* **2005**, *121*, 1085–1095. [CrossRef]
362. Zhao, X.; Heng, J.I.; Guardavaccaro, D.; Jiang, R.; Pagano, M.; Guillemot, F.; Iavarone, A.; Lasorella, A. The HECT-domain ubiquitin ligase Huwe1 controls neural differentiation and proliferation by destabilizing the N-Myc oncoprotein. *Nat. Cell Biol.* **2008**, *10*, 643–653. [CrossRef]
363. Forget, A.; Bihannic, L.; Cigna, S.M.; Lefevre, C.; Remke, M.; Barnat, M.; Dodier, S.; Shirvani, H.; Mercier, A.; Mensah, A.; et al. Shh signaling protects Atoh1 from degradation mediated by the E3 ubiquitin ligase Huwe1 in neural precursors. *Dev. Cell* **2014**, *29*, 649–661. [CrossRef]
364. Urbán, N.; van den Berg, D.L.; Forget, A.; Andersen, J.; Demmers, J.A.; Hunt, C.; Ayrault, O.; Guillemot, F. Return to quiescence of mouse neural stem cells by degradation of a proactivation protein. *Science* **2016**, *353*, 292–295. [CrossRef]
365. Garcia-Prat, L.; Martinez-Vicente, M.; Muñoz-Cánoves, P. Autophagy: A decisive process for stemness. *Oncotarget* **2016**, *7*, 12286–12288. [CrossRef]
366. Leeman, D.S.; Hebestreit, K.; Ruetz, T.; Webb, A.E.; McKay, A.; Pollina, E.A.; Dulken, B.W.; Zhao, X.; Yeo, R.W.; Ho, T.T.; et al. Lysosome activation clears aggregates and enhances quiescent neural stem cell activation during aging. *Science* **2018**, *359*, 1277–1283. [CrossRef]
367. García-Prat, L.; Martínez-Vicente, M.; Perdiguero, E.; Ortet, L.; Rodríguez-Ubreva, J.; Rebollo, E.; Ruiz-Bonilla, V.; Gutarra, S.; Ballestar, E.; Serrano, A.L.; et al. Autophagy maintains stemness by preventing senescence. *Nature* **2016**, *529*, 37–42. [CrossRef]
368. Oliver, L.; Hue, E.; Priault, M.; Vallette, F.M. Basal autophagy decreased during the differentiation of human adult mesenchymal stem cells. *Stem Cells Dev.* **2012**, *21*, 2779–2788. [CrossRef]
369. Salemi, S.; Yousefi, S.; Constantinescu, M.A.; Fey, M.F.; Simon, H.U. Autophagy is required for self-renewal and differentiation of adult human stem cells. *Cell Res.* **2012**, *22*, 432–435. [CrossRef]
370. Eijkelenboom, A.; Burgering, B.M. FOXOs: Signalling integrators for homeostasis maintenance. *Nat. Rev. Mol. Cell Biol.* **2013**, *14*, 83–97. [CrossRef]
371. Warr, M.R.; Binnewies, M.; Flach, J.; Reynaud, D.; Garg, T.; Malhotra, R.; Debnath, J.; Passegué, E. FOXO3A directs a protective autophagy program in haematopoietic stem cells. *Nature* **2013**, *494*, 323–327. [CrossRef]
372. Liu, F.; Lee, J.Y.; Wei, H.; Tanabe, O.; Engel, J.D.; Morrison, S.J.; Guan, J.L. FIP200 is required for the cell-autonomous maintenance of fetal hematopoietic stem cells. *Blood* **2010**, *116*, 4806–4814. [CrossRef]
373. Mortensen, M.; Ferguson, D.J.; Edelmann, M.; Kessler, B.; Morten, K.J.; Komatsu, M.; Simon, A.K. Loss of autophagy in erythroid cells leads to defective removal of mitochondria and severe anemia in vivo. *Proc. Natl. Acad. Sci. USA* **2010**, *107*, 832–837. [CrossRef]
374. Mortensen, M.; Watson, A.S.; Simon, A.K. Lack of autophagy in the hematopoietic system leads to loss of hematopoietic stem cell function and dysregulated myeloid proliferation. *Autophagy* **2011**, *7*, 1069–1070. [CrossRef]
375. Ho, T.T.; Warr, M.R.; Adelman, E.R.; Lansinger, O.M.; Flach, J.; Verovskaya, E.V.; Figueroa, M.E.; Passegué, E. Autophagy maintains the metabolism and function of young and old stem cells. *Nature* **2017**, *543*, 205–210. [CrossRef] [PubMed]

376. Vázquez, P.; Arroba, A.I.; Cecconi, F.; de la Rosa, E.J.; Boya, P.; de Pablo, F. Atg5 and Ambra1 differentially modulate neurogenesis in neural stem cells. *Autophagy* **2012**, *8*, 187–199. [CrossRef] [PubMed]
377. Zhang, J.; Liu, J.; Huang, Y.; Chang, J.Y.; Liu, L.; McKeehan, W.L.; Martin, J.F.; Wang, F. FRS2α-mediated FGF signals suppress premature differentiation of cardiac stem cells through regulating autophagy activity. *Circ. Res.* **2012**, *110*, e29–e39. [CrossRef]
378. Zhang, J.; Liu, J.; Liu, L.; McKeehan, W.L.; Wang, F. The fibroblast growth factor signaling axis controls cardiac stem cell differentiation through regulating autophagy. *Autophagy* **2012**, *8*, 690–691. [CrossRef] [PubMed]
379. Wang, C.; Liang, C.C.; Bian, Z.C.; Zhu, Y.; Guan, J.L. FIP200 is required for maintenance and differentiation of postnatal neural stem cells. *Nat. Neurosci.* **2013**, *16*, 532–542. [CrossRef]
380. Fiacco, E.; Castagnetti, F.; Bianconi, V.; Madaro, L.; De Bardi, M.; Nazio, F.; D'Amico, A.; Bertini, E.; Cecconi, F.; Puri, P.L.; et al. Autophagy regulates satellite cell ability to regenerate normal and dystrophic muscles. *Cell Death Differ.* **2016**, *23*, 1839–1849. [CrossRef] [PubMed]
381. Fortini, P.; Ferretti, C.; Iorio, E.; Cagnin, M.; Garribba, L.; Pietraforte, D.; Falchi, M.; Pascucci, B.; Baccarini, S.; Morani, F.; et al. The fine tuning of metabolism, autophagy and differentiation during in vitro myogenesis. *Cell Death Dis.* **2016**, *7*, e2168. [CrossRef]
382. Pietras, E.M.; Warr, M.R.; Passegué, E. Cell cycle regulation in hematopoietic stem cells. *J. Cell Biol.* **2011**, *195*, 709–720. [CrossRef]
383. Sage, J. The retinoblastoma tumor suppressor and stem cell biology. *Genes Dev.* **2012**, *26*, 1409–1420. [CrossRef]
384. Matsumoto, A.; Nakayama, K.I. Role of key regulators of the cell cycle in maintenance of hematopoietic stem cells. *Biochim. Biophys. Acta* **2013**, *1830*, 2335–2344. [CrossRef] [PubMed]
385. Nakamura-Ishizu, A.; Takizawa, H.; Suda, T. The analysis, roles and regulation of quiescence in hematopoietic stem cells. *Development* **2014**, *141*, 4656–4666. [CrossRef] [PubMed]
386. Popov, B.; Petrov, N. pRb-E2F signaling in life of mesenchymal stem cells: Cell cycle, cell fate, and cell differentiation. *Genes Dis.* **2014**, *1*, 174–187. [CrossRef] [PubMed]
387. Dumont, N.A.; Wang, Y.X.; Rudnicki, M.A. Intrinsic and extrinsic mechanisms regulating satellite cell function. *Development* **2015**, *142*, 1572–1581. [CrossRef]
388. Kuerbitz, S.J.; Plunkett, B.S.; Walsh, W.V.; Kastan, M.B. Wild-type p53 is a cell cycle checkpoint determinant following irradiation. *Proc. Natl. Acad. Sci. USA* **1992**, *89*, 7491–7495. [CrossRef] [PubMed]
389. Harper, J.W.; Elledge, S.J.; Keyomarsi, K.; Dynlacht, B.; Tsai, L.H.; Zhang, P.; Dobrowolski, S.; Bai, C.; Connell-Crowley, L.; Swindell, E.; et al. Inhibition of cyclin-dependent kinases by p21. *Mol. Biol. Cell* **1995**, *6*, 387–400. [CrossRef]
390. Vousden, K.H.; Lane, D.P. p53 in health and disease. *Nat. Rev. Mol. Cell Biol.* **2007**, *8*, 275–283. [CrossRef] [PubMed]
391. TeKippe, M.; Harrison, D.E.; Chen, J. Expansion of hematopoietic stem cell phenotype and activity in Trp53-null mice. *Exp. Hematol.* **2003**, *31*, 521–527. [CrossRef]
392. Chen, J.; Ellison, F.M.; Keyvanfar, K.; Omokaro, S.O.; Desierto, M.J.; Eckhaus, M.A.; Young, N.S. Enrichment of hematopoietic stem cells with SLAM and LSK markers for the detection of hematopoietic stem cell function in normal and Trp53 null mice. *Exp. Hematol.* **2008**, *36*, 1236–1243. [CrossRef]
393. Akala, O.O.; Park, I.K.; Qian, D.; Pihalja, M.; Becker, M.W.; Clarke, M.F. Long-term haematopoietic reconstitution by Trp53-/-p16Ink4a-/-p19Arf-/- multipotent progenitors. *Nature* **2008**, *453*, 228–232. [CrossRef]
394. Liu, Y.; Elf, S.E.; Miyata, Y.; Sashida, G.; Liu, Y.; Huang, G.; Di Giandomenico, S.; Lee, J.M.; Deblasio, A.; Menendez, S.; et al. p53 regulates hematopoietic stem cell quiescence. *Cell Stem Cell* **2009**, *4*, 37–48. [CrossRef]
395. Asai, T.; Liu, Y.; Di Giandomenico, S.; Bae, N.; Ndiaye-Lobry, D.; Deblasio, A.; Menendez, S.; Antipin, Y.; Reva, B.; Wevrick, R.; et al. Necdin, a p53 target gene, regulates the quiescence and response to genotoxic stress of hematopoietic stem/progenitor cells. *Blood* **2012**, *120*, 1601–1612. [CrossRef]
396. Yamashita, M.; Nitta, E.; Suda, T. Regulation of hematopoietic stem cell integrity through p53 and its related factors. *Ann. N. Y. Acad. Sci.* **2016**, *1370*, 45–54. [CrossRef]
397. Meletis, K.; Wirta, V.; Hede, S.M.; Nistér, M.; Lundeberg, J.; Frisén, J. p53 suppresses the self-renewal of adult neural stem cells. *Development* **2006**, *133*, 363–369. [CrossRef]
398. Weinberg, R.A. The retinoblastoma protein and cell cycle control. *Cell* **1995**, *81*, 323–330. [CrossRef]
399. Giacinti, C.; Giordano, A. RB and cell cycle progression. *Oncogene* **2006**, *25*, 5220–5227. [CrossRef]

400. Harbour, J.W.; Dean, D.C. The Rb/E2F pathway: Expanding roles and emerging paradigms. *Genes Dev.* **2000**, *14*, 2393–2409.
401. Viatour, P.; Somervaille, T.C.; Venkatasubrahmanyam, S.; Kogan, S.; McLaughlin, M.E.; Weissman, I.L.; Butte, A.J.; Passegué, E.; Sage, J. Hematopoietic stem cell quiescence is maintained by compound contributions of the retinoblastoma gene family. *Cell Stem Cell* **2008**, *3*, 416–428. [PubMed]
402. Hosoyama, T.; Nishijo, K.; Prajapati, S.I.; Li, G.; Keller, C. Rb1 gene inactivation expands satellite cell and postnatal myoblast pools. *J. Biol. Chem.* **2011**, *286*, 19556–19564. [CrossRef] [PubMed]
403. Cheng, T.; Rodrigues, N.; Shen, H.; Yang, Y.; Dombkowski, D.; Sykes, M.; Scadden, D.T. Hematopoietic stem cell quiescence maintained by p21cip1/waf1. *Science* **2000**, *287*, 1804–1808. [CrossRef]
404. Kippin, T.E.; Martens, D.J.; van der Kooy, D. p21 loss compromises the relative quiescence of forebrain stem cell proliferation leading to exhaustion of their proliferation capacity. *Genes Dev.* **2005**, *19*, 756–767. [CrossRef]

5

Codex (Cognitive Disorders Examination) Decision Tree Modified for the Detection of Dementia and MCI

Besa Ziso and Andrew J. Larner *

Cognitive Function Clinic, Walton Centre for Neurology and Neurosurgery, Liverpool L9 7LJ, UK; besa.Ziso@thewaltoncentre.nhs.uk

* Correspondence: A.J.Larner@thewaltoncentre.nhs.uk

Abstract: Many cognitive screening instruments are available to assess patients with cognitive symptoms in whom a diagnosis of dementia or mild cognitive impairment is being considered. Most are quantitative scales with specified cut-off values. In contrast, the cognitive disorders examination or Codex is a two-step decision tree which incorporates components from the Mini-Mental State Examination (MMSE) (three word recall, spatial orientation) along with a simplified clock drawing test to produce categorical outcomes defining the probability of dementia diagnosis and, by implication, directing clinician response (reassurance, monitoring, further investigation, immediate treatment). Codex has been shown to have high sensitivity and specificity for dementia diagnosis but is less sensitive for the diagnosis of mild cognitive impairment (MCI). We examined minor modifications to the Codex decision tree to try to improve its sensitivity for the diagnosis of MCI, based on data extracted from studies of two other cognitive screening instruments, the Montreal Cognitive Assessment and Free-Cog, which are more stringent than MMSE in their tests of delayed recall. Neither modification proved of diagnostic value for mild cognitive impairment. Possible explanations for this failure are considered.

Keywords: Codex; decision tree; dementia; Free-Cog; MoCA; mild cognitive impairment; sensitivity and specificity

---

1. Introduction

The cognitive disorders examination or Codex for the detection of dementia described by Belmin et al. [1,2] is a two-step decision tree for diagnostic prediction, developed by identifying independent variables related to dementia using a multivariable logistic model. Binary recursive partitioning incorporated the three-word recall and spatial orientation components from the Mini-Mental State Examination (MMSE) [3] along with a simplified clock drawing test (sCDT, scored 1 or 0, respectively, normal and abnormal) to produce four terminal nodes, the endpoint values having different probabilities of dementia diagnosis (categories A–D, respectively, with very low, low, high, and very high probability of dementia; Figure 1a). Codex takes around three minutes to perform. In the index study, Codex had both high sensitivity and specificity for the diagnosis of dementia (0.92 and 0.85, respectively) [1].

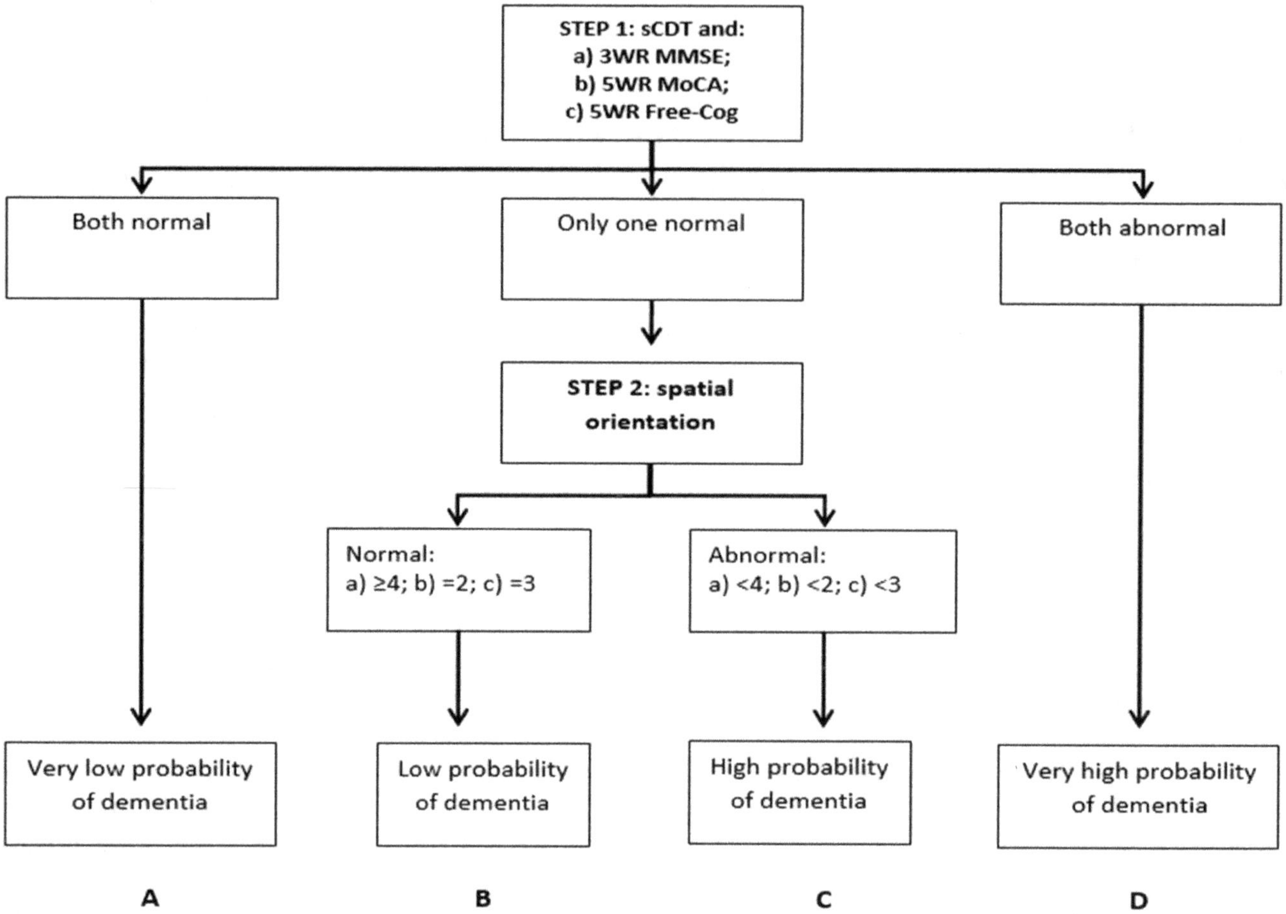

Figure 1. Codex decision tree: (**a**) Original Codex categories (from Belmin et al. 2007 [1]); (**b**) modified Codex categories from MoCA; (**c**) modified Codex categories from Free-Cog.

An independent pragmatic test accuracy study of Codex, undertaken by Ziso and Larner in a dedicated cognitive disorders clinic in a secondary care setting [4–6], confirmed good sensitivity and specificity for dementia diagnosis (0.84 and 0.82, respectively), as did a proof of concept study of a Greek translation of Codex based in a primary care setting (sensitivity 0.94, specificity 0.89) [7].

Codex has also found other applications, for example, in predicting postoperative delirium in patients undergoing femoral fracture repair [8] and in monitoring cognitive impairment before and after cochlear implantation surgery [9]. Codex was included as part of the protocol of the EVATEM study for the detection of cognitive disorders amongst community-dwelling elderly people with memory complaints [10].

Despite the excellent metrics for dementia detection, Codex performance in detecting mild cognitive impairment (MCI), often a prodrome to dementia, is less certain. Ziso and Larner found that for a diagnosis of any cognitive impairment, dementia or MCI, Codex sensitivity was lower (0.68) whilst specificity was improved (0.91) compared to dementia detection [5,6]. In the EVATEM study (see Table 4 in [11]), Codex was found to have low sensitivity (0.32) but high specificity (0.85) for the detection of cognitive impairment (MCI and dementia, of which MCI patients made up a large majority, 176/182). These data suggest that Codex as originally formulated may be insufficiently sensitive for the detection of MCI.

We reasoned that minor modifications to the Codex decision tree might improve its screening utility for MCI. Specifically, since most MCI, whether of single or multiple domain type, includes an amnestic component, the use of a more stringent delayed recall paradigm might result in an instrument more sensitive to lesser degrees of cognitive impairment. Both the Montreal Cognitive Assessment (MoCA) [12] and the recently described Free-Cog (Professor Alistair Burns, Manchester, UK, personal communication, 2017) have a delayed recall test of five words rather than three words as in the MMSE [3]. Deriving a modified Codex from these instruments might therefore increase sensitivity for MCI, as shown in head to head studies of MoCA and MMSE [12,13], even allowing for the fewer spatial orientation components in these tests (MoCA 2, Free-Cog 3, versus MMSE 5).

We analysed data from pragmatic test accuracy studies of MoCA [14] and Free-Cog [15] and also reanalyzed data from a previous Codex test accuracy study [5,6] to examine whether a modified Codex might improve diagnostic utility for MCI.

2. Materials and Methods

Data from consecutive patient cohorts, referred to a dedicated cognitive function clinic based in secondary care and who were administered either MoCA (June 2015–May 2016 inclusive) [14] or Free-Cog (November 2017–October 2018 inclusive) [15], were analysed. Data from a previous consecutive patient cohort, referred to the same clinic and who were administered MMSE and sCDT (February–November 2012 inclusive) [5,6], were reanalysed. Standard diagnostic criteria for dementia (DSM-IV) and MCI [16] were used in these studies. Criterion diagnosis was by the judgment of an experienced clinician based on diagnostic criteria.

In the modified Codex decision tree derived from MoCA (Figure 1b), there were five delayed recall components but only two spatial orientation components [12], whereas in modified Codex derived from Free-Cog (Figure 1c), there were five delayed recall components but only three spatial orientation components. Both MoCA and Free-Cog incorporate clock drawing tests, unlike the MMSE, the scoring for which was simplified to 1 or 0 depending on whether or not all elements were completed correctly, as per the original Codex [1].

Categorical data were derived from the decision trees with differing probabilities of diagnosis (A = very low, B = low, C = high, D = very high), with categories C and D taken to be indicators of cognitive impairment [1]. Codex categories were not used in reference diagnosis to avoid review bias.

Dependent on the date of the study, either STARD or STARDdem guidelines for reporting diagnostic test accuracy studies in dementia [17,18] were observed. Standard summary measures of discrimination were calculated: sensitivity and specificity, false positive and false negative rates, Youden index (Y), positive and negative predictive values (PPV, NPV), predictive summary index (PSI), accuracy, net reclassification improvement (NRI), positive and negative likelihood ratios (LR+, LR−), diagnostic odds ratio (DOR), and clinical utility indexes (CUI+, CUI−). The recently described "likelihood to be diagnosed or misdiagnosed" (LDM) metric, the ratio of number needed to misdiagnose (NNM = 1/(1 − Accuracy)) to either number needed to diagnose (NND = 1/Y) or number needed to predict (NNP = 1/PSI), was also calculated; desirably, tests have LDM >1 [19].

3. Results

Baseline demographic data from the studies examining original Codex and modified Codex derived from MoCA or Free-Cog are shown in Table 1, along with the distribution of observed Codex categories versus diagnosis for each formulation of the decision tree (Figure 2).

Table 1. Study demographics and base category data.

Codex	N	Gender F:M (% Female)	Age Range (Median)	Diagnosis Dementia/MCI/SMC (%)	Codex Category			
					A (%)	B (%)	C (%)	D (%)
Original	162	79:83 (49)	20–89 (61)	44/26/92 (27/16/57)	42 (25.9)	63 (38.8)	5 (3.1)	52 (32.1)
Modified from MoCA	257	116:141 (45)	22–89 (59)	43/75/139 (17/29/54)	15 (5.8)	159 (61.8)	9 (3.5)	74 (28.8)
Modified from Free-Cog	141	61:80 (43)	28–88 (62)	15/45/81 (11/32/57)	13 (9.2)	66 (46.8)	24 (17.0)	38 (26.9)

Abbreviations: MCI: mild cognitive impairment; SMC: subjective memory complaint; MoCA: Montreal Cognitive Assessment.

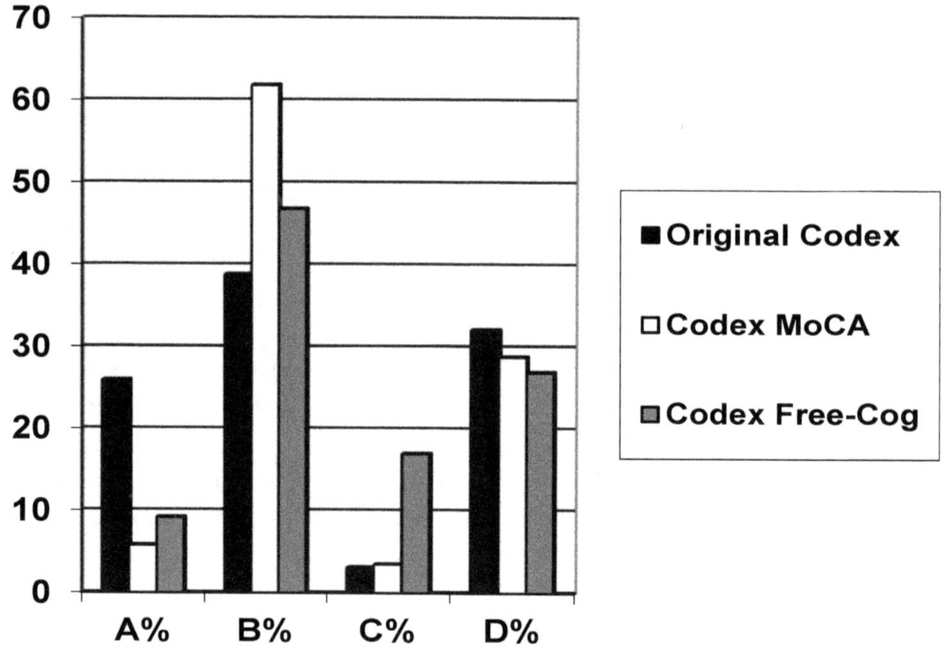

Figure 2. Codex categories versus patient diagnosis for each formulation of the decision tree; A = very low probability of dementia; B = low probability of dementia; C = high probability of dementia; D = very high probability of dementia (see Figure 1).

Measures of discrimination showed original Codex achieved very good sensitivity and specificity for the diagnosis of dementia versus no dementia, very good sensitivity for the diagnosis of dementia versus MCI, and very good specificity for the diagnosis of MCI versus no dementia (Table 2 and Figure 3a).

Table 2. Measures of discrimination for original Codex for the diagnosis of dementia and of MCI (with 95% confidence intervals).

	Diagnosis of Dementia vs. No Dementia (MCI + SMC)	**Diagnosis of Dementia vs. MCI**	**Diagnosis of MCI vs. No Cognitive Impairment (SMC)**
N	162 (44 vs. 118)	70 (44 vs. 26)	118 (26 vs. 92)
Prevalence (P = pre-test probability)	Dementia 0.27	Dementia 0.63	MCI 0.22
Pre-test odds (= P/1 − P)	Dementia 0.37	Dementia 1.69	MCI 0.28
Sensitivity (Se)	0.84 (0.73–0.95)	0.84 (0.73–0.95)	0.42 (0.23–0.61)
Specificity (Sp)	0.83 (0.76–0.90)	0.58 (0.39–0.77)	0.90 (0.84–0.96)
Y	0.67	0.42	0.32
PPV (= post-test probability)	0.65 (0.53–0.77)	0.77 (0.65–0.89)	0.55 (0.33–0.77)
NPV	0.93 (0.89–0.98)	0.68 (0.49–0.88)	0.85 (0.78–0.92)
PSI	0.58	0.45	0.40
Accuracy (Acc)	0.83 (0.78–0.89)	0.74 (0.64–0.85)	0.80 (0.72–0.87)
Net Reclassification Improvement (NRI = Acc − P)	0.56	0.11	0.58
LDM (= NNM/NND, NNM/NNP)	4.02, 3.48	1.63, 1.75	1.57, 1.97
LR+	4.96 (3.29–7.49) = moderate	1.99 (1.25–3.17) = slight	4.32 (2.01–9.30) = moderate
LR−	0.19 (0.13–0.29) = large	0.28 (0.17–0.44) = moderate	0.64 (0.30–1.38) = slight
DOR	25.9 (17.2–39.1)	7.21 (4.52–11.5)	6.76 (3.14–14.5)
Post-test odds (= pre-test odds × LR+)	Dementia 1.85	Dementia 3.36	MCI 1.21
CUI+ (= Se × PPV)	0.55 = adequate	0.65 = good	0.23 = very poor
CUI− (= Sp × NPV)	0.78 = good	0.39 = poor	0.76 = good

Abbreviations: MCI: mild cognitive impairment; SMC: subjective memory complaint; Y: Youden index; PPV: positive predictive value; NPV: negative predictive value; PSI: Predictive Summary Index; LDM: likelihood to diagnose or misdiagnose; NNM: number needed to misdiagnose; NND: number needed to diagnose; NNP: number needed to predict; LR+: positive likelihood ratio; LR−: negative likelihood ratio; DOR: diagnostic odds ratio; CUI+: positive clinical utility index; CUI−: negative clinical utility index.

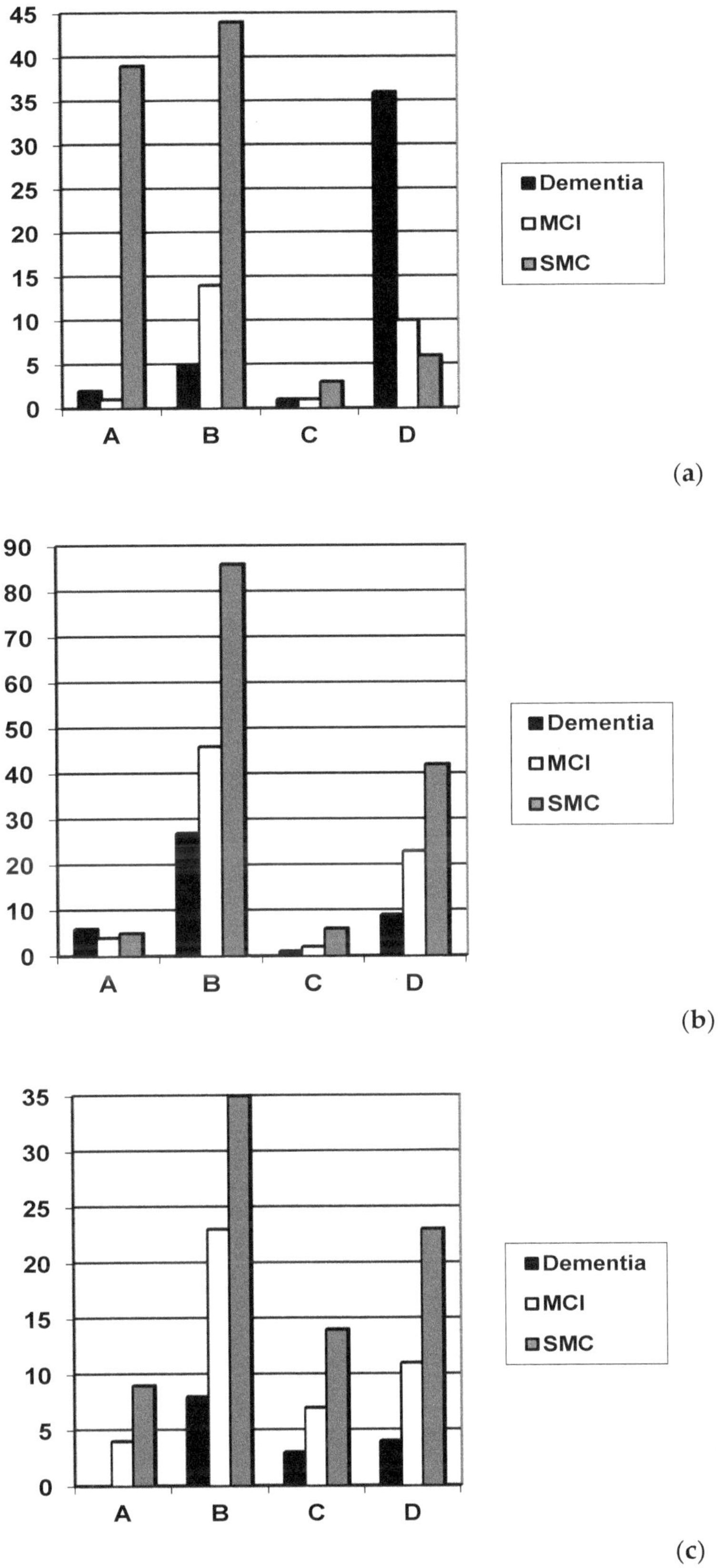

Figure 3. Diagnosis (dementia/MCI/SMC) plotted against: (**a**) Original Codex category (adapted from Ziso and Larner 2013 [5]); (**b**) Modified Codex category from MoCA; (**c**) Modified Codex category from Free-Cog; A = very low probability of dementia; B = low probability of dementia; C = high probability of dementia; D = very high probability of dementia (see Figure 1).

Measures of discrimination showed modified Codex derived from either MoCA (Table 3 and Figure 3b) or Free-Cog (Table 4 and Figure 3c) had lower sensitivity and specificity for both dementia and MCI diagnosis. For all parameters examined, original Codex performed better than either modified Codex.

Table 3. Measures of discrimination for modified Codex derived from MoCA for the diagnosis of dementia and of MCI (with 95% confidence intervals).

	Diagnosis of Dementia vs. No Dementia (MCI + SMC)	Diagnosis of Dementia vs. MCI	Diagnosis of MCI vs. No Cognitive Impairment (SMC)
N	257 (43 vs. 214)	118 (43 vs. 75)	214 (75 vs. 139)
Prevalence (P = pre-test probability)	Dementia 0.17	Dementia 0.36	MCI 0.35
Pre-test odds (= P/1 − P)	Dementia 0.20	Dementia 0.57	MCI 0.54
Sensitivity (Se)	0.23 (0.11–0.36)	0.23 (0.11–0.36)	0.33 (0.23–0.44)
Specificity (Sp)	0.66 (0.60–0.72)	0.67 (0.56–0.77)	0.65 (0.58–0.73)
Y	−0.11	−0.10	−0.02
PPV (= post-test probability)	0.12 (0.05–0.19)	0.29 (0.14–0.44)	0.34 (0.23–0.45)
NPV	0.81 (0.75–0.87)	0.60 (0.50–0.71)	0.65 (0.57–0.72)
PSI	−0.07	−0.11	−0.01
Accuracy (Acc)	0.59 (0.53–0.65)	0.51 (0.42–0.60)	0.54 (0.48–0.61)
Net Reclassification Improvement (NRI = Acc − P)	0.42	0.15	0.19
LDM (= NNM/NND, NNM/NNP)	−0.27, −0.17	−0.20, −0.22	−0.04, −0.02
LR+	0.68 (0.38–1.21) = slight	0.70 (0.37–1.31) = slight	0.97 (0.65–1.43) = slight
LR−	1.16 (0.66–2.07) = slight	1.15 (0.61–2.16) = slight	1.02 (0.69–1.51) = slight
DOR	0.59 (0.33–1.04)	0.61 (0.32–1.14)	0.95 (0.64–1.40)
Post-test odds (= pre-test odds × LR+)	Dementia 0.14	Dementia 0.40	MCI 0.52
CUI+ (= Se × PPV)	0.03 = very poor	0.07 = very poor	0.11 = very poor
CUI− (= Sp × NPV)	0.53 = adequate	0.40 = poor	0.42 = poor

Abbreviations: MCI: mild cognitive impairment; SMC: subjective memory complaint; Y: Youden index; PPV: positive predictive value; NPV: negative predictive value; PSI: Predictive Summary Index; LDM: likelihood to diagnose or misdiagnose; NNM: number needed to misdiagnose; NND: number needed to diagnose; NNP: number needed to predict; LR+: positive likelihood ratio; LR−: negative likelihood ratio; DOR: diagnostic odds ratio; CUI+: positive clinical utility index; CUI−: negative clinical utility index.

Table 4. Measures of discrimination for modified Codex derived from Free-Cog for the diagnosis of dementia and of MCI (with 95% confidence intervals).

	Diagnosis of Dementia vs. No Dementia (MCI + SMC)	Diagnosis of Dementia vs. MCI	Diagnosis of MCI vs. No Cognitive Impairment (SMC)
N	141 (15 vs. 126)	60 (15 vs. 45)	126 (45 vs. 81)
Prevalence (P = pre-test probability)	Dementia 0.11	Dementia 0.25	MCI 0.36
Pre-test odds (= P/1 − P)	Dementia 0.12	Dementia 0.33	MCI 0.56
Sensitivity (Se)	0.47 (0.21–0.72)	0.47 (0.21–0.72)	0.40 (0.26–0.54)
Specificity (Sp)	0.56 (0.48–0.65)	0.60 (0.47–0.74)	0.54 (0.43–0.65)
Y	0.03	0.07	−0.06
PPV (= post-test probability)	0.11 (0.03–0.19)	0.28 (0.10–0.46)	0.33 (0.20–0.45)
NPV	0.90 (0.83–0.97)	0.77 (0.63–0.91)	0.62 (0.51–0.73)
PSI	0.01	0.05	−0.05
Accuracy (Acc)	0.55 (0.47–0.64)	0.57 (0.44–0.69)	0.49 (0.40–0.58)
Net Reclassification Improvement (NRI = Acc − P)	0.44	0.32	0.13
LDM (= NNM/NND, NNM/NNP)	0.07, 0.02	0.63, 0.12	−0.12, −0.10
LR+	1.07 (0.60–1.91) = slight	1.17 (0.61–2.23) = slight	0.88 (0.57–1.35) = slight
LR−	0.95 (0.53–1.68) = slight	0.89 (0.46–1.70) = slight	1.10 (0.72–1.70) = slight
DOR	1.13 (0.63–2.01)	1.31 (0.69–2.51)	0.79 (0.52–1.22)
Post-test odds (= pre-test odds × LR+)	Dementia 0.13	Dementia 0.38	MCI 0.49
CUI+ (= Se × PPV)	0.05 = very poor	0.13 = very poor	0.13 = very poor
CUI− (= Sp × NPV)	0.51 = adequate	0.46 = poor	0.34 = very poor

Abbreviations: MCI: mild cognitive impairment; SMC: subjective memory complaint; Y: Youden index; PPV: positive predictive value; NPV: negative predictive value; PSI: Predictive Summary Index; LDM: likelihood to diagnose or misdiagnose; NNM: number needed to misdiagnose; NND: number needed to diagnose; NNP: number needed to predict; LR+: positive likelihood ratio; LR−: negative likelihood ratio; DOR: diagnostic odds ratio; CUI+: positive clinical utility index; CUI−: negative clinical utility index.

4. Discussion

The Codex decision tree proved easy to use, in both its original and modified forms. In particular, the ease of data extraction for modified Codex from both MoCA and Free-Cog required no extra sCDT step as required for original Codex derived from MMSE.

The performance of the original Codex for MCI diagnosis was very similar to that observed in the EVATEM study, namely, excellent specificity (0.90 vs. 0.85) and good NPV (0.85 vs 0.74) but poor sensitivity (0.42 vs 0.32) and modest PPV (0.55 vs 0.48). Original Codex therefore appears to be a test which is poor for ruling in a diagnosis of MCI.

The hope that minor modifications of the original Codex decision tree would afford better performance for MCI detection was not realized, with all parameters worse than for original Codex. Possible reasons for this failure might relate to the case mix in the various studies examined. There was an inversion in the frequency of dementia and MCI in the studies examining modified Codex compared to original Codex (see Table 1), reflecting changes in referral practice to the clinic. This changed the pretest odds of diagnosis in the different cohorts, specifically, in the latter cohorts examined with the modified forms of Codex, the pretest odds of MCI were higher than in the cohort administered original Codex. The typical shortcomings of clinic-based studies, such as the use of cross-sectional clinical diagnosis without delayed verification, are unlikely to explain the findings since this methodology was consistent between the study cohorts.

Many patients diagnosed clinically with subjective memory complaint were classified in category D (= very high probability of dementia) in the modified Codex decision trees (Figure 3b,c), hence false positives, suggesting inadequate test specificity. This might be anticipated if the modified Codex is, as hoped, more sensitive to cognitive impairment as a consequence of the changed (more stringent) delayed recall testing. However, some patients diagnosed clinically with dementia were nevertheless classified in category B (= low probability of dementia) in the modified Codex decision trees, hence false negatives, suggesting inadequate sensitivity. This might be a consequence of the changed (less stringent) spatial awareness testing.

Limitations of the study include the use of clinical diagnostic criteria for dementia and MCI, and the cross-sectional design which risks some miscategorisation of cases. The use of clinico-biological criteria incorporating imaging and CSF biomarkers [20] (not available to us) and longitudinal follow-up for the delayed verification of diagnosis might circumvent these problems. Moreover, "dementia" and "MCI" are broad categories which encompass a variety of neuropathological entities. Whilst Codex analysis by specific diagnosis might be desirable, this was not feasible with the small numbers of dementia and MCI cases (see Table 1). Furthermore, the goal of Codex, as for other cognitive screening instruments, is to identify those patients in whom additional testing is indicated to permit more fine-grained diagnostic classification. Screening tests can only screen for certain types of cognitive impairment related to dementia.

More broadly, this study poses questions about the value of decision trees and categorical data derived therefrom as opposed to the use of standard cognitive screening instruments (CSIs) generating quantitative data. Advantages of decision trees include the way in which they can facilitate medical decision making. The combination of choices from which the categories in a decision tree are derived may be taken to imply distinct management policies, hence in Codex, the categories A and B may result in patient reassurance, whilst categories C and D mandate further investigation, if necessary by onward referral to specialized services. However, medical decision-making policies may be less clear when using numerical cut-offs, although some CSIs, such as DemTect, further categorise cut-off scores in terms of suggested management policies [21]. In the future, the use of computerized techniques based on machine learning may provide better analyses than a decision tree [22,23].

The outcomes with modified Codex were less good than for the base tests (MoCA, Free-Cog), which generate quantitative data and from which Codex was extracted. The additional components in these CSIs may therefore add something which permits a more accurate diagnosis of MCI; data suggesting that CSI length (number of test items) correlates positively with measures of diagnostic accuracy have been presented [24]. Interestingly, in the EVATEM study, the best performance was found when all three tests examined (Codex, five-word test, and verbal fluency) were combined [11]. Whilst test brevity and the easy categorization of results is desirable in time-limited settings such as primary care, a different dispensation applies in dedicated cognitive disorders clinics based in secondary or tertiary care settings.

These data suggest that Codex, in either its original or modified form, is not sensitive for the diagnosis of MCI. Simple modifications of the decision tree which were anticipated to improve MCI detection did not produce the desired outcome, suggesting that tree impurity was not reduced, and that the modified tree was too shallow to identify MCI cases reliably. Hence, other instruments such as MoCA [12], MACE [14,25], and the Quick Mild Cognitive Impairment (Qmci) screen [26], some specifically designed for MCI identification, should be recommended for MCI diagnosis in preference to Codex.

5. Conclusions

Minor modifications to the Codex decision tree failed to improve diagnostic value, in particular sensitivity, for mild cognitive impairment.

Author Contributions: Data curation, A.J.L.; Formal analysis, A.J.L.; Investigation, B.Z. and A.J.L.; Methodology, B.Z. and A.J.L.; Project administration, B.Z.; Writing—original draft, A.J.L.; Writing—review & editing, B.Z. and A.J.L.

References

1. Belmin, J.; Pariel-Madjlessi, S.; Surun, P.; Bentot, C.; Feteanu, D.; Lefebvre des Noettes, V.; Onen, F.; Drunat, O.; Trivalle, C.; Chassagne, P.; et al. The cognitive disorders examination (Codex) is a reliable 3-minute test for detection of dementia in the elderly (validation study in 323 subjects). *Presse Med.* **2007**, *36*, 1183–1190. [CrossRef] [PubMed]
2. Belmin, J.; Oasi, C.; Folio, P.; Pariel-Madjlessi, S. Codex, un test ultra-rapide pour le repérage des démences chez les sujets âgés. *Revue Geriatr.* **2007**, *32*, 627–631.
3. Folstein, M.F.; Folstein, S.E.; McHugh, P.R. "Mini-Mental State." A practical method for grading the cognitive state of patients for the clinician. *J. Psychiatr. Res.* **1975**, *12*, 189–198. [CrossRef]
4. Larner, A.J. Codex (cognitive disorders examination) for the detection of dementia and mild cognitive impairment. Codex pour la détection de la démence et du mild cognitive impairment. *Presse Med.* **2013**, *42*, e425–e428. [CrossRef] [PubMed]
5. Ziso, B.; Larner, A.J. Codex (cognitive disorders examination) for the detection of dementia and mild cognitive impairment: Diagnostic utility. *J. Neurol. Neurosurg. Psychiatry* **2013**, *84*, e2. [CrossRef]
6. Larner, A.J. *Dementia in Clinical Practice: A Neurological Perspective. Pragmatic Studies in the Cognitive Function Clinic*, 3rd ed.; Springer: London, UK, 2018; pp. 89–90.
7. Avgerinou, C.; Koufogianni, K.; Solini-Kosti, E.; Belmin, J. Validation of the Greek translation of the Cognitive Disorders Examination (Codex) for the detection of dementia in primary care. *Ann. Hellenic Med.* **2017**, *34*, 334–342.
8. Mézière, A.; Paillaud, E.; Belmin, J.; Pariel, S.; Herbaud, S.; Canouï-Poitrine, F.; Le Thuautd, A.; Martyce, J.; Plaud, B. Delirium in older people after proximal femoral fracture repair: role of a preoperative screening cognitive test. *Ann. Fr. Anesth. Reanim.* **2013**, *32*, e91–e96. [CrossRef]
9. Ambert-Dahan, E.; Routier, S.; Marot, L.; Bouccara, D.; Sterkers, O.; Ferrary, E.; Mosnier, I. Cognitive evaluation of cochlear implanted adults using CODEX and MoCA screening tests. *Otol. Neurotol.* **2017**, *38*, e282–e284. [CrossRef] [PubMed]
10. Vannier-Nitenberg, C.; Dauphinot, V.; Bongue, B.; Sass, C.; Rouch, I.; Beuachet, O.; Krolak-Salmon, P.; Fantino, B. Early detection of memory impairment in people over 65 years old consulting at Health Examination Centers for the French health insurance: the EVATEM protocol. *BMC Geriatr.* **2013**, *13*, 55. [CrossRef]
11. Vannier-Nitenberg, C.; Dauphinot, V.; Bongue, B.; Sass, C.; Bathsavanis, A.; Rouch, I.; Deville, N.; Beauchet, O.; Krolak-Salmon, P.; Fantino, B. Performance of cognitive tests, individually and combined, for the detection

of cognitive disorders amongst community-dwelling elderly people with memory complaints: The EVATEM study. *Eur. J. Neurol.* **2016**, *23*, 554–561. [CrossRef]
12. Nasreddine, Z.S.; Phillips, N.A.; Bédirian, V.; Charbonneau, S.; Whitehead, V.; Collin, I.; Cummings, J.L.; Chertkow, H. The Montreal Cognitive Assessment, MoCA: A brief screening tool for mild cognitive impairment. *J. Am. Geriatr. Soc.* **2005**, *53*, 695–699. [CrossRef]
13. Larner, A.J. Comparing diagnostic accuracy of cognitive screening instruments: A weighted comparison approach. *Dement. Geriatr. Cogn. Disord. Extra* **2013**, *3*, 60–65. [CrossRef] [PubMed]
14. Larner, A.J. MACE versus MoCA: equivalence or superiority? Pragmatic diagnostic test accuracy study. *Int. Psychogeriatr.* **2017**, *29*, 931–937. [CrossRef] [PubMed]
15. Larner, A.J. Free-Cog: Pragmatic test accuracy study. *Dement. Geriatr. Cogn. Disord.* **2019**, *48*. accepted.
16. Winblad, B.; Palmer, K.; Kivipelto, M.; Jelic, V.; Fratiglioni, L.; Wahlund, L.-O.; Nordberg, A.; Bäckman, L.; Albert, M.; Almkvist, O.; et al. Mild cognitive impairment – beyond controversies, towards a consensus: report of the International Working Group on Mild Cognitive Impairment. *J. Intern. Med.* **2004**, *256*, 240–246. [CrossRef] [PubMed]
17. Bossuyt, P.M.; Reitsma, J.B.; Bruns, D.E.; Gatsonis, C.A.; Glasziou, P.P.; Irwig, L.M.; Moher, D.; Rennie, D.; de Vet, H.C.W.; Lijmer, J.G. The STARD statement for reporting studies of diagnostic accuracy: explanation and elaboration. *Clin. Chem.* **2003**, *49*, 7–18. [CrossRef]
18. Noel-Storr, A.H.; McCleery, J.M.; Richard, E.; Ritchie, C.W.; Flicker, L.; Cullum, S.J.; Davis, D.; Quinn, T.J.; Hyde, C.; Rutjes, A.W.; et al. Reporting standards for studies of diagnostic test accuracy in dementia: The STARDdem Initiative. *Neurology* **2014**, *83*, 364–373. [CrossRef] [PubMed]
19. Larner, A.J. Evaluating cognitive screening instruments with the "likelihood to be diagnosed or misdiagnosed" measure. *Int. J. Clin. Pract.* **2019**, *73*, e13265. [CrossRef]
20. Albert, M.S.; DeKosky, S.T.; Dickson, D.; Dubois, B.; Feldman, H.H.; Fox, N.C.; Gamst, A.; Holtzman, D.M.; Jagust, W.J.; Petersen, R.C.; et al. The diagnosis of mild cognitive impairment due to Alzheimer's disease: Recommendations from the National Institute on Aging-Alzheimer's Association workgroups on diagnostic guidelines for Alzheimer's disease. *Alzheimers Dement.* **2011**, *7*, 270–279. [CrossRef]
21. Kalbe, E.; Kessler, J. DemTect. In *Cognitive Screening Instruments. A Practical Approach*, 2nd ed.; Larner, A.J., Ed.; Springer: London, UK, 2017; pp. 197–208.
22. Pellegrini, E.; Ballerini, L.; Hernandez, M.D.C.V.; Chappell, F.M.; Gonzalez-Castro, V.; Anblagan, D.; Danso, S.; Muñoz-Maniega, S.; Job, D.; Pernet, C.; et al. Machine learning of neuroimaging for assisted diagnosis of cognitive impairment and dementia: A systematic review. *Alzheimers Dement. (Amst)* **2018**, *10*, 519–535. [CrossRef]
23. Chiu, P.Y.; Tang, H.; Wei, C.Y.; Zhang, C.; Hung, G.U.; Zhou, W. NMD-12: A new machine-learning derived screening instrument to detect mild cognitive impairment and dementia. *PLoS ONE* **2019**, *14*, e0213430. [CrossRef] [PubMed]
24. Larner, A.J. Performance-based cognitive screening instruments: an extended analysis of the time versus accuracy trade-off. *Diagnostics (Basel)* **2015**, *5*, 504–512. [CrossRef] [PubMed]
25. Hsieh, S.; McGrory, S.; Leslie, F.; Dawson, K.; Ahmed, S.; Butler, C.R.; Rowe, J.B.; Mioshi, E.; Hodges, J.R. The Mini-Addenbrooke's Cognitive Examination: A new assessment tool for dementia. *Dement. Geriatr. Cogn. Disord.* **2015**, *39*, 1–11. [CrossRef] [PubMed]
26. O'Caoimh, R.; Gao, Y.; McGlade, C.; Henry, L.; Gallagher, P.; Timmons, S.; Molloy, D.W. Comparison of the quick mild cognitive impairment (Qmci) screen and the SMMSE in screening for mild cognitive impairment. *Age Ageing* **2012**, *41*, 624–629. [CrossRef] [PubMed]

6

The Who, When, Why and How of PET Amyloid Imaging in Management of Alzheimer's Disease

Subapriya Suppiah [1,2], Mellanie-Anne Didier [3,4] and Sobhan Vinjamuri [3,*]

[1] Centre for Diagnostic Nuclear Imaging, University Putra Malaysia, Serdang 43400, Selangor, Malaysia; subapriya@upm.edu.my

[2] Department of Imaging, Faculty of Medicine and Health Sciences, University Putra Malaysia, Serdang 43400, Selangor, Malaysia

[3] The Royal Liverpool and Broadgreen University Hospitals NHS Trusts, Prescot St, Liverpool L7 8XP, UK; mellanie-anne.didier@rlbuht.nhs.uk

[4] Section of Nuclear Medicine, Department of Surgery, Radiology, Anaesthesia & Intensive Care, The University Hospital of The West Indies, The University of The West Indies, Mona Campus, Kingston 7, Jamaica

* Correspondence: Sobhan.Vinjamuri@rlbuht.nhs.uk

Abstract: Amyloid imaging using positron emission tomography (PET) has an emerging role in the management of Alzheimer's disease (AD). The basis of this imaging is grounded on the fact that the hallmark of AD is the histological detection of beta amyloid plaques (Aβ) at post mortem autopsy. Currently, there are three FDA approved amyloid radiotracers used in clinical practice. This review aims to take the readers through the array of various indications for performing amyloid PET imaging in the management of AD, particularly using 18F-labelled radiopharmaceuticals. We elaborate on PET amyloid scan interpretation techniques, their limitations and potential improved specificity provided by interpretation done in tandem with genetic data such as apolipiprotein E (APO) 4 carrier status in sporadic cases and molecular information (e.g., cerebral spinal fluid (CSF) amyloid levels). We also describe the quantification methods such as the standard uptake value ratio (SUVr) method that utilizes various cutoff points for improved accuracy of diagnosing AD, such as a threshold of 1.122 (area under the curve 0.894), which has a sensitivity of 92.3% and specificity of 90.5%, whereas the cutoff points may be higher in APOE ε4 carriers (1.489) compared to non-carriers (1.313). Additionally, recommendations for future developments in this field are also provided.

Keywords: Alzheimer's disease; diagnostic imaging; molecular imaging; precision medicine; quantification; nuclear medicine; ^{18}F-FDG; PET; neurocognitive disorder

---

1. Introduction and Role of [^{18}F]FDG PET

Diagnostic imaging has always played an important role in the management of Alzheimer's disease (AD). Conventionally, neurologists and psychiatrists depended on magnetic resonance imaging (MRI) to help diagnose probable AD, particularly in atypical cases, by identifying typical anatomical changes that are characteristic of AD [1]. This type of structural imaging, however, has its limitations due to naturally occurring variations in brain volume caused by the aging process and co-existing conditions that can cause medial temporal lobe atrophy, such as depression [2]. Hence, functional imaging such as positron emission tomography (PET) offers an irresistible enticement for increased accuracy of diagnosis. PET is very important in providing a one-stop solution and its function is not limited only to the oncology field [3].

There are two main categories of radiopharmaceuticals that are utilized for PET/CT imaging in patients suspected with AD. Initially, 2-Deoxy-2-[^{18}F]fluorodeoxyglucose ([^{18}F]FDG), a glucose analog, was utilized for PET brain imaging for the management of AD. Healthy brain cells avidly take up the substance, as they highly metabolize glucose, but the substance is relatively reduced in uptake in the temporo-parietal cortical regions that are affected by AD. Although the role of [^{18}F]FDG has been established for making the diagnosis of AD, the accuracy of the scan interpretations can decline markedly when it involves older patients. In a younger cohort with a mean age of 64 years of age, the sensitivity of [^{18}F]FDG PET was reported to be 100%, with a specificity of 75% (accuracy 84%), whereas a study with older patients has reported 20% lower accuracy in late-onset AD [4]. Consequently, this limitation was the catalyst for the development of more specific biomarkers for the detection of AD, namely amyloid precursors. The detection of amyloid precursors is said to be able to predict the conversion of at risk subjects to full blown AD 10 years prior to the onset of AD symptoms [5].

Amyloid precursors for PET imaging such as the short radioactive half-life (20 minutes) Pittsburgh compound B ([^{11}C]PiB), by crossing the blood brain barrier (BBB) and selectively binding to beta amyloid plaques (Aβ), are able to provide a virtual ante mortem histopathological portrait of the brain. Similar but newer radiopharmaceuticals include ^{18}F-labeled Aβ targeting tracers, such as [^{18}F]Florbetapir (Amyvid, Eli Lilly, USA) ([^{18}F]FBP), [^{18}F]Florbetaben (Neuraceq, Piramal, Mumbai) ([^{18}F]FBB), and [^{18}F]Flutemetamol (Vizamyl GE Healthcare, USA) ([^{18}F]FMT) [6–9]. These amyloid radiotracers are more suited for clinical settings and have high specificity for the detection of Aβ plaques [10]. These are relatively novel radiopharmaceuticals used in the management of AD as they also enable the quantification of Aβ plaque burden in the brain cortices, which is a hallmark of AD.

Previous research has focused on [^{18}F]FDG PET studies as it is a widely available radiotracer for various imaging indications and has well established cutoff points for standardized uptake values (SUVs) utilized for disease process quantification. More specifically, [^{18}F]FDG PET is used to differentiate AD from other clinical diagnoses by normalizing the uptake intensity to the mean metabolic rate for glucose utilization in the whole brain (CMR_{glc}) or the cerebellar glucose consumption, as these areas allow for accurate distinction of AD, by being maximally stable in subjects but minimally affected by external stimuli and are relatively unaffected by the disease of interest [11]. Nevertheless, many factors influence the value of the measured glucose uptake, namely patient related factors such as fasting blood glucose levels and altered bio-distribution of [^{18}F]FDG [12]. Additionally, an inverse relationship has been noted between cortical retention of amyloid compared with cerebral glucose metabolism determined with [^{18}F]FDG, which was detected to be most robust in the posterior temporoparietal lobes [13]. This pathognomonic finding on [^{18}F]FDG PET, however, may be absent in certain cases and regional fibrillary amyloid depositions have been noted to have little to nil significant association with regional cortical FDG hypometabolism, but rather the impaired FDG metabolism is more influenced by global amyloid burden [14].

AD, which is a major neurocognitive disorder (NCD), was first described by Alois Alzheimer in 1906, by discovering intracerebral neuritic plaques and neurofibrillary tangles (NFTs) in the post mortem study of a patient with chronic mental illness [15]. AD is currently the most common NCD, with more than 36 million cases worldwide and nearly catastrophic in its prevalence among older adults [16]. As a matter of fact, the prevalence of AD after the age of 85 years old is 85 per 1000 population. Approximately 1% of AD is autosomal dominant inheritance due to mutations on chromosomes 21 (APP), 14 (presenilin 1), and 1 (presenilin 2), which leads to early onset familial Alzheimer's disease (oeFAD). Nevertheless, most cases are idiopathic and often the diagnosis is elusive until a later stage in the disease progression. There are several subtypes of neurocognitive disorders (NCDs) which include Alzheimer's disease (AD), dementia with Lewy bodies (DLB), vascular dementia (VaD), and fronto-temporal dementia (FTD). Some sufferers have mixed type of NCDs; however, AD is the commonest subtype with over 60% of subjects suffering from this disorder.

Diagnosis of AD is made primarily on the basis of clinical criteria using the Diagnostic and Statistical Manual, 4th and 5th editions (DSM-IV and DSM-5) [17]. This method is combined with neuropsychiatric testing to objectively assess for cognitive impairment, i.e., Mini Mental State Examination (MMSE) or the Montreal Cognitive Assessment (MoCA) scoring [18]. For instance, in the absence of secondary causes, using MMSE scoring helps to grade the severity of cognitive decline with subjects scoring < 15/30 as having severe AD, < 24/30 being more likely to have mild AD, as well as subjects with reported memory deficits, and normal or slightly low scores but preserved ADL (activities of daily living), of having mild cognitive impairment (MCI) [17]. Moreover, subject education level has to be factored in when interpreting the assessment score. A set of standards created in 1984 by the National Institute of Neurological and Communicative Disorders and Stroke (NINCDS) and the Alzheimer's disease and Related Disorders Association (ADRDA) known as the NINCDS-ADRDA criteria had a sensitivity of 81% and specificity of 70% of diagnosing AD [19]. However, due to new developments in the field, Knopman et al., proposed recommendations in 2001 [20], which were later revised in 2011 [21].

The National Institute on Aging-Alzheimer's Association (NIA-AA) workgroups involved in preparation of diagnostic guidelines for AD, set a revised guideline that took into account distinguishing features of other dementing/neurocognitive deficit causing conditions that occur in a similarly aged population, which were not completely recognized in the past [21]. These criteria could help differentiate NCD subtypes such as DLB, VaD, and FTD from AD, as they have inherently different clinical characteristics, as well as unique pathophysiological features. The criteria propose the use of two classes of biomarkers to help diagnose AD, namely biomarkers for brain amyloid Aβ protein deposition detection and the biomarkers for downstream neuronal injury identification [21]. The former class includes two major biomarkers namely detection of reduced cerebrospinal fluid (CSF) $A\beta_{42}$ levels and positive PET amyloid imaging, whereas the latter includes three major biomarkers, namely elevated CSF tau, reduced [^{18}F]FDG uptake on PET in the temporoparietal lobes, and disproportionate atrophy at the medial, basal, and lateral temporal lobes on structural MRI scans [21]. Nevertheless, the criteria have their limitations with regards to absolute classification of subtypes due to the presence of certain inherent heterogeneity within the groups. For example, it is difficult to differentiate NCD subjects who have tauopathy disorders such as FTD, progressive supranuclear palsy (PSP), and cortico-basal degeneration [22].

In addition, the International Working Group (IWG) and the US NIA-AA have contributed criteria for the diagnosis of AD that better define clinical phenotypes and integrate the role of neuroimaging, genetic profiling, and CSF biomarkers [23]. Some of the recommendations are stated as a guideline and others are given as an option to be utilized at the discretion of the clinician. At present it is accepted that a good clinical assessment yields fairly good sensitivity and specificity to diagnose the different subtypes of NCDs and is reasonably on par with other types of investigations to diagnose AD. The IWG has proposed revisions to the diagnostic algorithm for defining typical and atypical AD, identifying mixed type of AD and preclinical states of AD [23].

The objective of this review is to expound on the various arrays of indications for performing amyloid PET imaging in the management of AD, how to interpret the scans, and the limitations of the test. PET quantification methods used to assess Aβ plaque load in the brain will also be clarified.

2. The Role of PET Amyloid Imaging in the Management of AD

There are various radiotracers that have been experimented with to enable in vivo detection of amyloid depositions in the brain. Among the main indications for performing an amyloid scan is to confirm the diagnosis in indeterminate or atypical cases, to aid in early detection of AD among subjects with mild cognitive impairment (MCI) and to enable quantification of progressive changes in brain amyloid load in response to anti-amyloid therapy. Currently, there are several compounds detected to have a high affinity to bind with fibrillary Aβ plaques that have received FDA approval. There is also a newer benzofuran derivative for the imaging of Aβ in vivo, i.e., [18F]FPYBF-2 (5-(5-(2-(2-(2-18F-fluoroethoxy)ethoxy)ethoxy)benzofuran-2-yl)-N-methylpyridin-2-amine), which is chemically stable, does not photodegrade, and has been tested for feasibility in distinguishing AD patients [24].

2.1. [^{11}C]Pittsburgh Compound-B

In January 2004, Klunk et al. published the first human amyloid PET study using ^{11}C-labeled Pittsburgh Compound-B ([^{11}C]PiB), also known as 2-(4-N-[^{11}C]methylaminophenyl)-6-hydroxybenzothiazole. This compound, which is radiolabeled to ^{11}C, has approximately 20-minutes half-life. Therefore, its use is restricted to centres that have an on-site cyclotron facility. Compared with healthy controls, AD patients typically showed marked retention of [^{11}C]PiB in areas of cerebral cortex that have been identified to contain substantial amounts of deposition of fibrillar Aβ plaques in AD patients [25]. Interestingly, an inverse relationship was noted between [^{11}C]PiB cortical retention with cerebral glucose metabolism determined with [^{18}F]FDG, which was most prominent in the parietal lobes [25].

Using distribution volume ratio (DVR) method, Rowe et al. demonstrated that there was higher [^{11}C]PiB binding in neocortical areas in AD and DLB patients when compared with healthy control subjects, and no cortical binding in FTD [26]. Although almost all AD patients have significantly positive [^{11}C]PiB scans, especially in later stages of the disease, even healthy adults can have falsely positive scan results, e.g., up to 12% of adults in their 60s, 30% of adults in their 70s, and a minimum of 50% of adults in their 80s [26]. The annual incidence of healthy subjects to develop [^{11}C]PiB positivity, as reported in a publication from the Mayo Clinic, evaluating elderly population, was estimated to be 13% per year [27].

2.2. [^{18}F]Florbetapir Scan

[^{18}F]Florbetapir ([^{18}F]FBP), which is also known as ^{18}F-AV-45 or 4-{(E)-2-[6-(2-{2-[2-(18F)Fluoroethoxy]ethoxy}ethoxy)-3-pyridinyl]vinyl}-N-methylaniline, is an ^{18}F-labelled amyloid PET ligand that has high accuracy in detecting brain amyloid deposition [28]. It is taken up rapidly through the BBB, and rapidly washed out from grey matter tissue that does not contain amyloid. It has a high affinity to aggregated Aβ, good separation between the radiotracer amyloid retention and background signal, and a long, stable pseudo-equilibrium allowing flexibility in the timing of image acquisition [29]. [^{18}F]FBP received the U.S. FDA approval in 2012, to be the initial nuclear medicine imaging radiotracer allowed to be utilized for subjects who are being investigated for AD or other causes of cognitive decline [30]. It has an advantage over [^{11}C]PiB because it has a longer half-life, which is approximately 110 min that makes it possible to transport it from site of production to regional PET scanner facilities.

It also demonstrates excellent specificity to Aβ detection and has favorable pharmacokinetics, whereby it is quickly cleared from the blood circulation with approximately 10% of the radiotracer remaining at 20 min post injection. The radiotracer readily enters the brain and 20 min post injection, a clear separation can be seen between individuals with and without significant cerebral amyloid deposition (Figure 1).

[^{18}F]FBP is maximally taken up in the brains of subjects with presumed presence of aggregated fibrillar Aβ after 30 min post injection. Furthermore, its biodistribution is stable for up to 60 min of being introduced intravenously. This allows a wide time window to facilitate the recommended imaging protocol of 10 min. Radiation dosimetry assessments in humans have indicated that the highest organ exposures to the introduced amyloid radioligand occur in the liver, gallbladder, urinary bladder, and the gut [28].

It is noteworthy that a significant amount of amyloid burden has been detected in [^{18}F]FBP scans among even cognitively normal elderly patients who have uncontrolled hypertension and underlying risk factors such as the presence of one or more APOE ε4 alleles [31]. Nevertheless, [^{18}F]FBP is widely used as a research biomarker in the Alzheimer's Disease Neuroimaging Initiative (ADNI) project and in several phase III clinical trials of experimental AD drugs.

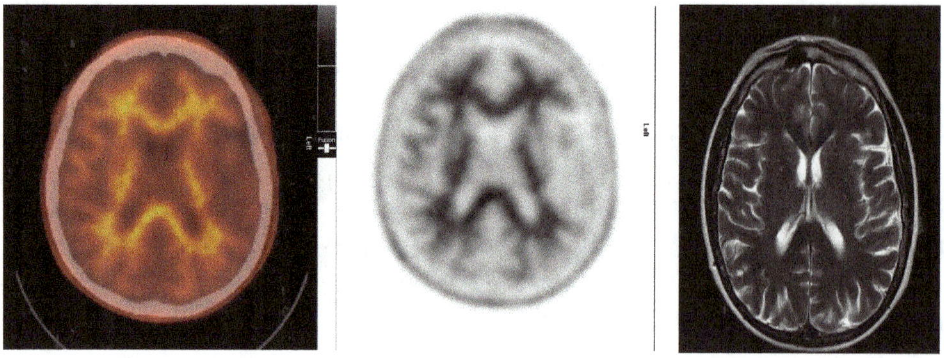

a b c

Figure 1. Normal study. Sixty-seven year old female patient with deteriorating cognition and multiple vascular risk factors for assessment for vascular dementia. (**a**) and (**b**) [18F]FBP shows good contrast between grey and white matter in all sections of the brain with no obvious evidence of beta amyloid plaque disease. This suggests that the diagnosis/development of Alzheimer's disease is less likely. (**c**) MRI brain scan (multiplanar and multi sequence acquisitions) shows no significant T2 signal abnormality or restricted diffusion to suggest space occupying lesion, infarction, or ischemic change. (figures are courtesy RLBUHT Hospital database).

2.3. [^{18}F]Florbetaben

[^{18}F]Florbetaben ([^{18}F]FBB) is another radiotracer used in amyloid PET imaging. In a study carried out in 2012 by Villemagne et al. [^{11}C]PiB and [^{18}F]FBB images were co-registered so that the selection of regions of interest (ROIs) were similar in both scans [32]. This was followed by utilizing the cerebellar cortex as a region of reference to calculate the standard uptake value ratios (SUVr). This gave good concordance of elevated SUVr using [^{18}F]FBB in subjects with AD compared to healthy controls [32].

2.4. [^{18}F]Flutemetamol

[^{18}F]Flutemetamol ([^{18}F]FMT) is a PET radiotracer with an extended half-life, which enables it to be distributed in vivo for a longer duration compared to [^{18}F]FBP. The data indicate that, as an amyloid imaging agent, the performance of [^{18}F]FMT is similar to that of [^{11}C]PiB in AD and AD-associated MCI [32]. Furthermore, a comparison made among amyloid radiotracers [^{11}C]PiB, [^{18}F]FBP, and [^{18}F]FMT revealed good contrast between composite amyloid retention ratio that was normalized by whole cerebellum, along with consistent detection of Aβ positivity in the scans [33].

3. The Role of PET Using Tau Imaging Radioligands

PET imaging that detects tau proteins is able to differentiate AD from other types of NCDs, namely DLB. The PET ligand [^{18}F]AV-1451 (formerly known as T807) binds to a broad spectrum of tau-positive inclusions, but not to tau-negative aggregates in autopsy samples from NCDs other than AD. In 2015, Rabinovici et al. reported preliminary in vivo results applying [^{18}F]AV-1451 PET imaging to patients with NCDs other than AD, which were associated with positive or negative tau pathology with promising results [34]. Additionally, [^{18}F]Florbenazine (^{18}F-AV-133), which is a biomarker for vesicular monamine type 2 transporters (VMAT2), has been noted to be significantly decreased in the Parkinson's disease/DLB group compared to AD patients, and can help to differentiate the two conditions in atypical cases. Neurocognitive impairment in DLB patients is significantly associated with VMAT2 density. Furthermore, significant differences have been detected in consecutive [^{18}F]AV-133 and [18F]FBP scans that are consistent with expected NCD pathology, i.e., greater amyloid depositions in AD and DLB as compared with Parkinson's disease and controls [35].

4. Enabling Early and Accurate Diagnosis of AD

In as much as AD progression is attributed to three cardinal neuropathological features, i.e., deposition of senile plaques in the extracellular matrix, neurofibrillary tangles (NFTs) accumulated in the intracellular compartment and synaptic degeneration, it is believed that it is actually the fibrillary Aβ particles that are crucial for the ultimate dysfunction of neurons and development of AD [36]. Although Aβ pathology is consistently detected in post mortem studies of AD patients, it has been reported to be present in 25–45% of normal elderly individuals [37]. This finding depends on the age of the cohort and the pathological criteria employed. It has been suggested that the presence of this pathology reflects the earliest stage in the development of AD [38]. Proving this hypothesis is a real challenge, caused by limitations inherent in post mortem analysis. Fortunately, recent developments of functional amyloid imaging that binds to fibrillar Aβ plaques, provides a unique opportunity to quantify this pathology in the ante mortem state.

[^{18}F]FBP, [^{18}F]FBB, and [^{18}F]FMT all have good affinity to bind with Aβ plaques, and are potentially excellent non-invasive tools for in vivo imaging of NCDs. In familial hereditary AD, significant brain amyloid burden appears years before symptoms of NCD [39], plus accumulation of amyloid deposits may start earlier than in sporadic AD. Amyloid imaging, particularly using the cerebellar grey matter or cerebral grey matter, has the potential clinical utility for aiding in differential diagnosis in early-onset AD and to support the clinical diagnosis of subjects with probable AD with improved diagnostic accuracy [1,40–44] (Table 1).

Alzheimer's Association and the Society of Nuclear Medicine and Molecular Imaging convened the Amyloid Imaging Taskforce (AIT) to gather empirical evidence that can help support the clinical utility of amyloid imaging. The AIT agreed upon a set of specific appropriate use criteria (AUC), ultimately empowering authorized medical practitioners to identify the types of patients and clinical circumstances in which amyloid PET could be used. It is recommended that patients who have persistent unexplained MCI, patients with atypical presentations of AD, and patients at an atypically early age who develop progressive NCD symptoms are more likely to benefit from this test [45]. As it is a very sub-specialized imaging tool, it is recommended that AD experts decide on the patients that would best benefit from an amyloid scan. The expert for this purpose should be self-identified as a physician trained and board-certified in neurology, psychiatry, or geriatric medicine who actively devotes a substantial proportion (≥25%) of patient contact time to the evaluation and care of adults with acquired mild cognitive impairment (MCI) or AD, as confirmed by peer recognition [45].

Although almost all AD patients have significantly positive amyloid scans, especially in the later stages of life, even cognitively normal elderly adults can have falsely positive scan results, which acts as a caveat for the interpretation of positive amyloid scans. Notably, the annual incidence of healthy subjects becoming amyloid scan positive, as reported in a recent study from the Mayo Clinic, evaluating elderly subjects, was estimated to be 13% per year [27].

5. Prognostication of Disease and Detecting Potential MCI Converters

In patients who are diagnosed with MCI, it may be beneficial to perform amyloid PET imaging to assess the plaque burden. This imaging has been known to detect high plaque burden, which can indicate a higher chance of the individual to convert to AD. Furthermore, many recent studies postulate that perhaps imaging is not a stand-alone test and the addition of CSF biomarkers, genetic information, and glucose metabolism to aid in the diagnosis may help improve the accuracy of interpretation of results [24,46–49] (Table 2). The role of amyloid PET imaging in MCI subjects has been extensively researched with variable results. Nevertheless, it is important to note that amyloid imaging is contraindicated in asymptomatic individuals because there are potentially more harmful than beneficial effects on the subject due to inaccurate assumptions made about the risks of developing AD and future outcomes on the basis of scan results per se.

Table 1. Clinical utility of amyloid positron emission tomography (PET) scans in diagnosing Alzheimer's disease (AD).

Author (Year)	Amyloid Tracer	Subjects	Age	Dose of Tracer (MBq)	Uptake Time (min)	Clinical Ref.	Reference Standard	Findings
Chiang (2017) [40]	[^{11}C]PiB	Cognitively healthy older adults	63 ± 5	555	60	DSM-5	MRS at hippocampus PiB: Cerebellar GM	Corrected for APOE ε3/ε4 positivity: ↓ glutathione levels associated with ↑ amyloid load at the hippocampus
Chiaravalloti (2018) [41]	[^{18}F]FBB, [^{18}F]FDG	AD: 38, Control FDG: 58	AD: 69 ± 8	[^{18}F]FBB: 295–320, FDG: 185–210	[^{18}F]FBB: 90	MMSE: 21.7 ± 5.9	ROI placed at selected cortical GM	FDG hypo-metabolism correlated with Amyloid positivity at temporal, parietal and limbic regions. Mean normalised SUVr: 1.28 +/− 0.1
Ciarmiello (2019) [42]	[^{18}F]FBB	66 (MCI)	75.97 ± 6.59	306 ± 29	86 ± 8	MMSE 25.4 ± 3.07	cerebellar GM	SUVr 1.3 = positive scan, 54% of positive scans correlated with AD neuropathology among MCI
Miki (2017) [43]	[^{18}F]FMT	Total: 70 AD: 25 MCI: 20 Controls: 25	75 ± 6	Single dose: 185 Cumulative dose: 240	90	NINCDS-ARDRA DSM-IV	Cerebellar GM	Visual reads: PPV: 88–92% NPV: 96–100%
Pothier (2019) [44]	[^{18}F]FBP	Cognitively normal older adults: 65 (MCI: 31, Controls: 34)	76.11 years old ± 4.73	4 MBq/kg body weight	50	MMSE, CDR	cerebellar GM	visual reads: Aβ+ > 1.21, SUVr cutoffs: Aβ+ > 1.17, Aβ− < 1.10, equivocal amyloid load as in between range. no significant difference in cognitive decline in Aβ+ and Aβ− groups
Suppiah (2018) [1]	[^{18}F]FBP	47 (Probable AD: 17, Possible AD: 30)	Probable AD: 63.5 ± 9.2, Possible AD: 62.7 ± 10.7	370	30	DSM-5, MMSE	visual reads of global cortical uptake compared with cerebellar GM	sensitivity: 62.5%, specificity: 77.4%, PPV: 58.8%, NPV:80.0%, severity of amyloid load was not correlated with diagnosis of probable AD

[^{18}F]FBB: Florbetaben, APOE: apolipoprotein genotype, AD: Alzheimer's disease, MCI: mild cognitive impairment (particularly amnestic type), CDR: Clinical Dementia Rating scale, Aβ+: amyloid beta positive PET scans, Aβ−: amyloid beta negative PET scans, NINCDS-ADRDA: National Institute of Neurological and Communicative Disorders and Stroke and the Alzheimer 's disease and Related Disorders Association, WM: white matter, GM: grey matter, Aβ42/40: CSF amyloid beta 42/40 ratio, ROI: region of interest, SUVr: standardized uptake value ratio, ref.: reference, DSM: Diagnostic and Statistical Manual, PPV: positive predictive value, NPV: negative predictive value, MRS: MRI spectroscopy.

Table 2. Amyloid PET findings correlated with other biomarkers of AD and mild cognitive impairment (MCI).

Author (Year)	Amyloid Tracer	Other Biomarkers	Subjects	Age (Years)	Dose of Tracer (MBq)	Uptake Time (min)	Clinical Reference	Reference Standard	Findings
Alongi (2019) [46]	[^{18}F]FBB	CSF amyloid levels	44 (neuro-cognitive deficit)	AD: 72.3, Controls: 68	269 ± 10%	90	ENS-EFNS criteria, MMSE	cerebellar WM	SUVr highest at precuneus, Amyloid PET: sens: 90.9% spec: 78.9%, CSF amyloid < 750 pg/mL: sens: 81.5% spec: 75.9%
Bouter (2019) [47]	[^{18}F]FBB	CSF amyloid levels	33 (neuro-cognitive deficit)	68.4 ± 10.3	300	90	MMSE 25.2 ± 3.0	global cortex	↓Aβ42/40 & SUVr correlated with MMSE, mean SUVr: APOE ε4 carrier: 1.489, non-carriers: 1.313
Frings (2018) [48]	[^{11}C]PiB	[^{18}F]FDG	39 (MCI)	Converter: 69.8 ± 7.1 Non converter: 70.0 ± 6.4	[^{11}C]PiB: 393 ± 56 [^{18}F] FDG: 224 ± 36	[^{18}F]FDG: 50–70	NINCDS-ADRDA	cerebellar GM	[^{11}C]PiB PET predicted conversion from MCI to AD, HR for positive [^{11}C]PiB scan: 10.2 (95% CI 1.3–78.1)
Higashi (2018) [24]	[^{18}F]FPYBF-2	[^{11}C]PiB	Controls: 61, Cases with suspected AD: 55 (AD: 27, MCI: 16, CN: 3, other NCDs: 9)	Controls: 53.7 ± 13.1, Cases: 74.4 ± 9.4	200 ± 22	50–70	DSM-IV and DSM-5 NINCDS-ADRDA	cerebellar GM	good correlation of PiB with ^{18}F-FPYBF-2, Mean Cortical Index: early AD: 1.288 ± 0.134 moderate AD: 1.342 ± 0.191, PiB SUVr: 1.435 ± 0.474
Kim (2018) [49]	[^{18}F]FBB, [^{18}F]FMT	APOE	523 (MCI) Aβ+: 238 Aβ−: 285	Validation Set Aβ+: 71.4 ± 7.2 Aβ-: 69.7 ± 8.2	[^{18}F]FBB: 311.5 [^{18}F]FMT: 197.7	90	DSM-IV and DSM-5, Seoul Neuro-psycho-logical Screening Battery	Visuals reads based on uptake at selected ROI	Positivity for APOE ε4 (OR 4.14) among MCI is associated with PET Aβ+.

[^{18}F]FBB: Florbetaben, [^{18}F]FMT: [^{18}F]-Flutemetamol, APOE: apolipoprotein genotype, AD: Alzheimer's disease, MCI: mild cognitive impairment (particularly amnestic type), CN: cognitively normal by neurophychiatric tests, Aβ+: amyloid beta positive PET scans, Aβ−: amyloid beta negative PET scans, ENS-EFNS: European Federation of the Neurological Societies dementia Guidelines, NINCDS-ADRDA: National Institute of Neurological and Communicative Disorders and Stroke and the Alzheimer 's disease and Related Disorders Association, WM: white matter, GM: grey matter, Aβ42/40: CSF amyloid beta 42/40 ratio, ROI: region of interest, SUVr: standardized uptake value ratio, HR: hazard ratio, [^{18}F]FDG: ^{18}F Fluorodeoxyglucose, DSM: Diagnostic and Statistical Manual, [^{18}F]FPYBF-2: 5-(5-(2-(2-(2-^{18}F-fluoroethoxy)ethoxy)ethoxy)benzofuran-2-yl)-N-methylpyridin-2-amine.

6. Aiding in Treatment Planning and Monitoring

Amyloid PET neuroimaging can act as a surrogate biomarker for the assessment of neuronal function and integrity. It can be utilized to quantify the beta amyloid peptide plaque burden in the cortices of the brain [1]. The development of this radiotracer has enabled works related to the formulation of disease-modifying drugs that can dissolve the intracerebral amyloid plaques. Hence, this type of targeted neuroimaging can act as a quantitative biomarker for the assessment of treatment response.

7. Pharmacokinetics of Amyloid Tracers and Scanning Protocol

Amyloid radioligands demonstrate high affinity and specificity to Aβ and favorable pharmacokinetics. The tracer, particularly [^{18}F]FBP (approximately 370 Mbq or 10 mci), is injected intravenously [1], followed by approximately 30–50 min uptake time, some radioligands such as [18F]FMT may require 90 min and others such as [18F]FBB may require up to 130 min to achieve equilibrium [40]. The image acquisition time is commonly 10 min. The compounds are rapidly cleared from circulation with only 10% remaining 20 min after injection. The substances readily enter the brain and 20 min post injection, a clear separation can be seen between individuals with and without amyloid (Figures 2–4).

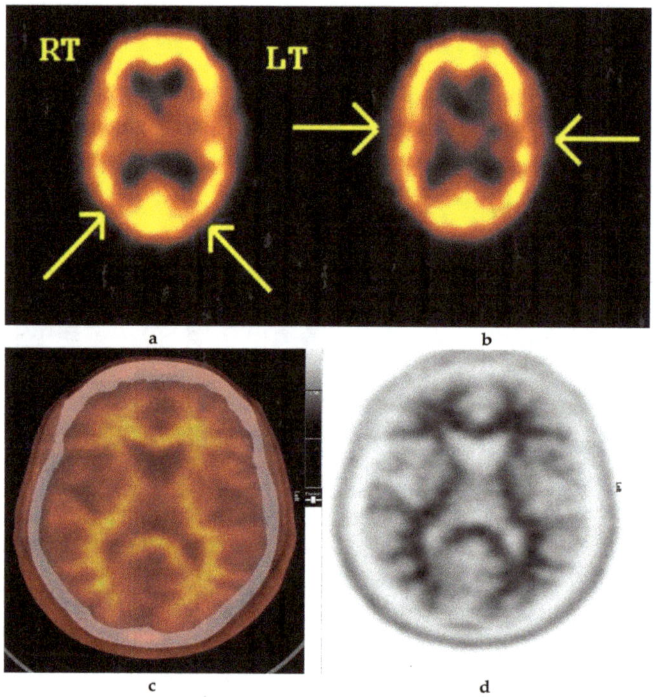

Figure 2. Normal study. Fifty-seven year old female patient memory problems/loss and confusion with a query of Alzheimer's disease. (**a**) and (**b**) Technetium-99m HMPAO-SPECT brain Scan [^{99m}Tc]HMPAO-SPECT brain scan. Brain scan showed mildly reduced perfusion to both temporal and both parietal lobes (yellow arrows) with relatively better perfusion anteriorly. Reduction of cerebral blood flow in these regions is commonly seen in patients with early Alzheimer's dementia rather than vascular dementia. However, in view of the subtle nature of the appearances on the [^{99m}Tc]HMPAO-SPECT brain scan, the [^{18}F]FBP brain scan was performed to identify beta amyloid plaque disease and to give a higher confidence for AD diagnosis or suggest vascular aetiology. (**c**) Color coded [^{18}F]FBP scan. (**d**) Grey scale [^{18}F]FBP scan shows good contrast between grey and white matter in sections of the brain and no obvious evidence of beta amyloid plaque disease. This means that the likelihood of developing AD is low and as such the overall findings are more suggestive of vascular aetiology rather than early AD. (Figures are courtesy RLBUHT Hospital database).

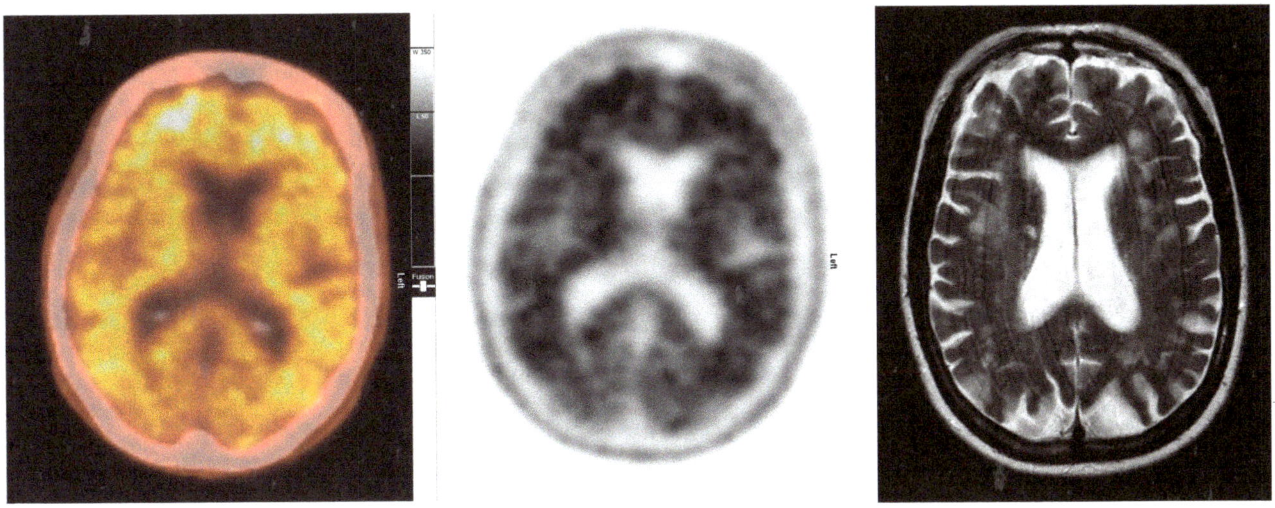

a b c

Figure 3. Abnormal study. Seventy-four year old male patient with a history of short term memory problems/gradual memory decline for some time and a query of dementing pathology. (**a**) and (**b**) [18F]FBP shows loss of contrast between grey and white matter in all sections of the brain. The scan is suggestive of beta-amyloid plaque deposition and in a patient with the above clinical presentation is suggestive of early AD. (**c**) MRI brain scan (multiplanar and multi sequence acquisitions) with some motion artefact shows generalised age appropriate cerebral atrophy, proportionate symmetrical temporal lobe atrophy, and corresponding dilatation of the cerebrospinal fluid (CSF) spaces. Moderate to marked periventricular T2 white matter hyperintensities likely to represent chronic small vessel ischemic changes. No diffusion restriction or space occupying lesions were identified. (Figures are courtesy RLBUHT Hospital database.).

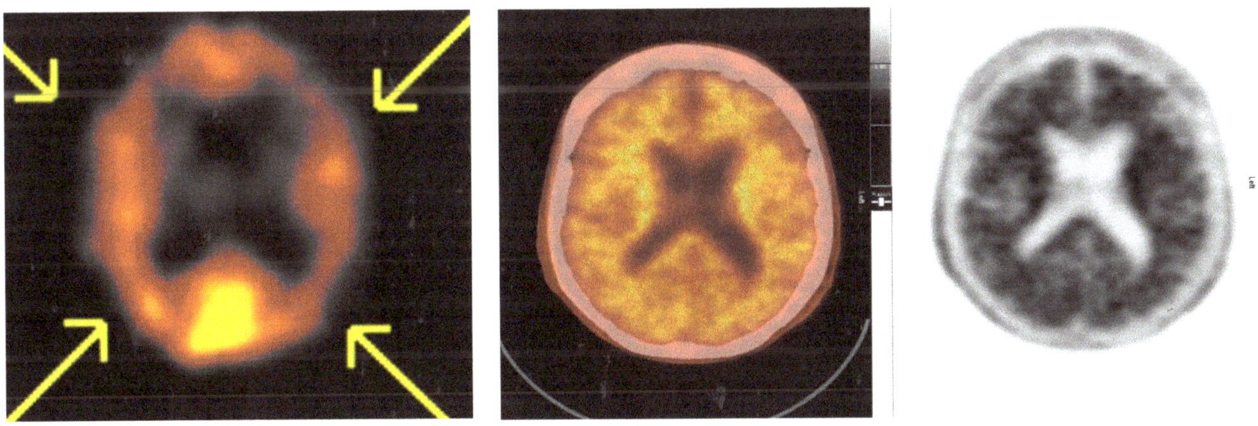

a b c

Figure 4. Abnormal study. Sixty-eight year old female patient with speech difficulties, deficits in memory, and visuospatial abilities. (**a**) [^{99m}Tc]HMPAO-SPECT brain scan shows asymmetrical heterogenous reduced perfusion to both parietal and temporal lobes (worse on the left side) as with involvement of the frontal lobes identified by the yellow arrows. Normal areas of temporal perfusion were noted in between the abnormal parietal and frontal areas. In a patient with cognitive impairment, the findings indicate patterns of cerebral blood flow commonly seen in patients with mixed dementia, i.e., Alzheimer's disease with vascular dementia. (**b**) Color coded [^{18}F]FBP scan. (**c**) Grey scale [^{18}F]FBP scans show loss of contrast between grey and white matter in all sections of the brain suggestive of beta-amyloid plaque deposition/disease. In conjunction with the [^{99m}Tc]HMPAO-SPECT brain scan, the overall findings are again suggestive of vascular as well as beta amyloid plaque disease (early AD), making the diagnosis mixed type AD. (Figures are courtesy RLBUHT Hospital database).

In brains presumed to have aggregated Aβ, maximum uptake of [^{18}F]FBP occurs approximately 30 min after injection and remains essentially unchanged for the subsequent 60 min, thus providing a wide time window to facilitate the 10-minute imaging protocol. Whole-body radiation dosimetry studies in humans indicate the pathway for excretion of the radioligand, with the gallbladder, intestines, liver, and urinary bladder demonstrating the highest exposure [28].

8. In Vivo Assessment and Measurement of Cerebral Amyloid Burden

The clinical use of amyloid PET commonly relies on visual assessment and interpretation (VA) of scans, in which the signal intensity of "target-rich" brain regions such as the frontal cortex is contrasted to that of "target-poor" regions such as subcortical white matter (Figure 2). VA can be used for assessing the likelihood of significant fibrillar Aβ burden in the brain. A systematic qualitative VA of images is necessary, so that evidence of standardized interpretation protocols that lead to acceptable levels of inter-rater agreement can be achieved. The interpretation of amyloid scans needs to be conducted by an imaging expert, to determine the presence or absence of Aβ plaque deposition. The imaging expert is usually a nuclear medicine specialist or radiologist with specific training in the interpretation of amyloid PET [45]. The amyloid PET data must be technically adequate and must be acquired at a fully qualified and certified facility for it to be of diagnostic quality.

The criteria for interpreting the [^{18}F]FBP scan as positive for AD by the VA method is identifying the presence of amyloid binding in the cortical regions relative to the cerebellum, which gives a poor grey-white matter contrast in the affected cerebral cortex. Among the brain areas affected by familial type of AD, which is related to the presence of amyloid precursor protein (APP) and Presenilin gene mutations, the striatal regions have been reported to have the highest amyloid depositions [50]. Sporadic type of AD that is related to APOE ε4 carrier status does not seem to have any regional predilection for amyloid burden; however, the amyloid deposition tends to have an earlier appearance in ApoE epsilon 4 carriers than non-carriers [50]. In a study performed by Newberg et al., [^{18}F]FDG PET scans were interpreted as positive if they displayed the classic pattern of hypometabolism in the temporo-parietal regions [51]. Based on that criterion, scans were classified as either positive or negative for AD. In addition, relative scoring systems have been used to assess the degree of either FDG hypometabolism or increased amyloid binding characteristic of specified regions based on a priori knowledge. Cluster analysis by La Joie et al. revealed distinct subsets of regions [52]:

1. in the hippocampus, atrophy exceeded hypometabolism, whereas Aβ load was minimal,
2. in posterior association areas, Aβ deposition was predominant, together with high hypometabolism and lower but still significant atrophy, and
3. in frontal regions, Aβ deposition was maximal, whereas detection of structural and metabolic alterations was low.

Atrophy and hypometabolism significantly correlated in the hippocampus and temporo-parietal cortex, whereas Aβ load was not significantly related to either atrophy or hypometabolism. Thus, they postulated that these findings probably reflect the differential involvement of region-specific pathological or protective mechanisms, such as the presence of neurofibrillary tangles (NFTs), disconnection, as well as compensation processes.

9. Quantitative Interpretation of Cortical Aβ

The quantitative assessment of amyloid plaques requires consistent efforts for standardization of protocols. The steps involved include proper subject selection and management, calibrated dosage of radiotracer administration, image analysis and quality control, selection of brain reference region, and optimization of various image processing and segmentation methods [50]. Technical factors can be attributed to lead to variability in measurements, and can affect interpretation of the scans, e.g., scanner parameters, injected dose, movement correction methods, and uptake time.

Among the regions of the brain that have the lowest fibrillary amyloid plaques are the cerebellar white matter and almost none in the cerebellar grey matter. Thus, these regions are preferentially used to calculate SUVr values. Particularly, the cerebellar cortex was selected as a reference standard for the very first clinical study using [^{11}C]PiB PET due to its absence of Congo red and thioflavin-S stained plaques [51]. In addition, the clearance of amyloid radiotracers from cerebellar grey matter is considered more similar to its clearance from the cerebral grey matter target regions [52]. Similarly, Schmidt et al. described quantitative assessment of cortical amyloid signal (reflecting amyloid plaque deposition) relative to a reference region that is believed not to accumulate amyloid (normal reference area), producing the SUVr measurement [50]. Wong et al. employed parametric reference region method or a simplified SUVr calculated from 10 min of scanning, 50–60 min after [^{18}F]FBP administration [29].

A step by step approach at assessment of amyloid scans is to scrutinize the CT scan images for abnormalities in the structure. Subsequently, ROIs will be selected to evaluate cortical regions associated with significant amyloid burden in MCI and AD patients. By using the Montreal Neurological Institute (MNI) atlas on SPM software the scans are normalized to the standard brain template and mean cortical and cerebellar values are calculated to give the SUVr data. Routinely, six (6) cortical grey matter regions are targeted for the ROI analysis, i.e., anterior and posterior cingulate, medial orbital frontal, temporal, and parietal lobes, and the precuneus [53].

There have been many preset threshold SUVr values that have been proposed to improve the sensitivity and specificity of amyloid PET scans (Table 1, column 8 and Table 2, column 9). Among the initially recommended preset cutoff points of SUVr $\geq$ 1.17 was indicated to reflect amyloid levels in the pathological range based on separate in vivo PET studies and autopsy reports from nineteen (19) end-of-life patients [54]. Hence, they were able to portray that [^{18}F]FBP PET SUVr values can potentially be used to characterize fibrillary amyloid levels in clinical cases having probable AD, MCI, and among cognitively normal older adults, by using continuous and binary visual read measures of Aβ load. Frequently, concurrent MRI scans are used to normalize the PET data and improve on the anatomical localization of AD pathology.

Conversely, qualitative visual reads assessment using amyloid PET scans have been noted to have a sensitivity of approximately 84.6% (95% CI 0.55–0.98) and a specificity of approximately 38.1% (95% CI 0.18–0.62) for differentiating AD patients from healthy control subjects [55]. Nevertheless, improved scan parameters and the combination of other biomarkers have aided in improving the test accuracy (Table 1; Table 2). Although the quantitative assessment of the global cortex SUVr—despite being more time consuming—is advocated to be more accurate, with improved sensitivity of 92.3% and specificity of 90.5% using a threshold value of 1.122 (area under the curve, AUC 0.894) [55], much work is needed for the standardization of scanning and the reporting techniques, the protocol for global regional uptake assessment, and the selection of the region of reference.

In view of visual assessment and SUVr assessment having a discrepancy of approximately 10%, it is evident that we need to look elsewhere for further improvements in the diagnostic confidence of interpreting amyloid PET scans. Quantification is particularly useful in equivocal cases and for the purpose of providing numerical data that can reflect the change in amyloid load that is related to anti-amyloid therapy.

Finally, it is important to be aware that AD occurs as a spectrum of impairment in various levels of cognitive function, sometimes with additional confounding neuropsychiatric symptoms, which makes it difficult to have a standardized tool or threshold for confirming the diagnosis. As a matter of fact, it is well known that there are discordant areas of sites of atrophy noted on structural MRI, regional hypometabolism noted on ^{18}F-FDG PET with areas of amyloid deposition detected by amyloid PET imaging. This phenomenon is likely due to the longitudinal evolution of hypometabolism, which occurs in the cerebral regions that are remotely located but connected by functionality with areas of increased amyloid burden [56]. Hence, it is evident that various imaging data, clinical, molecular, and genetic information are required to be evaluated in tandem as they provide complementary information for improved management of AD.

10. Limitations

The prevalence of amyloid PET positivity among healthy older adults is among the main limitations of this diagnostic imaging. It is speculated that age-specific positivity rates for amyloid PET are less than 5% in those 50–60 years old, 10–12% in those 60 to 70 years old, 25–30% in those 70–80 years old, and increases exponentially to more than 50% in persons aged 80–90 years [57].

Another major caveat is that a positive amyloid scan can also be seen not only in AD, but also in other medical conditions. For example, amyloid PET is frequently positive in DLB [58]. Nevertheless, [^{18}F]FDG scans can play a role in identifying the 'cingulate island sign' (CIS), which is present in DLB and demonstrates increased glucose metabolism in the posterior cingulate cortex [59,60]. The CIS is highly specific for DLB (97–100%) but with lower sensitivity (62–86%) [60]. The sensitivity of detecting DLB by neuroimaging can be improved by presynaptic dopaminergic imaging using [^{123}I]FP-CIT (DaTSCAN, GE Healthcare), which can give a pooled sensitivity of 86.5% (95% CI: 72–94.1%), but with relatively lower specificity of 93.6% (95% CI: 88.5–96.6%) [61]. Conversely, amyloid PET scans may, in certain instances, underestimate the brain amyloid plaque burden, especially in the setting of low cerebrospinal fluid (CSF) $A\beta_{42}$ levels and mild NCD of the AD type [62]. In cases of FTD, which has a similar insidious onset as AD but with predominantly language and behavioral abnormalities, [^{18}F]FDG PET may detect hypometabolism more frequent in the frontal, anterior cingulate, and anterior temporal regions, as opposed to the temporo-parietal and posterior cingulate regions in AD [63]. Although there can be some overlapping areas that demonstrate [^{18}F]FDG, PET amyloid scans often can differentiate FTD from AD as these cases demonstrate significantly lower amyloid uptake in frontal, temporo-parietal, and occipital lobes as well as in the putamen [64].

11. Conclusion

The aim of performing imaging scans in AD is to non-invasively aid in the diagnosis and provide objective confirmatory evidence of the cause of the neurocognitive deficit. This also aids the management of cognitive impairment, which includes prophylactic planning to anticipate future requirements of the patient. Overall, at present, PET amyloid imaging may promise a beneficial role to diagnose AD in inconclusive cases; however, there is an inherent limitation namely in its cost effectiveness and practical concerns for its execution due to many variations in protocols and cutoff values for interpretation of results.

12. Key Points

- Aβ deposition can be accurately detected by PET amyloid scans.
- AD subjects will usually have a positive amyloid scan.
- Caution needs to be exercised during interpretation and reporting of scan results, as positive amyloid scans can be seen in cognitively normal older adults, AD, and other subtypes of dementia such as DLB.
- The degree of amyloid deposition does not correlate with the severity of AD.
- Severity of amyloid deposition in young subjects (with increased genetic susceptibility) may be a prognostic factor for the development of early onset AD among them.
- Amyloid PET qualitative evaluation of cerebral amyloid presence can be made by binary visual assessment, with loss of grey white matter differentiation denoting a positive scan.
- Quantification of Aβ can be made using the whole cerebellum, cerebellar grey matter, and other regions of low to nil physiological amyloid deposition, as a reference point to calculate the standardised uptake value ratio (SUVr), using the assumption that these regions are usually spared in AD.

13. Recommendation

Future works should include recommendations for newer imaging radioligands, improved automated quantification of amyloid imaging, newer techniques for improved specificity in detecting subjects with Aβ deposition, and prognostication of at risk older adults for the possibility of developing Alzheimer's disease.

Author Contributions: S.S. and S.V. conceptualized this project. S.S. completed the original draft and M.-A.D. reviewed and edited the material. The entire project was done under S.V.'s supervision.

Acknowledgments: We would like to express our gratitude to the Nuclear Medicine Unit of the Royal Liverpool and Broadgreen University Hospitals NHS Trusts, (RLBUHT) Liverpool, UK for granting permission to use anonymised images from the database. We also thank Mr. Ian Hufton, Principle Physicist in Nuclear Medicine, RLBUHT, Liverpool, UK for his assistance in image retrieval from the hospital achieving system.

References

1. Suppiah, S.; Ching, S.M.; Nordin, A.J.; Vinjamuri, S. The role of PET/CT amyloid Imaging compared with Tc99m-HMPAO-SPECT imaging for diagnosing Alzheimer's disease. *Med. J. Malays.* **2018**, *73*, 141–146.
2. Dhikav, V.; Sethi, M.; Anand, K.S. Medial temporal lobe atrophy in Alzheimer's disease/mild cognitive impairment with depression. *Bri. J. Radiol.* **2014**, *87*, 20140150. [CrossRef] [PubMed]
3. Suppiah, S.; Andi Asri, A.A.; Ahmad Saad, F.F.; Hassan, H.A.; Mohtarrudin, N.; Chang, W.L.; Mahmud, R.; Nordin, A.J. One stop centre staging by contrast-enhanced 18F-FDG PET/CT in preoperative assessment of ovarian cancer and proposed diagnostic imaging algorithm: A single centre experience in Malaysia. *MJMHS* **2017**, *13*, 29–37.
4. Ng, S.; Villemagne, V.L.; Berlangieri, S.; Lee, S.T.; Cherk, M.; Gong, S.J.; Ackermann, U.; Saunder, T.; Tochon-Danguy, H.; Jones, G.; et al. Visual Assessment Versus Quantitative Assessment of 11C-PIB PET and 18F-FDG PET for Detection of Alzheimer's Disease. *J. Nucl. Med.* **2007**, *48*, 547–552. [CrossRef] [PubMed]
5. Morris, J.C.; Price, J.L. Pathologic correlates of nondemented aging, mild cognitive impairment, and early-stage Alzheimer's disease. *J. Mol. Neurosci.* **2001**, *17*, 101–118. [CrossRef]
6. Anand, K.; Sabbagh, M. Amyloid Imaging: Poised for Integration into Medical Practice. *Neurotherapeutics* **2017**, *14*, 54–61. [CrossRef]
7. Degenhardt, E.K.; Witte, M.M.; Case, M.G.; Yu, P.; Henley, D.B.; Hochstetler, H.M.; D'Souza, D.N.; Trzepacz, P.T. Florbetapir F18 PET Amyloid Neuroimaging and Characteristics in Patients with Mild and Moderate Alzheimer Dementia. *Psychosomatics* **2016**, *57*, 208–216. [CrossRef]
8. Daerr, S.; Brendel, M.; Zach, C.; Mille, E.; Schilling, D.; Zacherl, M.J.; Bürger, K.; Danek, A.; Pogarell, O.; Schildan, A.; et al. Evaluation of early-phase [(18)F]-florbetaben PET acquisition in clinical routine cases. *NeuroImage Clin.* **2016**, *14*, 77–86. [CrossRef]
9. Lowe, V.J.; Lundt, E.; Knopman, D.; Senjem, M.L.; Gunter, J.L.; Schwarz, C.G.; Bradley, J.K.; Clifford, R.J.; Ronald, C.P. Comparison of [18F]Flutemetamol and [11C]Pittsburgh Compound-B in cognitively normal young, cognitively normal elderly, and Alzheimer's disease dementia individuals. *NeuroImage Clin.* **2017**, *16*, 295–302. [CrossRef]
10. Salloway, S.; Gamez, J.E.; Singh, U.; Sadowsky, C.H.; Villena, T.; Sabbagh, M.N.; Thomas, G.B.; Ranjan, D.; Adam, S.F.; Kirk, A.F.; et al. Performance of [(18)F]flutemetamol amyloid imaging against the neuritic plaque component of CERAD and the current (2012) NIA-AA recommendations for the neuropathologic diagnosis of Alzheimer's disease. *Alzheimers Dement.* **2017**, *9*, 25–34. [CrossRef]
11. Dukart, J.; Mueller, K.; Horstmann, A.; Vogt, B.; Frisch, S.; Barthel, H.; Becker, G.; Möller, H.E.; Villringer, A.; Sabri, O.; et al. Differential effects of global and cerebellar normalization on detection and differentiation of dementia in FDG-PET studies. *NeuroImage* **2010**, *49*, 1490–1495. [CrossRef] [PubMed]
12. Azmi, N.H.M.; Suppiah, S.; Liong, C.W.; Noor, N.M.; Said, S.M.; Hanafi, M.H.; Chalermrat, K.; Fathinul, F.A.S.; Sobhan, V. Reliability of standardized uptake value normalized to lean body mass using the liver as a reference organ, in contrast-enhanced 18F-FDG PET/CT imaging. *Radiat. Phys. Chem.* **2018**, *147*, 35–39. [CrossRef]

13. Cohen, A.D.; Klunk, W.E. Early detection of Alzheimer's disease using PiB and FDG PET. *Neurobiol. Dis.* **2014**, *72*, 117–122. [CrossRef] [PubMed]
14. Altmann, A.; Ng, B.; Greicius, M.D.; Landau, S.M.; Jagust, W.J. Regional brain hypometabolism is unrelated to regional amyloid plaque burden. *Brain* **2015**, *138*, 3734–3746. [CrossRef]
15. Cipriani, G.; Dolciotti, C.; Picchi, L.; Bonuccelli, U. Alzheimer and his disease: A brief history. *Neurol. Sci.* **2011**, *32*, 275–279. [CrossRef]
16. Prince, M.; Bryce, R.; Albanese, E.; Wimo, A.; Ribeiro, W.; Ferri, C.P. The global prevalence of dementia: A systematic review and metaanalysis. *Alzheimers Dement.* **2013**, *9*, 63–75.e62. [CrossRef]
17. American Psychiatric Association. *Diagnostic and Statistical Manual of Mental Disorders*, 5th ed.; American Psychiatric Publishing: Arlington, VA, USA, 2013; p. 947.
18. Trzepacz, P.T.; Hochstetler, H.; Wang, S.; Walker, B.; Saykin, A.J. Relationship between the Montreal Cognitive Assessment and Mini-mental State Examination for assessment of mild cognitive impairment in older adults. *BMC Geriatr.* **2015**, *15*, 107. [CrossRef]
19. McKhann, G.; Drachman, D.; Folstein, M.; Katzman, R.; Price, D.; Stadlan, E.M. Clinical diagnosis of Alzheimer's disease: Report of the NINCDS-ADRDA Work Group under the auspices of Department of Health and Human Services Task Force on Alzheimer's Disease. *Neurology* **1984**, *34*, 939–944. [CrossRef]
20. Knopman, D.S.; DeKosky, S.T.; Cummings, J.L.; Chui, H.; Corey-Bloom, J.; Relkin, N.; Small, G.W.; Miller, B.; Stevens, J.C. Practice parameter: diagnosis of dementia (an evidence-based review). Report of the Quality Standards Subcommittee of the American Academy of Neurology. *Neurology* **2001**, *56*, 1143–1153. [CrossRef]
21. McKhann, G.M.; Knopman, D.S.; Chertkow, H.; Hyman, B.T.; Jack, C.R.; Kawas, C.H.; Klunk, W.E.; Koroshetz, W.J.; Manly, J.J.; Mayeux, R.; et al. The diagnosis of dementia due to Alzheimer's disease: Recommendations from the National Institute on Aging-Alzheimer's Association workgroups on diagnostic guidelines for Alzheimer's disease. *Alzheimers Dement.* **2011**, *7*, 263–269. [CrossRef]
22. Neary, D.; Snowden, J.; Mann, D. Frontotemporal dementia. *Lancet Neurol.* **2005**, *4*, 771–780. [CrossRef]
23. Dubois, B.; Feldman, H.H.; Jacova, C.; Hampel, H.; Molinuevo, J.L.; Blennow, K.; DeKosky, S.T.; Gauthier, S.; Selkoe, D.; Bateman, R.; et al. Advancing research diagnostic criteria for Alzheimer's disease: the IWG-2 criteria. *Lancet Neurol.* **2014**, *13*, 614–629. [CrossRef]
24. Higashi, T.; Nishii, R.; Kagawa, S.; Kishibe, Y.; Takahashi, M.; Okina, T.; Suzuki, N.; Hasegawa, H.; Nagahama, Y.; Ishizu, K.; et al. 18 F-FPYBF-2, a new F-18-labelled amyloid imaging PET tracer: First experience in 61 volunteers and 55 patients with dementia. *Ann. Nucl. Med.* **2018**, *32*, 206–216. [CrossRef] [PubMed]
25. Klunk, W.E.; Engler, H.; Nordberg, A.; Wang, Y.; Blomqvist, G.; Holt, D.P.; Bergström, M.; Savitcheva, I.; Huang, G.F.; Estrada, S.; et al. Imaging brain amyloid in Alzheimer's disease with Pittsburgh Compound-B. *Ann. Neurol.* **2004**, *55*, 306–319. [CrossRef] [PubMed]
26. Rowe, C.C.; Ng, S.; Ackermann, U.; Gong, S.J.; Pike, K.; Savage, G.; Cowie, T.F.; Dickinson, K.L.; Maruff, P.; Darby, D.; et al. Imaging beta-amyloid burden in aging and dementia. *Neurology* **2007**, *68*, 1718–1725. [CrossRef] [PubMed]
27. Jack, C.R., Jr.; Wiste, H.J.; Weigand, S.D.; Knopman, D.S.; Lowe, V.; Vemuri, P.; Mielke, M.M.; Jones, D.T.; Senjem, M.L.; Gunter, J.L.; et al. Amyloid-first and neurodegeneration-first profiles characterize incident amyloid PET positivity. *Neurology* **2013**, *81*, 1732–1740. [CrossRef] [PubMed]
28. Clark, C.M.; Schneider, J.A.; Bedell, B.J.; Beach, T.G.; Bilker, W.B.; Mintun, M.A.; Pontecorvo, M.J.; Hefti, F.; Carpenter, A.P.; Flitter, M.L.; et al. Use of florbetapir-PET for imaging beta-amyloid pathology. *JAMA* **2011**, *305*, 275–283. [CrossRef]
29. Wong, D.F.; Rosenberg, P.B.; Zhou, Y.; Kumar, A.; Raymont, V.; Ravert, H.T.; Dannals, R.F.; Nandi, A.; Brasić, J.R.; Ye, W.; et al. In vivo imaging of amyloid deposition in Alzheimer disease using the radioligand ^{18}F-AV-45 (florbetapir F 18). *J. Nucl. Med.* **2010**, *51*, 913–920. [CrossRef]
30. Filippi, L.; Chiaravalloti, A.; Bagni, O.; Schillaci, O. (18)F-labeled radiopharmaceuticals for the molecular neuroimaging of amyloid plaques in Alzheimer's disease. *Am. J. Nucl. Med. Mol. Imaging* **2018**, *8*, 268–281.
31. Rodrigue, K.M.; Rieck, J.R.; Kennedy, K.M.; Devous, M.D., Sr.; Diaz-Arrastia, R.; Park, D.C. Risk factors for β-amyloid deposition in healthy aging: vascular and genetic effects. *JAMA Neurol.* **2013**, *70*, 600–606. [CrossRef]

32. Villemagne, V.L.; Mulligan, R.S.; Pejoska, S.; Ong, K.; Jones, G.; O'Keefe, G.; Chan, J.G.; Young, K.; Tochon-Danguy, H.; Masters, C.L.; et al. Comparison of 11C-PiB and 18F-florbetaben for Abeta imaging in ageing and Alzheimer's disease. *Eur. J. Nucl. Med. Mol. Imaging* **2012**, *39*, 983–989. [CrossRef]
33. Ataka, S.; Takeda, A.; Mino, T.; Yamakawa, Y.; Yamamoto, K.; Tsutada, T.; Kawabe, J.; Wada, Y.; Shiomi, S.; Watanabe, Y.; et al. Comparison of [18F] Flutemetamol and [11C] PIB PET images. *Alzheimers Dement.* **2014**, *10*, P21. [CrossRef]
34. Rabinovici, G.D.; Schonhaut, D.; Baker, S.; Lazaris, A.; Ossenkoppele, R.; Lockhart, S.; Schöll, M.; Schwimmer, H.; Vogel, J.; Ayakta, N.; et al. Tau PET with [^{18}F]AV1451 in non-alzheimer's disease neurodegenerative syndromes. *Alzheimers Dement.* **2015**, *11*, P107–P109. [CrossRef]
35. Siderowf, A.; Pontecorvo, M.J.; Shill, H.A.; Mintun, M.A.; Arora, A.; Joshi, A.D.; Lu, M.; Adler, C.H.; Galasko, D.; Liebsack, C.; et al. PET imaging of amyloid with Florbetapir F18 and PET imaging of dopamine degeneration with 18F-AV-133 (florbenazine) in patients with Alzheimer's disease and Lewy body disorders. *BMC Neurol.* **2014**, *14*, 79. [CrossRef] [PubMed]
36. Sadigh-Eteghad, S.; Sabermarouf, B.; Majdi, A.; Talebi, M.; Farhoudi, M.; Mahmoudi, J. Amyloid-beta: A crucial factor in Alzheimer's disease. *Med. Princ. Pract.* **2015**, *24*, 1–10. [CrossRef] [PubMed]
37. Mormino, E.C.; Kluth, J.T.; Madison, C.M.; Rabinovici, G.D.; Baker, S.L.; Miller, B.L.; Koeppe, R.A.; Mathis, C.A.; Weiner, M.W.; Jagust, W.J. Episodic memory loss is related to hippocampal-mediated beta-amyloid deposition in elderly subjects. *Brain* **2009**, *132 Pt 5*, 1310–1323. [CrossRef]
38. Hardy, J.; Selkoe, D.J. The amyloid hypothesis of Alzheimer's disease: progress and problems on the road to therapeutics. *Science* **2002**, *297*, 353–356. [CrossRef]
39. Bateman, R.J.; Xiong, C.; Benzinger, T.L.; Fagan, A.M.; Goate, A.; Fox, N.C.; Marcus, D.S.; Cairns, N.J.; Xie, X.; Blazey, T.M.; et al. Clinical and biomarker changes in dominantly inherited Alzheimer's disease. *N. Engl. J. Med.* **2012**, *367*, 795–804. [CrossRef]
40. Chiang, G.C.; Mao, X.; Kang, G.; Chang, E.; Pandya, S.; Vallabhajosula, S.; Isaacson, R.; Ravdin, L.D. Relationships among cortical glutathione levels, brain amyloidosis, and memory in healthy older adults investigated in vivo with 1H-MRS and Pittsburgh compound-B PET. *Am. J. Neuroradiol.* **2017**, *38*, 1130–1137. [CrossRef]
41. Chiaravalloti, A.; Castellano, A.E.; Ricci, M.; Barbagallo, G.; Sannino, P.; Ursini, F.; Karalis, G.; Schillaci, O. Coupled Imaging with [18F]FBB and [18F]FDG in AD Subjects Show a Selective Association Between Amyloid Burden and Cortical Dysfunction in the Brain. *Mol. Imaging Biol.* **2018**, *20*, 659–666. [CrossRef]
42. Ciarmiello, A.; Tartaglione, A.; Giovannini, E.; Riondato, M.; Giovacchini, G.; Ferrando, O.; De Biasi, M.; Passera, C.; Carabelli, E.; Mannironi, A.; et al. Amyloid burden identifies neuropsychological phenotypes at increased risk of progression to Alzheimer's disease in mild cognitive impairment patients. *Eur. J. Nucl. Med. Mol. Imaging* **2019**, *46*, 288–296. [CrossRef] [PubMed]
43. Miki, T.; Shimada, H.; Kim, J.S.; Yamamoto, Y.; Sugino, M.; Kowa, H.; Heurling, K.; Zanette, M.; Sherwin, P.F.; Senda, M. Brain uptake and safety of Flutemetamol F 18 injection in Japanese subjects with probable Alzheimer's disease, subjects with amnestic mild cognitive impairment and healthy volunteers. *Ann. Nucl. Med.* **2017**, *31*, 260–272. [CrossRef] [PubMed]
44. Pothier, K.; Saint-Aubert, L.; Hooper, C.; Delrieu, J.; Payoux, P.; de Souto Barreto, P.; Vellas, B. MAPT/DSA Study Group. Cognitive changes of older adults with an equivocal amyloid load. *J. Neurol.* **2019**, *266*, 835–843. [CrossRef] [PubMed]
45. Johnson, K.A.; Minoshima, S.; Bohnen, N.I.; Donohoe, K.J.; Foster, N.L.; Herscovitch, P.; Karlawish, J.H.; Rowe, C.C.; Carrillo, M.C.; Hartley, D.M.; et al. Appropriate use criteria for amyloid PET: A report of the Amyloid Imaging Task Force, the Society of Nuclear Medicine and Molecular Imaging, and the Alzheimer's Association. *Alzheimers Dement.* **2013**, *9*, e-1-16. [CrossRef] [PubMed]
46. Alongi, P.; Sardina, D.S.; Coppola, R.; Scalisi, S.; Puglisi, V.; Arnone, A.; Raimondo, G.D.; Munerati, E.; Alaimo, V.; Midiri, F.; et al. 18F-Florbetaben PET/CT to Assess Alzheimer's Disease: A new Analysis Method for Regional Amyloid Quantification. *J. Neuroimaging* **2019**, *3*, 383–393. [CrossRef]
47. Bouter, C.; Vogelgsang, J.; Wiltfang, J. Comparison between amyloid-PET and CSF amyloid-β biomarkers in a clinical cohort with memory deficits. *Clin. Chim. Acta* **2019**, *492*, 62–68. [CrossRef]
48. Frings, L.; Hellwig, S.; Bormann, T.; Spehl, T.S.; Buchert, R.; Meyer, P.T. Amyloid load but not regional glucose metabolism predicts conversion to Alzheimer's dementia in a memory clinic population. *Eur. J. Nucl. Med. Mol. Imaging* **2018**, *45*, 1442–1448. [CrossRef]

49. Kim, S.E.; Woo, S.; Kim, S.W.; Chin, J.; Kim, H.J.; Lee, B.I.; Park, J.; Park, K.W.; Kang, D.Y.; Noh, Y.; et al. A nomogram for predicting amyloid PET positivity in amnestic mild cognitive impairment. *J. Alzheimers Dis.* **2018**, *66*, 681–691. [CrossRef]
50. Schmidt, M.E.; Chiao, P.; Klein, G.; Matthews, D.; Thurfjell, L.; Cole, P.E.; Margolin, R.; Landau, S.; Foster, N.L.; Mason, N.S.; et al. The influence of biological and technical factors on quantitative analysis of amyloid PET: Points to consider and recommendations for controlling variability in longitudinal data. *Alzheimers Dement.* **2015**, *11*, 1050–1068. [CrossRef]
51. Newberg, A.B.; Arnold, S.E.; Wintering, N.; Rovner, B.W.; Alavi, A. Initial clinical comparison of 18F-florbetapir and 18F-FDG PET in patients with Alzheimer disease and controls. *J. Nucl Med.* **2012**, *53*, 902–907. [CrossRef]
52. La Joie, R.; Perrotin, A.; Barre, L.; Hommet, C.; Mezenge, F.; Ibazizene, M.; Camus, V.; Abbas, A.; Landeau, B.; Guilloteau, D.; et al. Region-specific hierarchy between atrophy, hypometabolism, and beta-amyloid (Abeta) load in Alzheimer's disease dementia. *J. Neurosci.* **2012**, *32*, 16265–16273. [CrossRef] [PubMed]
53. Pfefferbaum, A.; Chanraud, S.; Pitel, A.-L.; Müller-Oehring, E.; Shankaranarayanan, A.; Alsop, D.C.; Rohlfing, T.; Sullivan, E.V. Cerebral blood flow in posterior cortical nodes of the default mode network decreases with task engagement but remains higher than in most brain regions. *Cereb. Cortex* **2011**, *21*, 233–244. [CrossRef] [PubMed]
54. Fleisher, A.S.; Chen, K.; Liu, X.; Roontiva, A.; Thiyyagura, P.; Ayutyanont, N.; Joshi, A.D.; Clark, C.M.; Mintun, M.A.; Pontecorvo, M.J.; et al. Using positron emission tomography and florbetapir F18 to image cortical amyloid in patients with mild cognitive impairment or dementia due to Alzheimer disease. *Arch. Neurol.* **2011**, *68*, 1404–1411. [CrossRef] [PubMed]
55. Camus, V.; Payoux, P.; Barré, L.; Desgranges, B.; Voisin, T.; Tauber, C.; La Joie, R.; Tafani, M.; Hommet, C.; Chételat, G.; et al. Using PET with 18F-AV-45 (florbetapir) to quantify brain amyloid load in a clinical environment. *Europ. J. Nucl. Medi. Mol. Imaging* **2012**, *39*, 621–631. [CrossRef] [PubMed]
56. Klupp, E.; Grimmer, T.; Tahmasian, M.; Sorg, C.; Yakushev, I.; Yousefi, B.H.; Drzezga, A.; Förster, S. Prefrontal hypometabolism in Alzheimer disease is related to longitudinal amyloid accumulation in remote brain regions. *J. Nucl. Med.* **2015**, *56*, 399–404. [CrossRef] [PubMed]
57. Marcus, C.; Mena, E.; Subramaniam, R.M. Brain PET in the diagnosis of Alzheimer's disease. *Clin. Nucl. Med.* **2014**, *39*, e413–e426. [CrossRef]
58. Kantarci, K.; Yang, C.; Schneider, J.A.; Senjem, M.L.; Reyes, D.A.; Lowe, V.J.; Barnes, L.L.; Aggarwal, N.T.; Bennett, D.A.; Smith, G.E.; et al. Antemortem amyloid imaging and β-amyloid pathology in a case with dementia with Lewy bodies. *Neurobiol. Aging* **2012**, *33*, 878–885. [CrossRef]
59. Iizuka, T.; Kameyama, M. Cingulate island sign on FDG-PET is associated with medial temporal lobe atrophy in dementia with Lewy bodies. *Ann. Nucl. Med.* **2016**, *30*, 421–429. [CrossRef]
60. Lim, S.M.; Katsifis, A.; Villemagne, V.L.; Best, R.; Jones, G.; Saling, M.; Bradshaw, J.; Merory, J.; Woodward, M.; Hopwood, M.; et al. The 18F-FDG PET cingulate island sign and comparison to 123I-beta-CIT SPECT for diagnosis of dementia with Lewy bodies. *J. Nucl. Med.* **2009**, *50*, 1638–1645. [CrossRef]
61. Papathanasiou, N.D.; Boutsiadis, A.; Dickson, J.; Bomanji, J.B. Diagnostic accuracy of 123I-FP-CIT (DaTSCAN) in dementia with Lewy bodies: A meta-analysis of published studies. *Parkinsonism Relat. Disord.* **2012**, *18*, 225–229. [CrossRef]
62. Lewczuk, P.; Matzen, A.; Blennow, K.; Parnetti, L.; Molinuevo, J.L.; Eusebi, P.; Kornhuber, J.; Morris, J.C.; Fagan, A.M. Cerebrospinal Fluid Abeta42/40 Corresponds Better than Abeta42 to Amyloid PET in Alzheimer's Disease. *J. Alzheimers Dis.* **2017**, *55*, 813–822. [CrossRef] [PubMed]
63. Foster, N.L.; Heidebrink, J.L.; Clark, C.M.; Jagust, W.J.; Arnold, S.E.; Barbas, N.R.; DeCarli, C.S.; Turner, R.S.; Koeppe, R.A.; Higdon, R.; et al. FDG-PET improves accuracy in distinguishing frontotemporal dementia and Alzheimer's disease. *Brain* **2007**, *130*, 2616–2635. [CrossRef] [PubMed]
64. Engler, H.; Santillo, A.F.; Wang, S.X.; Lindau, M.; Savitcheva, I.; Nordberg, A.; Lannfelt, L.; Långström, B.; Kilander, L. In vivo amyloid imaging with PET in frontotemporal dementia. *Eur. J. Nucl. Med. Mol. Imaging* **2008**, *35*, 100–106. [CrossRef] [PubMed]

7

Some Metabolites Act as Second Messengers in Yeast Chronological Aging

Karamat Mohammad, Paméla Dakik, Younes Medkour, Mélissa McAuley, Darya Mitrofanova and Vladimir I. Titorenko *

Department of Biology, Concordia University, 7141 Sherbrooke Street, West, SP Building, Room 501-13, Montreal, QC H4B 1R6, Canada; karamat.mohammad@concordia.ca (K.M.); pameladakik@gmail.com (P.D.); writetoyounes@gmail.com (Y.M.); melissa.mcauley@concordia.ca (M.M.); mitrofanova_darya@hotmail.com (D.M.)

* Correspondence: vladimir.titorenko@concordia.ca

Abstract: The concentrations of some key metabolic intermediates play essential roles in regulating the longevity of the chronologically aging yeast *Saccharomyces cerevisiae*. These key metabolites are detected by certain ligand-specific protein sensors that respond to concentration changes of the key metabolites by altering the efficiencies of longevity-defining cellular processes. The concentrations of the key metabolites that affect yeast chronological aging are controlled spatially and temporally. Here, we analyze mechanisms through which the spatiotemporal dynamics of changes in the concentrations of the key metabolites influence yeast chronological lifespan. Our analysis indicates that a distinct set of metabolites can act as second messengers that define the pace of yeast chronological aging. Molecules that can operate both as intermediates of yeast metabolism and as second messengers of yeast chronological aging include reduced nicotinamide adenine dinucleotide phosphate (NADPH), glycerol, trehalose, hydrogen peroxide, amino acids, sphingolipids, spermidine, hydrogen sulfide, acetic acid, ethanol, free fatty acids, and diacylglycerol. We discuss several properties that these second messengers of yeast chronological aging have in common with second messengers of signal transduction. We outline how these second messengers of yeast chronological aging elicit changes in cell functionality and viability in response to changes in the nutrient, energy, stress, and proliferation status of the cell.

Keywords: yeast; chronological aging; mechanisms of longevity regulation; metabolism; cell signaling; second messengers; mitochondria; interorganellar communications; proteostasis; regulated cell death

---

1. Introduction

Studies of the budding yeast *Saccharomyces cerevisiae* have led to the discovery of genes, signaling pathways, and small molecules that define the rate of cellular aging in this unicellular eukaryote [1–3]. Some of the genes, signaling pathways, and small molecules discovered in *S. cerevisiae* have been later found to play essential roles in cellular and organismal aging in diverse species of multicellular eukaryotes; it is believed, therefore, that the mechanisms underlying aging and longevity assurance have been conserved throughout the course of evolution [4–6]. Thus, the use of *S. cerevisiae* as a model organism is fundamental for the progress in aging research [2–4].

There are two different ways of studying aging in *S. cerevisiae*; each of these ways investigates a different mode of yeast aging.

A so-called replicative mode of yeast aging is monitored by counting the total number of asymmetric mitotic divisions—each producing a small daughter cell—that a mother cell could undergo on the surface of a solid nutrient-rich medium before it becomes senescent [2,7,8]. Yeast replicative aging has long been considered to resemble the aging of those cells in humans and other mammals that are able to divide mitotically; among these mitotically active cells are lymphocytes, monocytes, granulocytes, fibroblasts, and some stem cell types [2,4,6–8]. Recent studies have revealed that (1) many genes that modulate aging of post-mitotic cells in adults of the nematode *Caenorhabditis elegans* also influence yeast replicative aging [9–11]; and (2) many hallmarks of aging characteristic of post-mitotic cells in humans and other mammals are also cellular hallmarks of yeast replicative aging [12]. Hence, it is conceivable that the replicative mode of yeast aging may also mirror the aging of post-mitotic cells and even the aging of the entire organism in nematodes, humans, and other mammals [9–12].

A so-called chronological mode of yeast aging is monitored by determining how long a yeast cell cultured in a liquid medium can retain viability after it undergoes cell cycle arrest and enters a state of quiescence [2,13,14]. Yeast chronological aging is believed to model the aging of human and mammalian cells that lose the ability to divide mitotically; these post-mitotic cells include adipocytes, mature muscle cells, and mature neurons [2,14,15]. The chronological mode of yeast aging is also considered to be a simple model of organismal aging in multicellular eukaryotes [14,16].

Although the replicative and chronological modes of aging in yeast are usually examined separately from each other, recent evidence indicates that these two modes of yeast aging most likely converge into a single aging process [17–19].

Here, we review mechanisms through which the spatiotemporal dynamics of changes in the concentrations of some metabolites regulate the longevity of chronologically aging yeast. Based on the important advance in our understanding of these mechanisms, we conclude that a distinct group of metabolites act as second messengers that define the pace of yeast chronological aging.

2. Concentrations of Some Metabolites Define the Rate of Chronological Aging in Yeast

Recent studies have demonstrated that the intracellular and extracellular concentrations of some key metabolites play essential roles in regulating the longevity of chronologically aging *S. cerevisiae* [2–5,15,16,20–32]. These key metabolites are detected by certain protein sensors, which respond to concentration changes of the metabolites by altering the efficiencies of cellular processes known to define yeast chronological lifespan (CLS) [2–4,16,20–32]. In this section, we describe the metabolites whose concentration changes affect the pace of yeast chronological aging and discuss mechanisms through which these key metabolites influence yeast CLS.

2.1. NADPH

NADPH is generated in the Zwf1- and Gnd1-dependent reactions of the pentose phosphate pathway operating in the cytosol of *S. cerevisiae*, as well as in the Ald4-, Pos5-, Mae1-, and Idp1-driven reactions confined to yeast mitochondria [3,20,33]. NADPH is indispensable for the growth and viability of yeast cells because it serves as the major source of reducing equivalents for amino acid, fatty acid, and sterol synthesis [20,33]. In addition, NADPH has a specific role in longevity assurance of chronologically aging yeast because it provides electrons for thioredoxin and glutathione reductase systems (TRR and GTR, respectively) [34,35]. Both these NADPH-dependent reductase systems play essential roles in the maintenance of intracellular redox homeostasis, thereby decreasing the extent of oxidative damage to thiol-containing proteins that reside in the cytosol, nucleus, and mitochondria of yeast cells [34,35]. Such NADPH-driven, TRR- and GTR-dependent protection of many thiol-containing proteins from oxidative damage slows down yeast chronological aging (Figure 1A) [35].

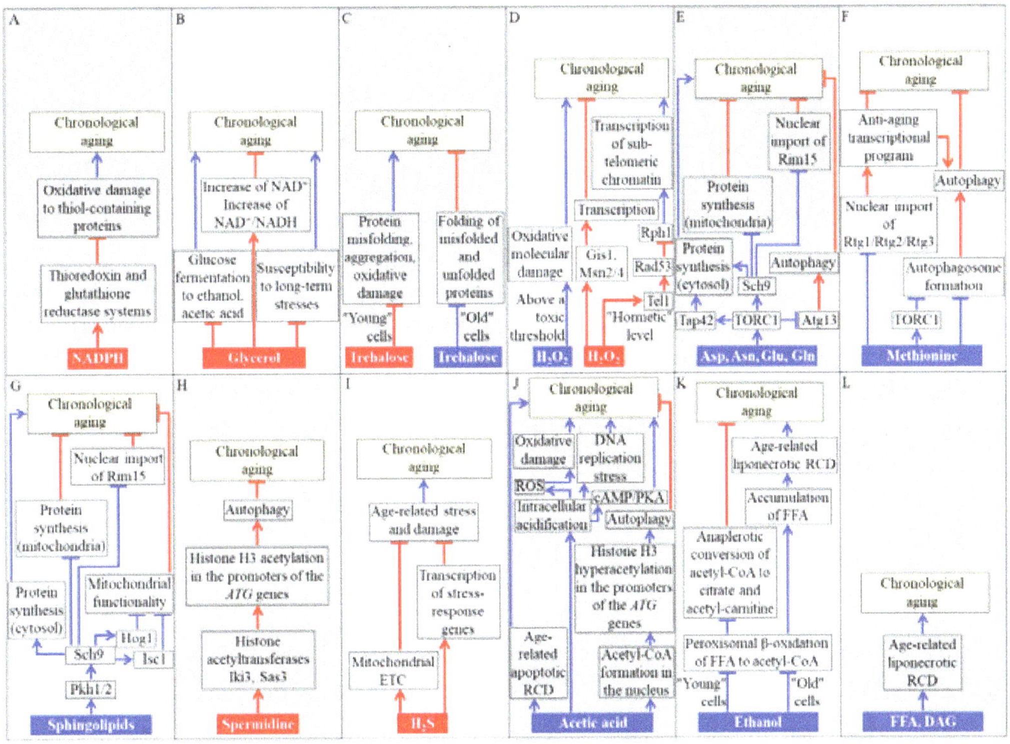

Figure 1. Mechanisms through which the concentrations of some key metabolites define the rate of chronological aging in the yeast *Saccharomyces cerevisiae*. These key metabolites include NADPH (**A**), glycerol (**B**), trehalose (**C**), H_2O_2 (**D**), the amino acids aspartate, asparagine, glutamate and glutamine (**E**), methionine (**F**), sphingolipids (**G**), spermidine (**H**), H_2S (**I**), acetic acid (**J**), ethanol (**K**), as well as FFA and DAG (**L**). These key metabolites are detected by a distinct set of ligand-specific protein sensors that respond to the concentration changes of the metabolites by altering the rates and efficiencies of longevity-defining cellular processes, thus creating a pro- or anti-aging cellular pattern and affecting the pace of yeast chronological aging. See text for more details. Activation arrows and inhibition bars denote pro-aging processes (displayed in blue color) or anti-aging processes (displayed in red color). Pro-aging or anti-aging metabolites are displayed in blue color or red color, respectively. Abbreviations: Asp, aspartate; Asn, asparagine; *ATG*, autophagy-related genes; ETC, electron transport chain; FFA, free (non-esterified) fatty acids; DAG, diacylglycerol; Glu, glutamate; Gln, glutamine; PKA, protein kinase A; RCD, regulated cell death; ROS, reactive oxygen species.

2.2. Glycerol

Glycerol is one of the products of glucose fermentation in the cytosol of *S. cerevisiae* cells [33]. An increase in the intracellular and extracellular concentrations of glycerol has been shown to decelerate yeast chronological aging [15,36]. Three mechanisms have been proposed to underlie such aging-delaying action of glycerol. These mechanisms are depicted in Figure 1B and outlined below. First mechanism: an increase in glucose fermentation to glycerol lowers metabolite flow into glucose fermentation to ethanol and acetic acid, both of which accelerate yeast chronological aging (Figure 1B) [3,15,36,37]. Second mechanism: glycerol decreases the susceptibility of yeast cells to long-term oxidative, thermal, and osmotic stresses; an age-related intensification of all these stresses is a potent pro-aging factor in chronologically aging yeast (Figure 1B) [3,36]. It is presently unknown if this second mechanism involves some protein sensors that respond to an increase in glycerol concentration by stimulating certain stress response processes in yeast cells. Third mechanism: an increase in glucose fermentation to glycerol allows an increase in both the intracellular concentration of NAD^+ and the intracellular $NAD^+/NADH$ ratio, thereby setting up a pro-longevity cellular pattern in chronologically aging *S. cerevisiae* (Figure 1B) [3,36].

2.3. Trehalose

Trehalose, a non-reducing disaccharide synthesized from glucose, has long been considered only as a reserve carbohydrate in *S. cerevisiae* cells [38]. However, recent evidence indicates that trehalose is also essential for regulating the longevity of chronologically aging yeast [37,39–45]. Depending on the chronological age of *S. cerevisiae*, trehalose exhibits either an anti-aging or pro-aging effect. Both these effects are due to the ability of trehalose to directly bind unfolded domains of proteins, thereby modulating various aspects of cellular proteostasis throughout CLS. In chronologically "young" yeast cells that proliferate, trehalose assists in sustaining an anti-aging pattern of cellular proteostasis. This is because trehalose binding to newly synthesized proteins in these cells helps to decrease the misfolding, aggregation, and oxidative damage of such proteins (Figure 1C) [37,41,46,47]. In chronologically "old" yeast cells that enter a non-proliferative state, trehalose contributes to the establishment of a pro-aging pattern of cellular proteostasis. This is because trehalose binding to hydrophobic amino acid side chains of misfolded, partially folded, and unfolded proteins in these cells shields extended patches of hydrophobic amino acid residues from the molecular chaperones needed for the folding of such proteins (Figure 1C) [37,41,46].

2.4. Hydrogen Peroxide (H_2O_2)

H_2O_2 is the major molecule of reactive oxygen species (ROS) [48]. In chronologically aging yeast, H_2O_2 and other ROS are initially generated in mitochondria and peroxisomes as by-products of mitochondrial respiration and peroxisomal oxidative metabolism, respectively [21–23]. After being made in mitochondria and peroxisomes, H_2O_2 is released from these two organelles and may play a dual role in regulating yeast CLS [21–23]. If the intracellular concentration of H_2O_2 exceeds a toxic threshold, it accelerates the process of chronological aging by eliciting oxidative damage to proteins, lipids, and nucleic acids in various locations within the yeast cell [21,48]. If the intracellular concentration of H_2O_2 is maintained at a "hormetic" level (i.e., a sub-lethal concentration of H_2O_2 that is insufficient to damage cellular macromolecules), this ROS can activate at least two signaling networks that extend yeast CLS by creating an anti-aging cellular pattern [2,3,27]. One of these hormetic H_2O_2-responsive signaling networks activates the Gis1, Msn2, and Msn4 transcription factors; after being activated, Gis1, Msn2, and Msn4 establish an anti-aging cellular pattern by stimulating the transcription of many genes involved in carbohydrate and lipid metabolism, nutrient sensing, cell cycle progression, autophagy, stress response and protection, and stationary phase survival (Figure 1D) [2,49,50]. Another hormetic H_2O_2-responsive signaling network is initiated when the DNA damage response (DDR) kinase Tel1 phosphorylates and activates the DDR kinase Rad53; Rad53 then phosphorylates and inactivates the histone demethylase Rph1, thus creating an anti-aging cellular pattern by suppressing the Rph1-driven transcription of sub-telomeric chromatin regions (Figure 1D) [51,52]. Mechanisms though which the Rad53-dependent suppression of sub-telomeric transcription prolongs yeast CLS remain unknown [51].

2.5. Amino Acids

The synthesis of the amino acids aspartate, asparagine, glutamate, and glutamine from tricarboxylic acid (TCA) cycle intermediates occurs in mitochondria of yeast cells [20,33]. These amino acids then exit mitochondria and activate protein kinase activity of the target of rapamycin complex 1 (TORC1), a pro-aging regulator confined to the surface of yeast vacuoles (Figure 1E) [53–56]. Active TORC1 orchestrates the establishment and maintenance of a pro-aging cellular pattern by phosphorylating at least three downstream protein targets and altering their activities. As outlined below, each of these downstream protein targets of TORC1 defines yeast CLS because it regulates one or more longevity-defining cellular processes.

One of the proteins phosphorylated by TORC1 is the nutrient-sensing protein kinase Sch9. Once phosphorylated by TORC1, Sch9 influences some longevity-defining cellular processes as follows: (1) it promotes ribosome assembly and stimulates translation initiation, thus activating the pro-aging process of protein synthesis in the cytosol [57–60]; (2) it slows down the anti-aging process of protein synthesis in mitochondria [55,56,61,62]; and (3) it inhibits nuclear import of Rim15, a nutrient-sensing protein kinase that elicits an anti-aging cellular pattern by stimulating the Gis1, Msn2, and Msn4 transcription factors in the nucleus [63–65]; this pro-aging effect of Sch9 is reinforced by the nutrient-sensing protein kinase A (PKA), which impedes nuclear import of Msn2 and Msn4 (Figure 1E) [65–67].

Another downstream phosphorylation target of active TORC1 is Tap42, a protein that (akin to Sch9) stimulates the pro-aging process of protein synthesis in the cytosol by promoting ribosome assembly and activating translation initiation (Figure 1E) [58,68].

The autophagy-initiating protein Atg13 is also a downstream phosphorylation target of active TORC1 [69,70]. The TORC1-driven phosphorylation of Atg13 suppresses the anti-aging process of autophagy by inhibiting autophagosome formation in the cytosol (Figure 1E) [71–73]. Atg13 can also be phosphorylated by PKA, which strengthens the pro-aging effect of TORC1 by further suppressing the formation of autophagosomes [69–73].

Like aspartate, asparagine, glutamate, and glutamine, the amino acid methionine is a pro-aging metabolite in yeast that ages chronologically (Figure 1F). A likely pro-aging effect of methionine consists in stimulating the methylation of tRNAs in the cytosol [74]. The resulting decline in the concentration of non-methylated tRNAs weakens nuclear import of the Rtg1/Rtg2/Rtg3 heterotrimeric transcription factor needed for driving an anti-aging transcriptional program (Figure 1F) [74]. Another pro-aging effect of methionine is manifested in its ability to inhibit autophagy by activating TORC1 and/or by suppressing autophagosome formation in a TORC1-independent manner (Figure 1F) [75]. This shortens yeast CLS by decreasing the acidity of the vacuole and by eliciting the accumulation of extracellular acetic acid, a potent pro-aging metabolite [74–77].

2.6. Sphingolipids

Sphingolipids are pro-aging metabolites in chronologically aging yeast because some genetic and pharmaceutical interventions that change the intracellular concentrations of certain sphingolipids have been shown to prolong yeast CLS [24,28,29,32]. Mechanisms underlying the essential role of sphingolipids in defining yeast CLS have begun to emerge; these mechanisms are outlined below.

After being synthesized in the endoplasmic reticulum (ER), the sphingolipid backbone base phytosphingosine stimulates protein kinase activities of Pkh1 and Pkh2 (Pkb-activating kinase homolog proteins 1 and 2) [78,79]. Pkh1 and Pkh2 then phosphorylate and activate the nutrient-sensing protein kinase Sch9 [24,80,81]. Such Pkh1/2-dependent phosphorylation of Sch9 establishes a Pkh1/2-Sch9 branch of a network that integrates nutrient and sphingolipid signaling (Figure 1G) [24,29,32,81]. As mentioned in Section 2.5, the phosphorylated and therefore active form of Sch9 in this signaling branch accelerates yeast chronological aging by stimulating the pro-aging process of protein synthesis in the cytosol [57–60], decelerating the anti-aging process of protein synthesis in mitochondria [55,56,61,62] and inhibiting nuclear import of the nutrient-sensing protein kinase Rim15 (Figure 1G) [63–65]. The Pkh1/2-dependent phosphorylation of Sch9 also elicits the Sch9-driven phosphorylation and activation of: (1) Hog1, a mitogen-activated protein kinase that attenuates mitochondrial functionality; and (2) Isc1, an inositol phosphosphingolipid phospholipase C that is involved in the formation of ceramides from complex sphingolipids in yeast mitochondria (Figure 1G) [24,28,29,32]. This ability of the Pkh1/2-Sch9 signaling branch to promote the phosphorylation of Hog1 and Isc1 allows it to coordinate mitochondrial functionality and sphingolipid metabolism, thus making an essential contribution to longevity regulation in chronologically aging yeast [24,28,29,32].

2.7. Spermidine

The natural polyamine spermidine is an aging-delaying metabolite that extends yeast CLS [82–84]. In yeast cells, spermidine is synthesized from the amino acids arginine and methionine in a series of reactions confined to mitochondria, the cytosol, and peroxisomes [84]. Spermidine delays yeast chronological aging because it inhibits the histone acetyltransferases Iki3 and Sas3 (Figure 1H) [82]. Although such spermidine-dependent inhibition of the two acetyltransferases attenuates transcription of many nuclear genes because it impairs histone H3 acetylation at their promoter regions, the extent of histone H3 acetylation at the promoter regions of several autophagy-related (*ATG*) genes is increased in yeast cells that exhibit high spermidine concentrations [82]. This selectively activates the transcription of the *ATG* genes, thus enhancing the cytoprotective process of autophagy and delaying yeast chronological aging (Figure 1H) [82,83].

2.8. Hydrogen Sulfide (H_2S)

H_2S is a metabolite that plays an essential role in the delay of yeast chronological aging by caloric restriction (CR) [85], a dietary regimen that delays aging, increases lifespan, and improves healthspan in evolutionarily distant eukaryotes [1,86,87]. In yeast, this water- and fat-soluble gas can be generated endogenously via two different metabolic pathways. One pathway of H_2S synthesis involves a unique yeast assimilation of exogenous inorganic sulfate [88]. Another pathway of H_2S synthesis is an evolutionarily conserved trans-sulfuration pathway (TSP) of transfer from methionine to cysteine [88]. In yeast cultured in a liquid synthetic medium, only H_2S that is endogenously synthesized via the TSP pathway and then released to the culture medium is responsible for yeast CLS extension under CR conditions [85]. Mechanisms through which an exogenous (extracellular) pool of H_2S delays chronological aging of yeast limited in calorie supply remain to be determined. It has been suggested that low, hormetic concentrations of H_2S may protect chronologically aging yeast from age-related stress and damage by accelerating the electron transport chain in mitochondria and/or by activating the transcription of many stress-response genes in the nucleus (Figure 1I) [85,88,89].

2.9. Acetic Acid

Acetic acid is one of the products of glucose fermentation by yeast cultured in a liquid medium under high oxygenation [2,15,33]. It is formed in the Ald6-dependent reaction that occurs in the cytosol and in the Ald4-driven reaction confined to mitochondria [3]. Acetic acid is a pro-aging metabolite that shortens yeast CLS [15,90].

Three mechanisms through which extracellular and/or intracellular pools of acetic acid may accelerate yeast chronological aging have been suggested, all based on known effects of these acetic acid pools. These mechanisms are outlined below.

First mechanism: acetic acid (and/or the acidification of the liquid culture medium it causes) may, directly or indirectly, elicit an age-related apoptotic mode of regulated cell death (Figure 1J) [15,90–94].

Second mechanism: extracellular acidification caused by the buildup of acetic acid in the culture medium may trigger intracellular acidification, which may then accelerate chronological aging by: (1) stimulating the pro-aging cyclic adenosine monophosphate (cAMP)/PKA signaling pathway; (2) increasing the concentration of ROS, thus eliciting oxidative damage to cellular macromolecules; and/or (3) enhancing DNA replication stress (Figure 1J) [2,90,92].

Third mechanism: nuclear transport of acetic acid and its subsequent Acs2-dependent conversion into acetyl-Coenzyme A (CoA) may suppress the transcription of nuclear *ATG* genes by causing histone H3 hyperacetylation at their promoter regions, thus slowing down the cytoprotective process of autophagy and accelerating yeast chronological aging (Figure 1J) [25,26,95,96].

It needs to be emphasized that exogenous acetic acid accelerates yeast chronological aging not only because it creates an acidic extracellular environment; indeed, neither other organic acids present in culture medium of aged yeast nor hydrochloric acid can shorten yeast CLS if added exogenously [15].

Moreover, only exogenous acetic acid at acidic pH, but not its conjugate base at neutral pH, exhibits the aging-accelerating effect in yeast [15]. It is conceivable, therefore, that only a combinatory action of acetic acid and an acidic extracellular environment is responsible for the acceleration of yeast chronological aging via the above mechanisms [15].

2.10. Ethanol

Yeast cells cultured in a liquid medium under low oxygenation produce ethanol as the main product of glucose fermentation in the Adh1-dependent reaction confined to the cytosol [2,3,13,14,33]. Ethanol is a pro-aging metabolite that shortens yeast CLS [37,97]. This pro-aging action of ethanol can be enhanced by the sirtuin deacetylase Sir2, which inhibits the Adh2-driven conversion of ethanol to acetaldehyde [97].

Ethanol accelerates yeast chronological aging via two different mechanisms. Both of these mechanisms are elicited in response to ethanol-dependent suppression of the Fox1-, Fox2-, and Fox3-driven peroxisomal β-oxidation of fatty acids to acetyl-CoA [21,37]. Each of these two mechanisms is specific to the chronological age of a yeast cell.

In chronologically "young" yeast, the ethanol-dependent suppression of acetyl-CoA formation in peroxisomes decreases its availability for anaplerotic conversion to citrate and acetyl-carnitine in these organelles [3,21,37]. This accelerates yeast chronological aging by weakening the longevity assurance process of supplying citrate and acetyl-carnitine to mitochondria for the replenishment of these two TCA cycle intermediates (Figure 1K) [3,21,37].

In chronologically "old" yeast, the ethanol-dependent suppression of peroxisomal β-oxidation of fatty acids leads to the excessive accumulation of free (non-esterified) fatty acids (FFA) [3,21,37]. Such build-up of FFA accelerates yeast chronological aging by increasing the risk of an age-related mode of regulated cell death (RCD) called "liponecrosis" (Figure 1K) [3,98–100].

2.11. FFA and Diacylglycerol (DAG)

The ethanol-driven excessive accumulation of unoxidized FFA in yeast peroxisomes (see Section 2.10) elicits several negative-feedback loops whose action causes a buildup of FFA and DAG in the ER and lipid droplets (LD) [3,100,101]. This buildup of FFA and DAG accelerates the onset of the liponecrotic mode of RCD, thereby increasing the risk of death and accelerating yeast chronological aging (Figure 1L) [3,21,98–100]. Thus, both FFA and DAG are pro-aging metabolites that shorten yeast CLS.

3. The Spatiotemporal Dynamics of Changes in Concentrations of Some Metabolites Define Yeast CLS

It is becoming increasingly evident that the concentrations of the key metabolites that influence the pace of yeast chronological aging are controlled spatially and temporally at different levels.

One level of the spatial control over the concentrations of these metabolites consists in regulating their intracellular and extracellular concentrations [3,102]. Some of the key metabolites can influence longevity-defining processes only within the cell they were produced; these metabolites: (1) define the pace of yeast chronological aging only via cell-autonomous mechanisms; (2) cannot act as low molecular weight transmissible longevity factors; and (3) include NADPH, trehalose, sphingolipids, FFA, and DAG [3,24,28,32,35,37,41,102]. In contrast, some of the key metabolites can influence longevity-defining processes both within the cell they were generated as well as within other cells in the yeast population; these metabolites: (1) define the pace of yeast chronological aging via both cell-autonomous and cell-non-autonomous mechanisms; (2) can act as low molecular weight transmissible longevity factors; and (3) include glycerol, H_2O_2, amino acids, spermidine, H_2S, acetic acid, and ethanol [3,15,36,50–52,54,71–73,82,85,93,94,97,102]. It is noteworthy that some of those metabolites that cannot act as low molecular weight transmissible longevity factors (and thus define the pace of yeast chronological aging only via cell-autonomous mechanisms) may change metabolism within the "host" cell so that this cell may respond by altering the production of acetic acid and/or other metabolites that can act via both cell-autonomous and cell-non-autonomous mechanisms.

Another level at which the concentrations of these key metabolites are controlled spatially consists in regulating their abundance in different organellar compartments within the cell. The effective concentrations of the metabolites that influence the pace of yeast chronological aging are established and maintained within an intricate network that involves the unidirectional and/or bidirectional flow of certain metabolites between mitochondria, the nucleus, vacuoles, peroxisomes, the ER, the plasma membrane, LD, and the cytosol [22,23,27].

In addition, the concentrations of the key metabolites that define yeast CLS are controlled temporally. Indeed, it has been found that: (1) these metabolite concentrations undergo age-related changes; and (2) the effects of these metabolites on their protein sensors are also subjected to age-related changes; these protein sensors respond to concentration changes of the key metabolites by altering the efficiencies of certain longevity-defining cellular processes [3,27]. It has been therefore proposed that the concentration changes of different key metabolites are temporally limited to certain longevity-defining periods called "checkpoints" [2,3,27,41,103]. Many of these checkpoints exist early in the life of chronologically aging yeast cultured in glucose-containing liquid media, during diauxic and post-diauxic growth phases [3,27]. NADPH, glycerol, H_2O_2, amino acids, sphingolipids, and spermidine are the key metabolites whose concentrations only at these "early" checkpoints play essential roles in defining the pace of yeast chronological aging [24,27,28,32,35,36,42,51–54,71–73,82]. Some of these checkpoints are the "late" checkpoints that occur after chronologically aging yeast cultured in glucose-containing liquid media undergoes cell cycle arrest and enters the non-proliferative stationary phase of culturing [3,27]. H_2S, acetic acid, FFA, and DAG are the key metabolites whose concentrations only at these "late" checkpoints make essential contributions to defining the pace of yeast chronological aging [15,27,37,85,93,94]. It is noteworthy that trehalose and ethanol are the two key metabolites whose concentrations affect the longevity of chronologically aging yeast at both the "early" and the "late" checkpoints; for each of these two metabolites, the longevity-defining effect at the "early" checkpoint differs from that at the "late" checkpoint (see Sections 2.3 and 2.10) [3,27,41]. It has been also proposed that at each of these "early" and "late" checkpoints, the concentration changes of the key metabolites are detected by a distinct set of checkpoint-specific protein sensors. These protein sensors have been called "master regulators" because their suggested common role consists in responding to the concentration changes of different key metabolites by altering the rates and efficiencies of various longevity-defining cellular processes throughout the chronological lifespan, thus establishing a pro- or anti-aging cellular pattern and defining yeast CLS [3,27].

4. Conclusions

Based on our analysis of how the spatiotemporal dynamics of changes in the concentrations of some metabolites influence yeast CLS, we conclude that a distinct group of metabolites can act as second messengers that define the pace of yeast chronological aging. Molecules that can operate both as intermediates of yeast metabolism and as second messengers of yeast chronological aging include NADPH, glycerol, trehalose, H_2O_2, amino acids, sphingolipids, spermidine, H_2S, acetic acid, ethanol, FFA, and DAG. Akin to second messengers of signal transduction [104,105], these second messengers of yeast chronological aging: (1) are generated and can undergo substantial concentration changes within a yeast cell in response to some extracellular stimuli (i.e., nutrients and hormetic stresses); these extracellular stimuli are detected by certain hierarchically organized proteins and protein complexes (i.e., the TORC1 and PKA signaling pathways) that then transduce the signal to some metabolic reactions involved in the generation of the intracellular second messengers; (2) differ from each other in their chemical properties and solubilities; these differences allow the second messengers to transduce the signal in the polar chemical environment of the cytosol or organelle interior, be distributed within the hydrophobic chemical environment of the cellular or organellar membrane, or be translocated across such membranes as a gas or free radical; (3) are subjected to stringent spatial control; indeed, the movement of these second messengers within the cell and their exit out of the cell are regulated in response to changes in the nutrient, energy, stress, and/or proliferation status of the cell; (4) are also controlled temporally, as their intracellular and extracellular concentrations at different periods of chronological lifespan vary significantly and are regulated by alterations in nutrient availability, stress intensity, and cell proliferation rate; and (5) are detected by a distinct set of ligand-specific protein sensors that respond to the concentration changes of different second messengers by altering the rates and efficiencies of longevity-defining cellular processes, thereby creating a pro- or anti-aging cellular pattern and affecting the pace of yeast chronological aging.

Of note, Pietrocola et al. [26] have recently concluded that acetyl-CoA can operate both as a metabolic intermediate and as a second messenger in regulating the delicate balance between cellular catabolism and anabolism in eukaryotic organisms across phyla. In conjunction with the demonstration that acetyl-CoA plays essential roles in regulating the longevity of chronologically aging yeast (see Sections 2.9 and 2.10; [21,25,37,95,96]), this important conclusion further supports the notion that intermediates of some metabolic pathways in eukaryotic cells can function as second messengers that orchestrate global changes in cell functionality in response to changes in the nutrient, energy, stress, and proliferation status of the cell.

Acknowledgments: We are grateful to current and former members of the Titorenko laboratory for discussions. This research was supported by grants from the NSERC of Canada and Concordia University Chair Fund to Vladimir I. Titorenko. Karamat Mohammad and Paméla Dakik were supported by the Concordia University Graduate Fellowship Awards. Younes Medkour was supported by the Concordia University Public Scholars Program Award. Vladimir I. Titorenko is a Concordia University Research Chair in Genomics, Cell Biology, and Aging.

Abbreviations

Asp	aspartate
Asn	asparagine
ATG	autophagy-related genes
ER	endoplasmic reticulum
ETC	electron transport chain
FFA	free (non-esterified) fatty acids
CLS	chronological lifespan
CR	caloric restriction
DAG	diacylglycerol
DDR	DNA damage response
Glu	glutamate
Gln	glutamine
GTR	glutathione reductase
LD	lipid droplets
PKA	protein kinase A
Pkh1	Pkb-activating kinase homolog protein 1
Pkh2	Pkb-activating kinase homolog protein 2
RCD	regulated cell death
ROS	reactive oxygen species
TCA	tricarboxylic acid
TORC1	target of rapamycin complex 1
TRR	thioredoxin reductase
TSP	transsulfuration pathway

References

1. Fontana, L.; Partridge, L.; Longo, V.D. Extending healthy life span—From yeast to humans. *Science* **2010**, *328*, 321–326. [CrossRef] [PubMed]
2. Longo, V.D.; Shadel, G.S.; Kaeberlein, M.; Kennedy, B. Replicative and chronological aging in *Saccharomyces cerevisiae*. *Cell Metab.* **2012**, *16*, 18–31. [CrossRef] [PubMed]
3. Arlia-Ciommo, A.; Leonov, A.; Piano, A.; Svistkova, V.; Titorenko, V.I. Cell-autonomous mechanisms of chronological aging in the yeast *Saccharomyces cerevisiae*. *Microb. Cell* **2014**, *1*, 163–178. [CrossRef] [PubMed]
4. Kaeberlein, M. Lessons on longevity from budding yeast. *Nature* **2010**, *464*, 513–519. [CrossRef] [PubMed]
5. Váchová, L.; Cáp, M.; Palková, Z. Yeast colonies: A model for studies of aging, environmental adaptation, and longevity. *Oxid. Med. Cell. Longev.* **2012**, *2012*. [CrossRef] [PubMed]
6. Denoth Lippuner, A.; Julou, T.; Barral, Y. Budding yeast as a model organism to study the effects of age. *FEMS Microbiol. Rev.* **2014**, *38*, 300–325. [CrossRef] [PubMed]
7. Steinkraus, K.A.; Kaeberlein, M.; Kennedy, B.K. Replicative aging in yeast: The means to the end. *Annu. Rev. Cell Dev. Biol.* **2008**, *24*, 29–54. [CrossRef] [PubMed]
8. Steffen, K.K.; Kennedy, B.K.; Kaeberlein, M. Measuring replicative life span in the budding yeast. *J. Vis. Exp.* **2009**, *28*, 1209. [CrossRef] [PubMed]
9. Smith, E.D.; Tsuchiya, M.; Fox, L.A.; Dang, N.; Hu, D.; Kerr, E.O.; Johnston, E.D.; Tchao, B.N.; Pak, D.N.; Welton, K.L.; et al. Quantitative evidence for conserved longevity pathways between divergent eukaryotic species. *Genome Res.* **2008**, *18*, 564–570. [CrossRef] [PubMed]
10. Ghavidel, A.; Baxi, K.; Ignatchenko, V.; Prusinkiewicz, M.; Arnason, T.G.; Kislinger, T.; Carvalho, C.E.; Harkness, T.A. A genome scale screen for mutants with delayed exit from mitosis: Ire1-independent induction of autophagy integrates ER homeostasis into mitotic lifespan. *PLoS Genet.* **2015**, *11*, e1005429. [CrossRef] [PubMed]
11. McCormick, M.A.; Delaney, J.R.; Tsuchiya, M.; Tsuchiyama, S.; Shemorry, A.; Sim, S.; Chou, A.C.; Ahmed, U.; Carr, D.; Murakami, C.J.; et al. A comprehensive analysis of replicative lifespan in 4698 single-gene deletion strains uncovers conserved mechanisms of aging. *Cell Metab.* **2015**, *22*, 895–906. [CrossRef] [PubMed]
12. Janssens, G.E.; Veenhoff, L.M. Evidence for the hallmarks of human aging in replicatively aging yeast. *Microb. Cell* **2016**, *3*, 263–274. [CrossRef] [PubMed]
13. Fabrizio, P.; Longo, V.D. The chronological life span of *Saccharomyces cerevisiae*. *Methods Mol. Biol.* **2007**, *371*, 89–95. [PubMed]
14. Longo, V.D.; Fabrizio, P. Chronological aging in *Saccharomyces cerevisiae*. *Subcell. Biochem.* **2012**, *57*, 101–121. [PubMed]
15. Burtner, C.R.; Murakami, C.J.; Kennedy, B.K.; Kaeberlein, M. A molecular mechanism of chronological aging in yeast. *Cell Cycle* **2009**, *8*, 1256–1270. [CrossRef] [PubMed]
16. Longo, V.D.; Kennedy, B.K. Sirtuins in aging and age-related disease. *Cell* **2006**, *126*, 257–268. [CrossRef] [PubMed]
17. Murakami, C.; Delaney, J.R.; Chou, A.; Carr, D.; Schleit, J.; Sutphin, G.L.; An, E.H.; Castanza, A.S.; Fletcher, M.; Goswami, S.; et al. pH neutralization protects against reduction in replicative lifespan following chronological aging in yeast. *Cell Cycle* **2012**, *11*, 3087–3096. [CrossRef] [PubMed]
18. Delaney, J.R.; Murakami, C.; Chou, A.; Carr, D.; Schleit, J.; Sutphin, G.L.; An, E.H.; Castanza, A.S.; Fletcher, M.; Goswami, S.; et al. Dietary restriction and mitochondrial function link replicative and chronological aging in *Saccharomyces cerevisiae*. *Exp. Gerontol.* **2013**, *48*, 1006–1013. [CrossRef] [PubMed]
19. Molon, M.; Zadrag-Tecza, R.; Bilinski, T. The longevity in the yeast *Saccharomyces cerevisiae*: A comparison of two approaches for assessment the lifespan. *Biochem. Biophys. Res. Commun.* **2015**, *460*, 651–656. [CrossRef] [PubMed]
20. Cai, L.; Tu, B.P. Driving the cell cycle through metabolism. *Annu. Rev. Cell Dev. Biol.* **2012**, *28*, 59–87. [CrossRef] [PubMed]
21. Titorenko, V.I.; Terlecky, S.R. Peroxisome metabolism and cellular aging. *Traffic* **2011**, *12*, 252–259. [CrossRef] [PubMed]
22. Beach, A.; Burstein, M.T.; Richard, V.R.; Leonov, A.; Levy, S.; Titorenko, V.I. Integration of peroxisomes into an endomembrane system that governs cellular aging. *Front. Physiol.* **2012**, *3*, 283. [CrossRef] [PubMed]

23. Leonov, A.; Titorenko, V.I. A network of interorganellar communications underlies cellular aging. *IUBMB Life* **2013**, *65*, 665–674. [CrossRef] [PubMed]
24. Huang, X.; Withers, B.R.; Dickson, R.C. Sphingolipids and lifespan regulation. *Biochim. Biophys. Acta* **2014**, *1841*, 657–664. [CrossRef] [PubMed]
25. Schroeder, S.; Zimmermann, A.; Carmona-Gutierrez, D.; Eisenberg, T.; Ruckenstuhl, C.; Andryushkova, A.; Pendl, T.; Harger, A.; Madeo, F. Metabolites in aging and autophagy. *Microb. Cell* **2014**, *1*, 110–114. [CrossRef] [PubMed]
26. Pietrocola, F.; Galluzzi, L.; Bravo-San Pedro, J.M.; Madeo, F.; Kroemer, G. Acetyl coenzyme A: A central metabolite and second messenger. *Cell Metab.* **2015**, *21*, 805–821. [CrossRef] [PubMed]
27. Dakik, P.; Titorenko, V.I. Communications between mitochondria, the nucleus, vacuoles, peroxisomes, the endoplasmic reticulum, the plasma membrane, lipid droplets, and the cytosol during yeast chronological aging. *Front. Genet.* **2016**, *7*, 177. [CrossRef] [PubMed]
28. Eltschinger, S.; Loewith, R. TOR complexes and the maintenance of cellular homeostasis. *Trends Cell Biol.* **2016**, *26*, 148–159. [CrossRef] [PubMed]
29. Teixeira, V.; Costa, V. Unraveling the role of the target of rapamycin signaling in sphingolipid metabolism. *Prog. Lipid Res.* **2016**, *61*, 109–133. [CrossRef] [PubMed]
30. Laxman, S. Conceptualizing eukaryotic metabolic sensing and signaling. *J. Indian Inst. Sci.* **2017**, *97*, 59–77. [CrossRef] [PubMed]
31. Li, X.; Handee, W.; Kuo, M.H. The slim, the fat, and the obese: Guess who lives the longest? *Curr. Genet.* **2017**, *63*, 43–49. [CrossRef] [PubMed]
32. Mitrofanova, D.; Dakik, P.; McAuley, M.; Medkour, Y.; Mohammad, K.; Titorenko, V.I. Lipid metabolism and transport define longevity of the yeast *Saccharomyces cerevisiae*. *Front. Biosci.* **2018**, *23*, 1166–1194.
33. Fraenkel, D.G. *Yeast Intermediary Metabolism*; Cold Spring Harbor Laboratory Press: Cold Spring Harbor, NY, USA, 2011; ISBN 978-0-87969-797-6.
34. Grant, C.M. Role of the glutathione/glutaredoxin and thioredoxin systems in yeast growth and response to stress conditions. *Mol. Microbiol.* **2001**, *39*, 533–541. [CrossRef] [PubMed]
35. Brandes, N.; Tienson, H.; Lindemann, A.; Vitvitsky, V.; Reichmann, D.; Banerjee, R.; Jakob, U. Time line of redox events in aging postmitotic cells. *Elife* **2013**, *2*, e00306. [CrossRef] [PubMed]
36. Wei, M.; Fabrizio, P.; Madia, F.; Hu, J.; Ge, H.; Li, L.M.; Longo, V.D. Tor1/Sch9-regulated carbon source substitution is as effective as calorie restriction in life span extension. *PLoS Genet.* **2009**, *5*, e1000467. [CrossRef] [PubMed]
37. Goldberg, A.A.; Bourque, S.D.; Kyryakov, P.; Gregg, C.; Boukh-Viner, T.; Beach, A.; Burstein, M.T.; Machkalyan, G.; Richard, V.; Rampersad, S.; et al. Effect of calorie restriction on the metabolic history of chronologically aging yeast. *Exp. Gerontol.* **2009**, *44*, 555–571. [CrossRef] [PubMed]
38. François, J.; Parrou, J.L. Reserve carbohydrates metabolism in the yeast *Saccharomyces cerevisiae*. *FEMS Microbiol. Rev.* **2001**, *25*, 125–145. [CrossRef] [PubMed]
39. Samokhvalov, V.; Ignatov, V.; Kondrashova, M. Reserve carbohydrates maintain the viability of *Saccharomyces cerevisiae* cells during chronological aging. *Mech. Ageing Dev.* **2004**, *125*, 229–235. [CrossRef] [PubMed]
40. Wang, J.; Jiang, J.C.; Jazwinski, S.M. Gene regulatory changes in yeast during life extension by nutrient limitation. *Exp. Gerontol.* **2010**, *45*, 621–631. [CrossRef] [PubMed]
41. Kyryakov, P.; Beach, A.; Richard, V.R.; Burstein, M.T.; Leonov, A.; Levy, S.; Titorenko, V.I. Caloric restriction extends yeast chronological lifespan by altering a pattern of age-related changes in trehalose concentration. *Front. Physiol.* **2012**, *3*, 256. [CrossRef] [PubMed]
42. Ocampo, A.; Liu, J.; Schroeder, E.A.; Shadel, G.S.; Barrientos, A. Mitochondrial respiratory thresholds regulate yeast chronological life span and its extension by caloric restriction. *Cell Metab.* **2012**, *16*, 55–67. [CrossRef] [PubMed]
43. Cao, L.; Tang, Y.; Quan, Z.; Zhang, Z.; Oliver, S.G.; Zhang, N. Chronological lifespan in yeast is dependent on the accumulation of storage carbohydrates mediated by Yak1, Mck1 and Rim15 kinases. *PLoS Genet.* **2016**, *12*, e1006458. [CrossRef] [PubMed]
44. Svenkrtova, A.; Belicova, L.; Volejnikova, A.; Sigler, K.; Jazwinski, S.M.; Pichova, A. Stratification of yeast cells during chronological aging by size points to the role of trehalose in cell vitality. *Biogerontology* **2016**, *17*, 395–408. [CrossRef] [PubMed]

45. Leonov, A.; Feldman, R.; Piano, A.; Arlia-Ciommo, A.; Lutchman, V.; Ahmadi, M.; Elsaser, S.; Fakim, H.; Heshmati-Moghaddam, M.; Hussain, A.; et al. Caloric restriction extends yeast chronological lifespan via a mechanism linking cellular aging to cell cycle regulation, maintenance of a quiescent state, entry into a non-quiescent state and survival in the non-quiescent state. *Oncotarget* **2017**, *8*, 69328–69350. [CrossRef] [PubMed]
46. Singer, M.A.; Lindquist, S. Multiple effects of trehalose on protein folding in vitro and in vivo. *Mol. Cell* **1998**, *1*, 639–648. [CrossRef]
47. Jain, N.K.; Roy, I. Effect of trehalose on protein structure. *Protein Sci.* **2009**, *18*, 24–36. [CrossRef] [PubMed]
48. Giorgio, M.; Trinei, M.; Migliaccio, E.; Pelicci, P.G. Hydrogen peroxide: A metabolic by-product or a common mediator of ageing signals? *Nat. Rev. Mol. Cell Biol.* **2007**, *8*, 722–728. [CrossRef] [PubMed]
49. Causton, H.C.; Ren, B.; Koh, S.S.; Harbison, C.T.; Kanin, E.; Jennings, E.G.; Lee, T.I.; True, H.L.; Lander, E.S.; Young, R.A. Remodeling of yeast genome expression in response to environmental changes. *Mol. Biol. Cell* **2001**, *12*, 323–337. [CrossRef] [PubMed]
50. Fabrizio, P.; Pozza, F.; Pletcher, S.D.; Gendron, C.M.; Longo, V.D. Regulation of longevity and stress resistance by Sch9 in yeast. *Science* **2001**, *292*, 288–290. [CrossRef] [PubMed]
51. Schroeder, E.A.; Raimundo, N.; Shadel, G.S. Epigenetic silencing mediates mitochondria stress-induced longevity. *Cell Metab.* **2013**, *17*, 954–964. [CrossRef] [PubMed]
52. Schroeder, E.A.; Shadel, G.S. Crosstalk between mitochondrial stress signals regulates yeast chronological lifespan. *Mech. Ageing Dev.* **2014**, *135*, 41–49. [CrossRef] [PubMed]
53. Crespo, J.L.; Powers, T.; Fowler, B.; Hall, M.N. The TOR-controlled transcription activators GLN3, RTG1, and RTG3 are regulated in response to intracellular levels of glutamine. *Proc. Natl. Acad. Sci. USA* **2002**, *99*, 6784–6789. [CrossRef] [PubMed]
54. Powers, R.W., 3rd; Kaeberlein, M.; Caldwell, S.D.; Kennedy, B.K.; Fields, S. Extension of chronological life span in yeast by decreased TOR pathway signaling. *Genes Dev.* **2006**, *20*, 174–184. [CrossRef] [PubMed]
55. Conrad, M.; Schothorst, J.; Kankipati, H.N.; Van Zeebroeck, G.; Rubio-Texeira, M.; Thevelein, J.M. Nutrient sensing and signaling in the yeast *Saccharomyces cerevisiae*. *FEMS Microbiol. Rev.* **2014**, *38*, 254–299. [CrossRef] [PubMed]
56. Swinnen, E.; Ghillebert, R.; Wilms, T.; Winderickx, J. Molecular mechanisms linking the evolutionary conserved TORC1-Sch9 nutrient signalling branch to lifespan regulation in *Saccharomyces cerevisiae*. *FEMS Yeast Res.* **2014**, *14*, 17–32. [CrossRef] [PubMed]
57. Urban, J.; Soulard, A.; Huber, A.; Lippman, S.; Mukhopadhyay, D.; Deloche, O.; Wanke, V.; Anrather, D.; Ammerer, G.; Riezman, H.; et al. Sch9 is a major target of TORC1 in *Saccharomyces cerevisiae*. *Mol. Cell* **2007**, *26*, 663–674. [CrossRef] [PubMed]
58. Huber, A.; Bodenmiller, B.; Uotila, A.; Stahl, M.; Wanka, S.; Gerrits, B.; Aebersold, R.; Loewith, R. Characterization of the rapamycin-sensitive phosphoproteome reveals that Sch9 is a central coordinator of protein synthesis. *Genes Dev.* **2009**, *23*, 1929–1943. [CrossRef] [PubMed]
59. Lee, J.; Moir, R.D.; Willis, I.M. Regulation of RNA polymerase III transcription involves SCH9-dependent and SCH9-independent branches of the target of rapamycin (TOR) pathway. *J. Biol. Chem.* **2009**, *284*, 12604–12608. [CrossRef] [PubMed]
60. Wei, Y.; Zheng, X.F. Sch9 partially mediates TORC1 signaling to control ribosomal RNA synthesis. *Cell Cycle* **2009**, *8*, 4085–4090. [CrossRef] [PubMed]
61. Bonawitz, N.D.; Chatenay-Lapointe, M.; Pan, Y.; Shadel, G.S. Reduced TOR signaling extends chronological life span via increased respiration and upregulation of mitochondrial gene expression. *Cell Metab.* **2007**, *5*, 265–277. [CrossRef] [PubMed]
62. Pan, Y.; Shadel, G.S. Extension of chronological life span by reduced TOR signaling requires down-regulation of Sch9p and involves increased mitochondrial OXPHOS complex density. *Aging* **2009**, *1*, 131–145. [CrossRef] [PubMed]
63. Roosen, J.; Engelen, K.; Marchal, K.; Mathys, J.; Griffioen, G.; Cameroni, E.; Thevelein, J.M.; de Virgilio, C.; de Moor, B.; Winderickx, J. PKA and Sch9 control a molecular switch important for the proper adaptation to nutrient availability. *Mol. Microbiol.* **2005**, *55*, 862–880. [CrossRef] [PubMed]
64. Wanke, V.; Cameroni, E.; Uotila, A.; Piccolis, M.; Urban, J.; Loewith, R.; de Virgilio, C. Caffeine extends yeast lifespan by targeting TORC1. *Mol. Microbiol.* **2008**, *69*, 277–285. [CrossRef] [PubMed]

65. Smets, B.; Ghillebert, R.; de Snijder, P.; Binda, M.; Swinnen, E.; de Virgilio, C.; Winderickx, J. Life in the midst of scarcity: Adaptations to nutrient availability in *Saccharomyces cerevisiae*. *Curr. Genet.* **2010**, *56*, 1–32. [CrossRef] [PubMed]
66. Medvedik, O.; Lamming, D.W.; Kim, K.D.; Sinclair, D.A. MSN2 and MSN4 link calorie restriction and TOR to sirtuin-mediated lifespan extension in *Saccharomyces cerevisiae*. *PLoS Biol.* **2007**, *5*, e261. [CrossRef] [PubMed]
67. Lee, P.; Cho, B.R.; Joo, H.S.; Hahn, J.S. Yeast Yak1 kinase, a bridge between PKA and stress-responsive transcription factors, Hsf1 and Msn2/Msn4. *Mol. Microbiol.* **2008**, *70*, 882–895. [CrossRef] [PubMed]
68. Broach, J.R. Nutritional control of growth and development in yeast. *Genetics* **2012**, *192*, 73–105. [CrossRef] [PubMed]
69. Laplante, M.; Sabatini, D.M. mTOR signaling in growth control and disease. *Cell* **2012**, *149*, 274–293. [CrossRef] [PubMed]
70. Alers, S.; Wesselborg, S.; Stork, B. ATG13: Just a companion, or an executor of the autophagic program? *Autophagy* **2014**, *10*, 944–956. [CrossRef] [PubMed]
71. Yorimitsu, T.; Zaman, S.; Broach, J.R.; Klionsky, D.J. Protein kinase A and Sch9 cooperatively regulate induction of autophagy in *Saccharomyces cerevisiae*. *Mol. Biol. Cell* **2007**, *18*, 4180–4189. [CrossRef] [PubMed]
72. Stephan, J.S.; Yeh, Y.Y.; Ramachandran, V.; Deminoff, S.J.; Herman, P.K. The Tor and PKA signaling pathways independently target the Atg1/Atg13 protein kinase complex to control autophagy. *Proc. Natl. Acad. Sci. USA* **2009**, *106*, 17049–17054. [CrossRef] [PubMed]
73. Stephan, J.S.; Yeh, Y.Y.; Ramachandran, V.; Deminoff, S.J.; Herman, P.K. The Tor and cAMP-dependent protein kinase signaling pathways coordinately control autophagy in *Saccharomyces cerevisiae*. *Autophagy* **2010**, *6*, 294–295. [CrossRef] [PubMed]
74. Johnson, J.E.; Johnson, F.B. Methionine restriction activates the retrograde response and confers both stress tolerance and lifespan extension to yeast, mouse and human cells. *PLoS ONE* **2014**, *9*, e97729. [CrossRef] [PubMed]
75. Ruckenstuhl, C.; Netzberger, C.; Entfellner, I.; Carmona-Gutierrez, D.; Kickenweiz, T.; Stekovic, S.; Gleixner, C.; Schmid, C.; Klug, L.; Sorgo, A.G.; et al. Lifespan extension by methionine restriction requires autophagy-dependent vacuolar acidification. *PLoS Genet.* **2014**, *10*, e1004347. [CrossRef] [PubMed]
76. Wu, Z.; Song, L.; Liu, S.Q.; Huang, D. Independent and additive effects of glutamic acid and methionine on yeast longevity. *PLoS ONE* **2013**, *8*, e79319. [CrossRef] [PubMed]
77. Ruckenstuhl, C.; Netzberger, C.; Entfellner, I.; Carmona-Gutierrez, D.; Kickenweiz, T.; Stekovic, S.; Gleixner, C.; Schmid, C.; Klug, L.; Hajnal, I.; et al. Autophagy extends lifespan via vacuolar acidification. *Microb. Cell* **2014**, *1*, 160–162. [CrossRef] [PubMed]
78. Liu, K.; Zhang, X.; Lester, R.L.; Dickson, R.C. The sphingoid long chain base phytosphingosine activates AGC-type protein kinases in *Saccharomyces cerevisiae* including Ypk1, Ypk2, and Sch9. *J. Biol. Chem.* **2005**, *280*, 22679–22687. [CrossRef] [PubMed]
79. Liu, K.; Zhang, X.; Sumanasekera, C.; Lester, R.L.; Dickson, R.C. Signalling functions for sphingolipid long-chain bases in *Saccharomyces cerevisiae*. *Biochem. Soc. Trans.* **2005**, *33*, 1170–1173. [CrossRef] [PubMed]
80. Huang, X.; Liu, J.; Dickson, R.C. Down-regulating sphingolipid synthesis increases yeast lifespan. *PLoS Genet.* **2012**, *8*, e1002493. [CrossRef] [PubMed]
81. Liu, J.; Huang, X.; Withers, B.R.; Blalock, E.; Liu, K.; Dickson, R.C. Reducing sphingolipid synthesis orchestrates global changes to extend yeast lifespan. *Aging Cell* **2013**, *12*, 833–841. [CrossRef] [PubMed]
82. Eisenberg, T.; Knauer, H.; Schauer, A.; Büttner, S.; Ruckenstuhl, C.; Carmona-Gutierrez, D.; Ring, J.; Schroeder, S.; Magnes, C.; Antonacci, L.; et al. Induction of autophagy by spermidine promotes longevity. *Nat. Cell Biol.* **2009**, *11*, 1305–1314. [CrossRef] [PubMed]
83. Morselli, E.; Galluzzi, L.; Kepp, O.; Criollo, A.; Maiuri, M.C.; Tavernarakis, N.; Madeo, F.; Kroemer, G. Autophagy mediates pharmacological lifespan extension by spermidine and resveratrol. *Aging* **2009**, *1*, 961–970. [CrossRef] [PubMed]
84. Minois, N.; Carmona-Gutierrez, D.; Madeo, F. Polyamines in aging and disease. *Aging* **2011**, *3*, 716–732. [CrossRef] [PubMed]
85. Hine, C.; Harputlugil, E.; Zhang, Y.; Ruckenstuhl, C.; Lee, B.C.; Brace, L.; Longchamp, A.; Treviño-Villarreal, J.H.; Mejia, P.; Ozaki, C.K.; et al. Endogenous hydrogen sulfide production is essential for dietary restriction benefits. *Cell* **2015**, *160*, 132–144. [CrossRef] [PubMed]

86. De Cabo, R.; Carmona-Gutierrez, D.; Bernier, M.; Hall, M.N.; Madeo, F. The search for antiaging interventions: From elixirs to fasting regimens. *Cell* **2014**, *157*, 1515–1526. [CrossRef] [PubMed]
87. Lee, C.; Longo, V. Dietary restriction with and without caloric restriction for healthy aging. *F1000Res.* **2016**, *5*. [CrossRef] [PubMed]
88. Hine, C.; Mitchell, J.R. Calorie restriction and methionine restriction in control of endogenous hydrogen sulfide production by the transsulfuration pathway. *Exp. Gerontol.* **2015**, *68*, 26–32. [CrossRef] [PubMed]
89. Shim, H.S.; Longo, V.D. A protein restriction-dependent sulfur code for longevity. *Cell* **2015**, *160*, 15–17. [CrossRef] [PubMed]
90. Burhans, W.C.; Weinberger, M. Acetic acid effects on aging in budding yeast: Are they relevant to aging in higher eukaryotes? *Cell Cycle* **2009**, *8*, 2300–2302. [CrossRef] [PubMed]
91. Burtner, C.R.; Murakami, C.J.; Olsen, B.; Kennedy, B.K.; Kaeberlein, M. A genomic analysis of chronological longevity factors in budding yeast. *Cell Cycle* **2011**, *10*, 1385–1396. [CrossRef] [PubMed]
92. Mirisola, M.G.; Longo, V.D. Acetic acid and acidification accelerate chronological and replicative aging in yeast. *Cell Cycle* **2012**, *11*, 3532–3533. [CrossRef] [PubMed]
93. Giannattasio, S.; Guaragnella, N.; Zdralević, M.; Marra, E. Molecular mechanisms of *Saccharomyces cerevisiae* stress adaptation and programmed cell death in response to acetic acid. *Front. Microbiol.* **2013**, *4*, 33. [CrossRef] [PubMed]
94. Falcone, C.; Mazzoni, C. External and internal triggers of cell death in yeast. *Cell. Mol. Life Sci.* **2016**, *73*, 2237–2250. [CrossRef] [PubMed]
95. Eisenberg, T.; Schroeder, S.; Andryushkova, A.; Pendl, T.; Küttner, V.; Bhukel, A.; Mariño, G.; Pietrocola, F.; Harger, A.; Zimmermann, A.; et al. Nucleocytosolic depletion of the energy metabolite acetyl-coenzyme A stimulates autophagy and prolongs lifespan. *Cell Metab.* **2014**, *19*, 431–444. [CrossRef] [PubMed]
96. Mariño, G.; Pietrocola, F.; Eisenberg, T.; Kong, Y.; Malik, S.A.; Andryushkova, A.; Schroeder, S.; Pendl, T.; Harger, A.; Niso-Santano, M.; et al. Regulation of autophagy by cytosolic acetyl-coenzyme A. *Mol. Cell* **2014**, *53*, 710–725. [CrossRef] [PubMed]
97. Fabrizio, P.; Gattazzo, C.; Battistella, L.; Wei, M.; Cheng, C.; McGrew, K.; Longo, V.D. Sir2 blocks extreme life-span extension. *Cell* **2005**, *123*, 655–667. [CrossRef] [PubMed]
98. Richard, V.R.; Beach, A.; Piano, A.; Leonov, A.; Feldman, R.; Burstein, M.T.; Kyryakov, P.; Gomez-Perez, A.; Arlia-Ciommo, A.; Baptista, S.; et al. Mechanism of liponecrosis, a distinct mode of programmed cell death. *Cell Cycle* **2014**, *13*, 3707–3726. [CrossRef] [PubMed]
99. Sheibani, S.; Richard, V.R.; Beach, A.; Leonov, A.; Feldman, R.; Mattie, S.; Khelghatybana, L.; Piano, A.; Greenwood, M.; Vali, H.; et al. Macromitophagy, neutral lipids synthesis, and peroxisomal fatty acid oxidation protect yeast from "liponecrosis", a previously unknown form of programmed cell death. *Cell Cycle* **2014**, *13*, 138–147. [CrossRef] [PubMed]
100. Mohammad, K.; Dakik, P.; Medkour, Y.; McAuley, M.; Mitrofanova, D.; Titorenko, V.I. Yeast cells exposed to exogenous palmitoleic acid either adapt to stress and survive or commit to regulated liponecrosis and die. *Oxid. Med. Cell. Longev.* **2018**, *2018*. [CrossRef]
101. Beach, A.; Titorenko, V.I. In search of housekeeping pathways that regulate longevity. *Cell Cycle* **2011**, *10*, 3042–3044. [CrossRef] [PubMed]
102. Medkour, Y.; Svistkova, V.; Titorenko, V.I. Cell-nonautonomous mechanisms underlying cellular and organismal aging. *Int. Rev. Cell Mol. Biol.* **2016**, *321*, 259–297. [PubMed]
103. Burstein, M.T.; Kyryakov, P.; Beach, A.; Richard, V.R.; Koupaki, O.; Gomez-Perez, A.; Leonov, A.; Levy, S.; Noohi, F.; Titorenko, V.I. Lithocholic acid extends longevity of chronologically aging yeast only if added at certain critical periods of their lifespan. *Cell Cycle* **2012**, *11*, 3443–3462. [CrossRef] [PubMed]
104. Cantley, L.; Hunter, T.; Sever, R.; Thorner, J. *Signal Transduction: Principles, Pathways, and Processes;* Cold Spring Harbor Laboratory Press: Cold Spring Harbor, NY, USA, 2014; ISBN 978-0-87969-901-7.
105. Lim, W.; Mayer, B.; Pawson, T. *Cell Signaling: Principles and Mechanisms*; Garland Science: New York, NY, USA, 2015; ISBN 978-0-8153-4244-1.

8

Aging, Melatonin and the Pro- and Anti-Inflammatory Networks

Rüdiger Hardeland

Johann Friedrich Blumenbach Institute of Zoology and Anthropology, University of Göttingen, 37073 Göttingen, Germany; rhardel@gwdg.de

Abstract: Aging and various age-related diseases are associated with reductions in melatonin secretion, proinflammatory changes in the immune system, a deteriorating circadian system, and reductions in sirtuin-1 (SIRT1) activity. In non-tumor cells, several effects of melatonin are abolished by inhibiting SIRT1, indicating mediation by SIRT1. Melatonin is, in addition to its circadian and antioxidant roles, an immune stimulatory agent. However, it can act as either a pro- or anti-inflammatory regulator in a context-dependent way. Melatonin can stimulate the release of proinflammatory cytokines and other mediators, but also, under different conditions, it can suppress inflammation-promoting processes such as NO release, activation of cyclooxygenase-2, inflammasome NLRP3, gasdermin D, toll-like receptor-4 and mTOR signaling, and cytokine release by SASP (senescence-associated secretory phenotype), and amyloid-β toxicity. It also activates processes in an anti-inflammatory network, in which SIRT1 activation, upregulation of Nrf2 and downregulation of NF-κB, and release of the anti-inflammatory cytokines IL-4 and IL-10 are involved. A perhaps crucial action may be the promotion of macrophage or microglia polarization in favor of the anti-inflammatory phenotype M2. In addition, many factors of the pro- and anti-inflammatory networks are subject to regulation by microRNAs that either target mRNAs of the respective factors or upregulate them by targeting mRNAs of their inhibitor proteins.

Keywords: circadian; immunosenescence; inflammaging; melatonin; microRNAs; sirtuin-1

---

1. Introduction

Aging is associated with manifold changes. These comprise declined secretion of hormones such as melatonin [1,2], reduced activities of aging-related factors such as sirtuin-1 (SIRT1) [3], deterioration of the circadian oscillator system [4,5], multiple alterations in the immune system that is frequently shifted toward the proinflammatory side [6–10], and many more deviations of cell biological relevance. Importantly, the changes specifically mentioned are interrelated in multiple ways [3,5,9,10]. This is largely based on the pleiotropy of both melatonin [11] and the circadian system [12–14]. However, these relationships are highly complex, include actions in opposite directions, and cannot be interpreted in reductionist ways.

For example, the effects of melatonin in the immune system can be either pro- or anti-inflammatory [15–17]. Generally, melatonin acts as an immune stimulatory agent and the direction into which the balance is shifted has turned out to be highly conditional. The influence of melatonin on SIRT1 expression has also revealed effects of either down- or upregulation, in this case, with a remarkable difference between tumor and non-tumor cells [5]. While being strongly suppressive in cancer, melatonin mainly stimulated SIRT1 in nontransformed cells, especially in the context of aging. However, a considerable problem exists concerning the, unfortunately, prevailing determination of SIRT1 expression rather than activity. Assuming a correlation between expression and activity, which is questionable, is a profound misconception in the case of sirtuins [18]. Sirtuin activities are not primarily determined by their protein levels but rather by NAD^+ concentration, which depends on the activity of nicotinamide phosphoribosyltransferase (NAMPT) [19–22]. The contrast between SIRT1 expression and activity has become evident in a study on the effect of BRCA1 (breast cancer 1, early onset) in ovarian cancer [23]. Suppression of BRCA1 reduced SIRT1 expression, but it increased NAD^+ concentration and, therefore, SIRT1 activity. Moreover, BRCA1 overexpression upregulated SIRT1 expression and decreased NAD^+ levels and SIRT1 activity. This divergence also seems to be relevant to aging. SIRT1 expression was not generally shown to be decreased in the course of aging, but rather, it was shown to often increase. Nevertheless, SIRT1 activity was found to be reduced because of lowered NAD^+ levels [24,25]. However, this does not yet mean that positive correlations between SIRT1 expression and activity are generally excluded in the context of aging. In senescence-accelerated SAMP8 mice, SIRT1 expression was found to be reduced relative to the widely isogenic control strain SAMR1 [26]. Moreover, a number of studies have shown that effects of melatonin that increased SIRT1 expression were suppressed by sirtuin inhibitors such as sirtinol or EX527 [27–39]. Therefore, mandatory requirements are to either determine SIRT1 activity and NAD^+ concentration (recommended) or to at least test the effects of sirtuin inhibitors [18].

The changes in melatonin secretion and SIRT1 activity also have a circadian dimension. Both of them are under circadian control and exhibit cycles of high amplitudes. Moreover, either of them can influence circadian oscillators. Apart from its known chronobiotic actions via the suprachiasmatic nucleus (SCN), melatonin also influences peripheral oscillators [40]. SIRT1 has been identified as an accessory oscillator component [19–21] that increases circadian amplitudes of both central and peripheral clocks [21,41]. At least one of the mechanisms described is of relevance for antagonizing age-related decreases in the amplitudes of the SCN output [41]. An additional aspect concerns the conclusion that SIRT1 acts as a partial mediator of melatonin effects [18,42]. Finally, it seems important to remain aware of the different phases of increases and decreases observed within a circadian cycle. It is basic knowledge of chronobiology that a specific treatment applied in different phases leads to different, often opposite, effects [5]. In the context of aging, additional difficulty results from the fact of non-identical changes observed between the populations of oscillators within the body. In a senescent mammal, some oscillators exhibit phase changes, others reduced amplitudes, in the extreme, down to arrhythmicity, whereas others remain widely unchanged [4]. Collectively, all these variabilities summarized here oppose any expectation of finding exclusively unidirectional relationships by applying melatonin, sirtuin overexpression, or other modulators of circadian rhythms.

These reservations also have to be kept in mind when considering the effects of melatonin and SIRT1 in the regulation of pro- and anti-inflammatory processes. These are of particular relevance to aging and age-related diseases, especially as proinflammatory mechanisms gain increasing importance in the course of senescence. The overlapping effects of melatonin and SIRT1 in the field of inflammation regulation will be discussed in this article.

2. Melatonin and the Proinflammatory Network

In the course of studies that revealed numerous effects of melatonin beyond the control of circadian oscillators, immunological actions of melatonin were also discovered [9,15,43–46]. However, the statement that melatonin possesses properties that exceed the control of oscillators does not mean that the resulting effects are independent of circadian rhythms. Both melatonin secretion and signaling are subjected to circadian control. Parameters affected, including immunological ones, are also influenced by the circadian system [11,47]. With regard to the immune system, the situation is somewhat more complicated as melatonin is also synthesized by several types of leukocytes [11,44,48,49].

Many of the earlier investigations on melatonin in the immune system revealed proinflammatory effects, as repeatedly summarized [11,15,17,44]. Notably, these actions were predominantly discovered in studies using isolated leukocytes or transformed leukocyte-derived cell lines [16,17,44]. Although such an approach appears to be reasonable in the beginning, it may not sufficiently reflect the complexity of the immune system and the additional participation of, in classical terms, non-immune cells in both proinflammatory responses and the regulation of the pro-/anti-inflammatory balance. Data obtained in humans also indicated proinflammatory actions of melatonin in rheumatoid arthritis [50–52]. These findings were regarded as a general caveat concerning the use of the immune stimulator melatonin in autoimmune diseases. This view has received partial support by a study in a multiple sclerosis model [53]. Most of the earlier findings on proinflammatory effects in cell cultures concerned the upregulation of proinflammatory cytokines (IL-1β, IL-2, IL-6, IL-8, IL-12, IFNγ, and TNFα) and downregulation of their anti-inflammatory counterpart (IL-10), as summarized elsewhere [15,16,44]. Additionally, melatonin was shown to counteract the inhibition of IL-2 production by prostaglandin E_2 in human lymphocytes [54].

However, this short overview of the inflammation-promoting effects does not yet sufficiently describe the actions of melatonin within the proinflammatory network. In fact, these actions also comprise numerous suppressive changes in this network and, thereby, can turn out to result in an anti-inflammatory balance. To appropriately judge the complex influences of melatonin, it is necessary to view it under these different, additional perspectives: (1) changes in tissues and their main cellular constituents; (2) cell specificity; (3) effects on clonal expansion, differentiation, and polarization in the immune system; (4) contributing proinflammatory effects of non-immune cells; and (5) conditionality, with regard to high-grade or low-grade inflammatory challenges that may occur in the progression of aging or by experimental procedures.

As recently summarized, melatonin-induced elevation of proinflammatory cytokines, such as IL-1β, IL-2, IL-6, IL-12, TNFα, and IFNγ, has been repeatedly observed in monocytes, monocyte-derived cell lines, and type 1 T-helper cells [17]. One can assume that similar responses occur in M1 macrophages, M1 microglia and, especially concerning IL-6, IL-8, and TNFα, also in epithelial cells and various other cell types. Notably, these findings can be seen in the context of pro-oxidant and cytotoxic effects exerted by melatonin in monocytes, as observed above an activation threshold as low as 50 pM [55]. Moreover, melatonin was found to increase another proinflammatory cytokine, IL-17A, in Th17 cells [56], an effect that spreads proinflammatory responses by inducing the release of other mediators, such as IL-1β, IL-6, TNFα, the neutrophil-attracting Il-8, and by upregulating cyclooxygenase-2 (COX-2) and iNOS (inducible NO synthase) [57–65]. This host of secondary effects by IL-17A has been shown to be involved in autoimmune diseases and in neuroinflammation and is, therefore, of relevance to age-related health problems and to adverse effects of melatonin, especially in autoimmunity. Additionally, melatonin was shown to upregulate IL-1β, TNFα, and IFNγ in splenocytes [66]. Several other effects of melatonin concern the upregulation of cytokines that are primarily involved in differentiation and clonal expansion, such as M-CSF (macrophage colony-stimulating factor) and SCF (stem cell factor) in macrophages and splenocytes, TGFβ (transforming growth factor) in macrophages and dendritic cells, and thymosin-α and thymulin in thymocytes, as summarized elsewhere [16]. Melatonin was shown to promote differentiation of progenitor cells to Th lymphocytes, NK lymphocytes, granulocytes, and macrophages [16,44, 45]. All these effects may have secondary consequences to the pro-/anti-inflammatory balance. In bone marrow, an upregulation of GM-CSF (granulocyte/monocyte colony-stimulating factor) may be interpreted in a similar way, but, on the other hand, melatonin-induced release of the immune-opioids MIO15 (melatonin-induced opioid) and MIO67 [16,67–69] can be expected to favor the anti-inflammatory side of the immune system.

The proinflammatory network comprises numerous components, which are regulated differently by melatonin. Moreover, the responses are often highly contextual. Findings obtained by applying pro-oxidant or proinflammatory challenges, such as administration of oxidotoxins, mitotoxins, bacterial lipopolysaccharides (LPS) or experimental sepsis, may not lead to results comparable to those found in aging. Therefore, it seems important to focus on changes that really occur in aging or age-related diseases and can be mostly classified as low-grade inflammation [10,17,70]. Several sources of aging-related inflammation shall be mentioned as being of foremost importance: (1) enhanced release of proinflammatory cytokines as a consequence of immunosenescence; (2) neuronal overexcitation in an $^{\bullet}$NO-mediated interplay with microglia and astrocytes; (3) amyloid-β (Aβ) toxicity; (4) brain insulin resistance; (5) diabetes and metabolic syndrome; (6) senescence-associated secretory phenotype (SASP) of non-immune cells with DNA damage response (DDR); (7) garb-aging; (8) reduced antioxidant protection by decreased melatonin; and, presumably, also (9) metabolic malfunction because of poorly coordinated and weakened circadian rhythms. Notably, all these pathophysiological alterations are associated with oxidative and nitrosative/nitrative stress and mitochondrial malfunction. They have multiple interconnections and, thereby, display the potential of forming vicious cycles [10,17,70].

Immunosenescence, which is primarily associated with thymic involution and, additionally, exhaustion of leukocyte subpopulations upon lifelong exposure to foreign antigens, typically leads to a shift toward a proinflammatory phenotype, which is evident by increased levels of proinflammatory cytokines that may result in a so-called immune risk profile [7,10,70–73]. Neuronal overexcitation causes increased formation of $^{\bullet}$NO, which can activate microglia, astrocytes, and other neurons that also release $^{\bullet}$NO at elevated rates. These responses contribute to a spreading of excitation and to the release of oxidants and proinflammatory mediators, especially by microglia. High levels of $^{\bullet}$NO and superoxide anions ($O_2^{\bullet-}$) generate the formation of their adduct, peroxynitrite ($ONOO^-$), a highly reactive intermediate that causes damage to mitochondria and additionally generates free radicals ($ONOO^- + H^+ \rightarrow ONOOH \rightarrow {}^{\bullet}NO_2 + {}^{\bullet}OH$; $ONOO^- + CO_2 \rightarrow ONOOCO_2^- \rightarrow {}^{\bullet}NO_2 + CO_3^{\bullet-}$) [74,75]. These radicals, their precursors, and several other reactive nitrogen species that can be formed from them interfere with the mitochondrial electron transport chain (ETC) [74,76,77]. As recently summarized, melatonin protects the ETC against these reactive intermediates [77], in addition to various other mitochondria-protecting actions [78–83]. Aβ peptides have, besides other effects, pro-oxidant and proinflammatory properties. The main toxicity is caused by Aβ monomers and oligomers, with an additional contribution by amyloid plaques. Peptides and oligomers induce microglia activation [84,85] and, additionally, responses by astrocytes [86] and neurons [86,87], which all upregulate NADPH oxidase, thereby elevating $O_2^{\bullet-}$ formation. Notably, the release of proinflammatory mediators in response to Aβ is not restricted to microglia. Even neurons have been shown to respond to Aβ peptides by upregulating TNFα, IL-1β, COX-2, and the T-cell and monocyte attractant chemokine CX3CL1 [87]. Aβ toxicity should not only be seen in the context of established Alzheimer's disease (AD), since these peptides also appear in the CSF (cerebrospinal fluid) of healthy subjects, but are normally widely removed by clearance of CSF and ISF (interstitial fluid), especially during sleep [88–91]. Sleep disturbance impairs Aβ clearance, which has been discussed as a contribution to the development of AD pathology [92]. Circadian disruption, a major source of sleep disturbances, indicates that changes in melatonin secretion may be involved. In fact, melatonin has been recently shown to increase Aβ clearance [93,94]. Numerous other anti-amyloidogenic effects of melatonin have been also described and repeatedly reviewed [70,95–98]. A recent overview [17] has particularly focused on the anti-inflammatory aspect and the suppression of Aβ secretion by melatonin. This includes, in cellular test systems, the reduction of βAPP (β-amyloid precursor protein) mRNA expression [99], inhibition of β- and γ-secretases [100], and the upregulation of α-secretase, an enzyme that competes with β- and γ-secretases and produces the nonamyloidogenic and neuroprotective fragment sAPPα [101]. The shift from β- and γ-secretases to α-secretase was recently also confirmed in the hippocampus of senescent mice [102,103]. In transgenic AD mouse models, melatonin was found to substantially delay the accumulation of Aβ and to extend lifespan [104,105]. However, this was only observed after an early onset of treatment in the first months of life, but not at later age [106], findings that leave a pessimistic perspective for the treatment of humans. Another, surprising nexus to AD pathology and inflammation emerged, when brain insulin resistance was shown to be an early sign of neuroinflammation at the onset of AD [107,108]. For further details and references, see [17,109]. This aspect remains to be studied in the context of melatonin, but would require a strict discrimination between nocturnal rodents and humans, since the disregard of this difference has led to substantial misinterpretations concerning the beneficial or detrimental role of melatonin in type 2 diabetes [5,16]. Also, beyond the CNS, type 2 diabetes and, in a broader sense, metabolic syndrome, are associated with low-grade inflammation, a phenomenon known under the term of metaflammation [110–112], which contributes to inflammaging [111,112]. Numerous beneficial effects of melatonin in metabolic syndrome have been recently summarized [113], which have been observed in both experimental animals and clinical studies and indicate a reduction of metaflammation.

Another aspect of proinflammatory effects concerns the role of non-immune cells in inflammaging. This comprises mainly three processes, SASP, garb-aging, and release of macromolecules from dying cells. In SASP, DNA-damaged cells are arrested in terms of proliferation, but continue to participate in the metabolism of the tissue. However, they release several signal molecules, including proinflammatory cytokines and chemokines, thereby inducing local, low-grade inflammation [114–118]. SASP has been observed in many cells of peripheral tissues, but also in astrocytes and is, therefore, relevant to the CNS [70,119,120]. Notably, SASP has also been shown to be induced by sleep disruption [121]. As this was associated with increased oxidative stress, the observed changes may comprise a chronodisruption-related nocturnal loss of protection by melatonin. Studies on direct effects of melatonin against SASP are still in their infancy, but recent initial results have described this [122–124]. In mechanistic terms, melatonin was shown to suppress the PARP-1 [poly(ADP-ribose) polymerase-1]-induced expression of SASP genes [122]. Whether or not this role of PARP-1 can be generalized remains to be clarified, since this regulator, which is an indicator of DNA damage, has also been interpreted as an epigenomic safeguard that interferes with SASP-associated microRNAs [125]. In another context, melatonin was reported to suppress SASP by downregulating NF-κB and upregulating Nrf2 (nuclear factor erythroid 2-related factor 2) [124], i.e., two known effects of melatonin that are typically observed in mechanisms of antioxidative and anti-inflammatory protection [17,126]. Other sources of low-grade inflammation by non-immune cells, such as garb-aging [127] and release of components of dying cells such as histone H1 [128] and molecules of mitochondrial origin (nucleic acids, *N*-formylated peptides and proteins) to the cytosol [129–132], are presumably also of substantial relevance to inflammaging, but have not been sufficiently studied in relation to melatonin. Nevertheless, this connection exists with high likelihood with regard to mitochondrial DNA (mtDNA), especially if it is damaged or oxidized. Activation of the NLRP3 inflammasome by mtDNA has been repeatedly described, whereas counteractions by melatonin have been multiply documented and reviewed, as summarized elsewhere [133]. Melatonin administration was shown to be as effective as NLRP3 deficiency [134]. Unfortunately, the important proinflammatory pathway of cGAS/STING (cyclic GMP-AMP synthase/stimulator of IFN genes) signaling has, to date, been poorly considered in melatonin research. This would be of particular interest, as cGAS is a cytosolic DNA detector. Moreover, the depletion of cGAS and STING counteracted cell senescence and prevented SASP in human and murine fibroblasts [135]. cGAS appears as a mediator of cell stress reactions and has been assumed to be involved in aging-related diseases [131]. This interpretation has received support by recent findings on a human *Sting* gene polymorphism that is associated with low-risk of aging-related diseases, presumably by reducing inflammaging [136].

Activation of the NLRP3 inflammasome in various systems, under different conditions and counteractions by melatonin, have been recently reviewed [17]. These findings were widely related to the suppression of NF-κB signaling by melatonin, which is likewise important in the attenuation of oxidative damage [126]. NF-κB was also reported to induce pyroptosis via gasdermin D (GSDMD) in adipose tissue, which was likewise inhibited by melatonin [137]. Other inflammation-related and melatonin-sensitive effects of NF-κB concern the upregulation of iNOS and COX-2 [138–141]. Moreover, in the context of presenilin-1 upregulation and pathogenic βAPP processing, a pathway involving PIN1 (peptidyl-prolyl cis-trans isomerase NIMA-interacting 1) and GSK3β (glycogen synthase kinase 3β) was shown to activate NF-κB, which was, in accordance with many other findings on NF-κB suppression, inhibited by melatonin [142].

Another proinflammatory route is based on TLR4 (toll-like receptor 4) activation, e.g., via the IFNγ adaptor protein, TRIF (toll-receptor-associated activator of interferon). In the macrophage-like cell line RAW264.7, melatonin has been shown to suppress the release of proinflammatory cytokines, such as TNFα, IL-1β, IL-6, and IL-8, by TRIF and TLR4 inhibition [143]. As TLR4 also mediates pro-oxidant actions via NF-κB, more general effects by melatonin on this pathway may be assumed. This conclusion is supported by several pertinent findings describing protection by melatonin [17]. Similar anti-inflammatory effects were also obtained in an in vivo model of ovarian cancer [144]. Information on melatonin effects concerning other TLR subforms is still scarce. No effects were found in a single study on TLR2 [144], whereas inhibition of TLR3 was reported [145,146].

A further possible proinflammatory pathway that is inhibited by melatonin concerns mTOR (mechanistic target of rapamycin) activation. However, most respective information is not directly related to inflammation, but rather to mitophagy or apoptosis. Interestingly, an mTOR inhibiting action by melatonin was also shown to be suppressed by inhibition of PIN1 [123]. Moreover, the attenuation of microglial activation and neuroinflammation after traumatic brain injury by melatonin was also interpreted on the basis of interference with mTOR [147]. This route will be of further interest in the specific context of melatonin's anti-inflammatory actions.

3. Melatonin, SIRT1, and the Anti-Inflammatory Network

While melatonin is partially acting by either stimulating or inhibiting components of the proinflammatory network, it also upregulates molecules of an anti-inflammatory network. Some of them are negatively correlated with proinflammatory agents. For instance, NF-κB, a transcription factor involved in prooxidant and, thereby, proinflammatory responses, is inversely coupled to antioxidant and anti-inflammatory regulators, in particular, Nrf2 [17,126,139,148–151]. A similar correlation seems to exist in the case of PARK7 (parkinsonism associated deglycase; also known as DJ-1) [149,150], a protein that acts, beside other effects, as a redox-sensitive chaperone and stress sensor. In Parkinson's disease (PD), it has been shown to be neuroprotective [152].

An especially important anti-inflammatory regulator under control by melatonin is SIRT1. It has been classified as a secondary signaling molecule that mediates several effects of melatonin [18,42]. In non-tumor cells, it has been shown to be upregulated by melatonin and effects by melatonin have been repeatedly reported to be suppressed by sirtuin inhibitors or *Sirt1* siRNA [5], notably also in an anti-inflammatory context [17]. The relationship between melatonin and SIRT1 may be regarded as a mutual one, since SIRT1 can enhance circadian amplitudes in the SCN [41] and may, thereby, influence the melatonin rhythm [3]. With this background, the functional overlap of described melatonin and SIRT1 actions seems worthwhile to be recalled.

This overlap becomes obvious from two lines of evidence, (1) the interference of sirtuin-related agents with melatonin effects, and (2) similar actions of melatonin and SIRT1. In the former context, reductions of NLRP3 inflammasome activation and IL-1β levels by melatonin were blocked by the sirtuin inhibitor EX527 in a rat COPD (chronic obstructive pulmonary disease) model [39]. The same inhibitor also blocked anti-inflammatory actions of melatonin such as downregulation of TNFα and IL-1β in acute kidney injury of rats [36]. Several other results on sirtuin inhibition of melatonin treatment were obtained under conditions of more severe inflammation. This was observed in cardiac ischemia/reperfusion of normal [30] and diabetic rats [31], correspondingly in ER stress of H9C2 cardiomyocytes [31], in LPS-treated microglial cell lines [37], and in brain injury by cecal ligation/puncture in mice [32]. Further studies, without measurement of inflammatory parameters, in which melatonin effects were blunted by sirtuin inhibitors or *Sirt1* siRNA, are summarized elsewhere [5,17].

Numerous studies have demonstrated antioxidant and anti-inflammatory actions by SIRT1 that are also known from melatonin [17]. This concerns the suppression of NF-κB activation [153–156], the upregulation of Nrf2 [157–161], suppression of NLRP3 inflammasome activation [39,162–165], and inhibition of TLR4 signaling [166–168]. An important player in TLR4 activation is HMGB1 (high mobility group box-1), an inflammatory signaling molecule released by monocytes and macrophages, and also by other cells (e.g., endothelial). SIRT1 is known to deacetylate HMGB1 [169,170], to inhibit its nucleocytoplasmic transfer, and to prevent its release [167,171–176]. Importantly, HMGB1 also favors the polarization of macrophages and microglia towards the proinflammatory M1 type [177–181]. With regard to the melatonin–SIRT1 relationship, it is of interest that anti-inflammatory actions via HMGB1 inhibition have been also reported for melatonin, as recently summarized [17]. Again, SIRT1 may mediate melatonin effects in this case, an assumption to be experimentally confirmed.

SIRT1 also displays several additional anti-inflammatory effects, which cannot yet be matched with corresponding data from melatonin treatment. As mentioned in the previous section, some reports on melatonin effects on mTOR signaling have not been directly related to inflammation. Other studies on actions of melatonin on mTORC1 (mTOR complex 1) activity in cancer cells led to contradictory results [182–184] and, therefore, do not provide a reliable basis for comparison. However, SIRT1 has been shown to counteract adipose inflammation by suppressing mTORC1 signaling [185]. Another investigation on liver steatosis reported an increase of mTORC1 activity upon hepatocyte-specific deletion of SIRT1 [186]. Under conditions of sepsis, SIRT1 was also reported to deacetylate and, thereby, inhibit NICD (intracellular domain of Notch) [187,188]. Apart from its developmental roles, Notch is known to act in a proinflammatory way by promoting M1 polarization of macrophages or related cells. Conversely, SIRT1 knockdown upregulated Notch1 in stellate cells at both mRNA and protein levels [189]. However, the relationship to melatonin remains unclear because beneficial effects of Notch signaling were reported in studies on protection against ischemia/reperfusion and Aβ toxicity by melatonin [190–192], in spite of the fact that Notch activation is known to cause inflammatory responses. Either the endpoints studied were unrelated to macrophages or microglia, respectively, or Notch signaling may be a case in which SIRT1 does not mediate melatonin effects. This would be surprising, as melatonin was shown to upregulate SIRT1 under conditions of ischemia/reperfusion, and as some of the melatonin effects were blocked by EX527 or *Sirt1* siRNA [5,30,31].

Another recently reported anti-inflammatory action of SIRT1 has been observed in macrophages after treatment with LPS. The lncRNA-CCL2, which is related to the gene locus of the chemokine CCL2 and stimulates the release of proinflammatory cytokines, was downregulated by SIRT1 [193]. No corresponding data on changes of lncRNA-CCL2 expression by melatonin are actually available.

Despite the fact that many proinflammatory effects of melatonin are mediated by lymphocytes [15,44,49,54,56], such responses were also obtained in monocytes and monocyte-derived cells [11,15,44]. However, as macrophages and related cells represent major executive players in inflammation, their polarization into proinflammatory M1 or anti-inflammatory M2 phenotypes is of utmost importance for the pro-/anti-inflammatory balance. In fact, melatonin is capable of shifting this balance toward the anti-inflammatory side by favoring M2 and disfavoring M1 polarization, as recently reviewed [194]. One of the major anti-inflammatory effects in the inhibition of M1 function consists in the MT_1 receptor-mediated activation of JAK2 (Janus kinase 2), which phosphorylates STAT3 (signal transducer and activator of transcription 3) [194–197]. In the nucleus, pSTAT3 dimers activate SOCS1 (suppressor of cytokine signaling 1), which favors NF-κB degradation by virtue of its property as an E3 ubiquitin ligase and, thus, inhibits NF-κB actions at the chromatin [194,198–200]. Additionally, suppression of NF-κB actions has been reported for RORα [194,201]. This relationship is highly convincing, since RORα knockout causes strong upregulations of proinflammatory cytokines [202]. However, as RORα has been definitely shown to be incapable of binding melatonin [203,204], actions of melatonin via this transcription factor have to be of indirect nature [18,194]. A possibility of particular interest concerns an effect of SIRT1 on RORα, in its function as a partial mediator of melatonin effects. As far as melatonin upregulates SIRT1, a known mechanism can become effective, which comprises deacetylation of PGC-1α (peroxisome proliferator-activated receptor-γ coactivator-1α) and facilitates the binding of RORα to its response elements (ROREs) [41]. With regard to the number of documented anti-inflammatory actions of SIRT1 summarized above, this idea is insofar attractive as SIRT1 was shown to suppress NF-κB signaling, as likewise reported for RORα [153–155]. This does not exclude additional actions of SIRT1, which was also found to be involved in SOCS1 signaling [205].

M2 polarization of macrophages, and presumably in similar ways of microglial cells, is largely promoted by STAT6 phosphorylation, in pathways regulated by melatonin and anti-inflammatory cytokines, especially IL-4 and IL-13 [194]. A key step in these processes is tyrosine phosphorylation of IRS-2 (insulin receptor substrate 2), which can be achieved in multiple ways [194]: (1) via IL-4 or IL-13 binding to IL-4 receptor-α, phosphorylation of JAK1/3 or JAK1/Tyk2 (tyrosine kinase-2), which may cause tyrosine phosphorylation of STAT6 directly or, alternately, IRS-2, followed by GRB2 (growth factor receptor bound-2) activation and STAT6 phosphorylation, or (2) via melatonin and an $MT_{1/2}$-dependent cascade of pIRS-2, GRB2, and pSTAT6. pSTAT6 dimers are responsible for M2-specific gene expressions, partially in conjunction with KLF4 (krüppel-like factor 4), which interacts with pSTAT6. Additional effects of melatonin seem to contribute, such as $MT_{1/2}$-dependent inhibition of PI3K (phosphoinositide 3-kinase), thereby blocking the proinflammatory Akt/mTORC1 cascade [194]. Moreover, this inhibitory effect of melatonin can be assumed to prevent two other negative modulatory actions, (1) by the mTORC1 downstream factor GRB10 and (2) by p70S6K (p50S-6-kinase). Tyrosine phosphorylation of IRS-2 and expression of M2 genes were found to be substantially increased by GBR10 knockdown [206]. Serine phosphorylation of IRS-2 by p70S6K was shown to counteract M2 polarization [206].

4. Modulation of the Networks by Noncoding RNAs, an Emerging Field

The discovery of countless noncoding RNAs (ncRNAs) with regulatory properties has substantially changed our understanding of regulation. Many of these RNAs interfere with posttranscriptional processes. This is especially the case in most microRNAs (miRNAs), which target mRNAs, and snoRNAs (small nucleolar RNAs), which are involved in RNA processing [207,208]. Other categories of RNAs such as eRNAs (enhancer RNAs) or super-enhancer lncRNAs (super enhancer long noncoding RNAs) directly interact with the chromatin and even with DNA [209]. piRNAs (PIWI-interacting RNAs) silence transposable elements via both transcriptional and posttranscriptional mechanisms [210]. Multiple functions are known for lncRNAs, in addition to enhancer properties. They may either positively or negatively regulate gene expression, which has been even observed in their subgroup of asRNAs (antisense RNAs). Moreover, various lncRNAs are precursors of miRNAs or snoRNAs [209]. Moreover, many lncRNAs and circRNAs (circular RNAs) serve as miRNA sponges and gain particular relevance in the transmission of intercellular signals by exosomes and ectosomes [209,211,212]. With regard to melatonin, numerous ncRNAs of different categories were shown to be influenced by this pleiotropic regulator [209,213–215]. As ncRNAs also modulate inflammation, macrophage activities, and NF-κB signaling [216–219], the relationship to melatonin is of particular interest and will certainly gain increasing future importance.

A complete consideration of all ncRNAs with positive or negative actions on inflammation would go beyond the scope of this article. A comprehensive list of miRNAs that affect pro- or anti-inflammatory cytokines has been recently published [220]. With regard to the melatonin-related task of this review, only those ncRNAs shall be discussed that are influenced by melatonin or change its downstream factors or interfere with major regulatory parts of the networks, especially if they concern areas of action known to be a matter of beneficial actions by melatonin, such as sepsis, ischemia/reperfusion, aging, or neurodegeneration. Findings obtained in the field of microRNAs are summarized in Table 1. Only those miRNAs have been considered that are related to the field of inflammation regulation. Many additional studies have revealed effects of melatonin on other miRNAs [214,221,222]. However, the outcome in a non-inflammatory context cannot be expected to be the same. This concerns especially the situation in cancer, although cancer can also have an inflammatory aspect. The major difference between non-tumor and tumor cells concerns the inverse relationship between melatonin and SIRT1 and the pro-apoptotic activity of melatonin in tumor cells [5,16,17]. One of the most extensive studies on melatonin effects on miRNAs [221] that has been omitted from Table 1 has been conducted in breast cancer cell lines. The determinations revealed 12 miRNAs that were upregulated by melatonin and 10 others that were downregulated. The analysis of their 5′-utr sequences indicated that these 22 miRNAs might target 2029 mRNAs.

Table 1. Regulation of microRNA expression by melatonin and effects of microRNAs on SIRT1, Nrf2, and NF-κB in the context of inflammation.

miRNA	Change by Melatonin	Effect on Sirt1	Effect on Nrf2	Nrf2-Related Target	Effect on NF-κB	NF-κB-Related Target
miR-7		↓? [223]	↑ [224]	Keap1	↓ [225,226]	
miR-7-5p					↓ [227]	
miR-9		↓ [228–236]			↓ [236–242]	
miR-9					↑ [243,244]	MCPIP1, TRIM56
miR-20a					↑ [245,246]	CYLD
miR-21		↓ [247]				
miR-23a	↓ [194,248]	↓ [249–251]	↑ [252]	Keap1	↑ [194]	
miR-23a-3p		↓ [253]				
miR-23b		↓ [249]				
miR-23b-3p		↓ [155,254]				
miR-24	↓ [255]	↑ [256]				
miR-24-3p			↑ [257]	Keap1		
miR-26a					↓ [258]	
miR-27b					↓ [259]	
miR-29		↓ [260]	↑ [261,262]	Keap1		
miR-30a	↑ [263]	↓ [264]			↓ [265]	
miR-30a-3p		↓ [266,267]				
miR-30e-5p	↓ [268]					
miR-31					↓ [269]	TRADD
miR-34a	↓ [270]	↓ [271–275]				
miR-34a-5p		↓ [276]				
miR-101			↓ [277]			
miR-106a/b		↓ [278]				
miR-124a		↓ [279]				
miR-125a/b					↑ [280–284]	A20
miR-125b					↓ [285–289]	TRAF, MIP-1α
miR-126	↑ [270]	↑ [290]			↑ [291–293]	TOM1, IκB
miR-128		↓ [294–296]			↑ [297,298]	IκB
miR-132		↓ [249]				
miR-135a		↓ [228]				
miR-142-3p	↑ [299]					
miR-144			↓ [300]			
miR-145-5p		↓ [276]				
miR-146a	↑ [270]		↓ [301]		↑ [302–305]	TRAF6, IRAK1
miR-150					↓ [306–309]	
miR-152	↓ [310]	↓ [256]				
miR-153			↓ [300]			
miR-155	↓ [194,310]	↓ [279,311,312]	↑ [313,314]			
miR-181a-c		↓ [228,230,315]				
miR-182		↓ [316]			↑ [317–320]	CYLD, TCEAL7
miR-195-5p		↓ [276]				
miR-199b		↓ [228]				
miR-200a	↑ [321,322]	↓ [189,323–327]	↑ [328–336]	Keap1	↑ [337]	
miR-200a-3p		↓ [276,338,339]				
miR-204		↓ [228]				

Table 1. *Cont.*

miRNA	Change by Melatonin	Effect on Sirt1	Effect on Nrf2	Nrf2-Related Target	Effect on NF-κB	NF-κB-Related Target
miR-210					↓ [340,341]	DR6
miR-212	↓ [299]	↓ [249,267,342–344]				
miR-217		↓ [345]				
miR-301a					↑ [346–350]	NKRF
miR-326					↑ [351]	BCL2A1
miR-340			↓ [352]			
miR-340-5p			↓ [155,300,353]			
miR-495		↓ [354]				
miR-675	↑ [355]					
miR-675-3p	↑ [322]					
Let-7					↑ [356]	A20
Let-7a	↑ [357]					
Let-7e					↑ [358]	IκBβ
Let-7f					↑ [359]	A20
Let-7g					↑ [360]	
Let-7i		↓ [361]			↑ [361]	SIRT1

Abbreviations: A20, ubiquitin-editing enzyme A20 (=TNFAIP3, tumor necrosis factor alpha-induced protein 3); BCL2A1, B-cell lymphoma 2A1; CYLD, cylindromatosis; DR6, death receptor 6; IRAK1, interleukin-1 receptor-associated kinase 1; KEAP1, Kelch-like ECH-associated protein 1; MCPIP1, monocyte chemotactic protein-induced protein 1; MIP-1α, macrophage inflammatory protein-1α ; NKRF, NF-κB repressing factor; TCEAL7, Transcription elongation factor A protein-like 7; TOM1, target of Myb1; TRADD, tumor necrosis factor receptor type 1-associated DEATH domain protein; TRAF6, tumor necrosis factor receptor-associated factor 6; TRIM56, tripartite-motif-containing protein 56. ↓↑ indicate down- or upregulations, respectively.

The pleiotropic targeting of various mRNAs by a single miRNA does not only open the possibility of jointly downregulating several mRNAs that are functionally connected, but may also reflect multiple functions in different contexts. This problem of overlapping actions of miRNAs with roles in both inflammation and cancer is also evident in the findings summarized in Table 1. Although the miRNAs were selected because of their modulation of inflammation, several of them exhibited other, perhaps independent, actions related to tumor promotion and progression. In fact, several molecules listed have been classified as oncomiRs, such as miR-21, miR-23a, miR-29, miR-106b, miR-125b, miR-155, and miR-182 [316,362–364].

The examples in Table 1, in which changes of miRNA expression by melatonin have been combined with actions of inflammation-related miRNAs on expression of SIRT1, Nrf2, and NF-κB, do not show a uniform picture. One of the reasons concerns the differences in context, cell types, and conditions, under which the studies have been performed. In many cases, changes by melatonin and effects on SIRT1, Nrf2, and NF-κB have been investigated in different systems. In a few cases, opposite effects have been obtained. In addition to organ specificity of melatonin actions, the difference between pro- and anti-inflammatory actions of melatonin has to be considered. The main purpose of this table is to provide information to investigators on which miRNAs they may focus on when studying melatonin effects in inflammation, especially in those cases where actions of melatonin on miRNAs have not yet been analyzed.

A few special types of connections between melatonin and the three possible downstream factors shall be briefly discussed. The levels of miR-7 have been shown to increase during aging, and it was assumed that it may downregulate SIRT1 [223]. On the other hand, the upregulation of Nrf2 and downregulation of NF-κB in the non-aging context of training athletes, which jointly indicate an antioxidant and anti-inflammatory action, is not easily compatible with reduced SIRT1 in senescence. In other cases of reduced SIRT1 expression, the reservation has to be made that decreased SIRT1 expression may be associated with elevated SIRT1 activity [23], as long as NAD^+ levels or inhibition by sirtuin inhibitors have not been determined. In reports in which upregulation by melatonin was associated with downregulation of SIRT1 (miR-30a) or Nrf2 and upregulation of NF-κB (miR-146a), this combination may be interpreted as a route of melatonin's proinflammatory arm. The example of miR-24, which is suppressed by melatonin, but enhances SIRT1 expression, may be taken as a tumor-specific relationship, because this would conform to melatonin's known suppression of SIRT1 in cancer cells [5,365]. Therefore, this may not be applicable to inflammation control. The presence of miR-126, which is upregulated by melatonin and increases SIRT1 expression, indicates a role of this sirtuin as a mediator of melatonin and may appear, at first glance, as an example of the anti-inflammatory route. However, this contrasts strongly with the upregulation of NF-κB and would require clarification by studying all these factors in the same system. A number of SIRT1-targeting miRNAs is downregulated by melatonin, such as miR-23a, miR-34a, miR-152, miR-155, miR-212, and, according to some but not all data, miR-200a. This reduction of SIRT1-suppressing miRNAs would, again, be compatible with findings on SIRT1-mediated melatonin effects [17,18]. Unfortunately, the findings concerning miRNA-mediated changes of NF-κB are, to date, often not generally compatible with the alterations in the other factors. Further studies will be required for obtaining a coherent picture. However, this reservation concerns only the participation of miRNAs, whereas the effects of melatonin and SIRT1 on Nrf2 and NF-κB have been unequivocally demonstrated [17].

Available information concerning melatonin effects on other noncoding RNAs is, unfortunately, limited. A few publications have addressed such actions on lncRNAs. In the case of the lncRNA *H19*, a relationship to miR-675 (cf. Table 1) exists, which is a derivative of the former. The effects of melatonin on H_2O_2-exposed cardiac progenitor cells correspond to those of the microRNA and, consequently, *H19* knockdown abolishes the action of miR-675 [355]. The molecule miR-675 was shown to target *USP10* (ubiquitin carboxyl-terminal hydrolase 10) mRNA, which was concluded to cause downregulation of p53 and p21, thereby inhibiting premature senescence by oxidative stress [355]. Upregulation of *H19* and miR-675 by melatonin was also observed in protection experiments against brain injury after subarachnoid hemorrhage [357]. In a study on pulmonary hypertension, melatonin reduced *H19* expression and, therefore, also that of miR-675-3p, whereas *H19* was shown to suppress miR-200a [322]. Meanwhile, numerous other studies have confirmed the role of *H19* in inflammatory processes (not cited), however, they did not consider melatonin. Another type of interaction between lncRNA and miRNA was based on sponging. The lncRNA *MEG3* was reported to enhance pyroptosis in atherosclerotic models, such as human aortic endothelial cells exposed to oxidized LDL (low density lipoprotein). *MEG3* was found to sponge miR-223 and to activate NLRP3, whereas melatonin was shown to reduce pyroptosis by suppressing NLRP3 activation and downstream factors, such as NF-κB, gasdermin D, IL-1β, and IL-18 [366]. In hair follicle fibroblasts of cashmere goats, melatonin upregulated the lncRNA *MTC*, which was associated with proliferation and also NF-κB activation [367]. This finding was in contrast to many other results on NF-κB suppression by melatonin obtained in the context of antioxidant actions. Two other reports have dealt with melatonin's actions in hepatocellular carcinomas. In one study, melatonin was shown to reduce cancer progression by upregulating FoxA2, which induced the lncRNA *CPS1-IT1*, with a downstream effect of reduced HIF-1α activity [368]. In another investigation, melatonin suppressed DNA repair capacity by upregulating the antisense lncRNA *RAD51-AS1*, which interacts with *RAD51* mRNA, and the findings were interpreted as a sensitization to chemotherapeutic drugs [369]. A functionally different lncRNA, *TERRA* (telomeric repeat-containing RNA), has been investigated in the context of melatonin. This RNA interacts with PARP-1 (polyADP-ribose polymerase-1), a sensor of DNA damage. This interaction was shown to stimulate SASP, but melatonin suppressed SASP-related gene expression and, therefore, an important aging-promoting process [122].

Work on the mediation of melatonin effects on lncRNAs can be expected to become highly important in the future [198,370], although this line of investigation is still in its infancy. This assumption is also based on the increasing body of evidence in related fields, in particular, the circadian system [209,371] and gerontology [372,373]. Numerous lncRNAs, e.g., over 600 in murine liver, were found to vary in a circadian fashion, often at very high amplitudes [371]. It would be a surprise if the chronobiotic regulator melatonin would not modulate at least a fraction of them. Among the lncRNAs, particular attention should be paid to subforms of a different functionality, such as asRNAs, eRNAs and, importantly, super-enhancer lncRNAs, all of which contain numerous species under circadian control [209,371]. The prominent role of lncRNAs in the control of inflammation has also become evident and has been reviewed multiple times [374–380]. In this context, more research on melatonin is desired. A further category of RNAs that will gain importance in the melatonin field, but are still devoid of pertinent investigations, are the circRNAs, which are known to sponge miRNAs [211,381–383]. With regard to a miRNA discussed above, miR-7, which is sponged by the circRNA *CDR1as* (alias *ciRS-7*), a few recent publications indicate relationships to NF-κB signaling [384–386] and to Aβ secretion [384], and they also demonstrate the profoundness of *CDR1as* deficiency in the brain [387].

5. Conclusions

The decrease of melatonin in aging and in various aging-related diseases [1,2] has different, potentially opposite, consequences. The same is valid for melatonin replacement therapies. This results from the dual roles of melatonin as both a pro- and anti-inflammatory regulator [15–17]. The conditionality that determines whether melatonin promotes the one or the other mode of immunological response should be a precondition for appropriately judging what kind of change has to be expected. Unfortunately, to date, this conditionality is not completely understood. Tendentially, one can conclude that anti-inflammatory actions of melatonin are mostly prevailing [17], however, with the important exception of autoimmune diseases, in which the immune stimulatory properties of melatonin may turn out to be detrimental. This concerns especially rheumatoid arthritis [50–52] and multiple sclerosis [53]. Whether melatonin may be unfavorable in type 2 diabetes of humans, in spite of its clearly antidiabetic actions in rodents, remains to be clarified in detail and may partially depend on age [5]. The difference between humans and rodents has to be seen in the contrasting associations of melatonin with food consumption and related metabolic activities in diurnality vs. nocturnality [5,16]. The inflammatory aspect of type 2 diabetes extends to brain insulin resistance, which has been identified as a proinflammatory change in early AD [107–109]. Whether or not melatonin may be detrimental in PD has been a matter of controversy [388–390]. The reported improvements by melatonergic antagonists in PD [390] should at least be regarded as a caveat [391].

Under other conditions, melatonin has been shown to preferentially exert anti-inflammatory, antioxidant, and other beneficial actions in aging [10,26,70,74,93–98,392–394]. Concerning anti-inflammatory effects, melatonin suppresses various processes that lead to enhanced formation of reactive oxygen and nitrogen species and to proinflammatory signaling, as summarized in Section 2. Moreover, it also stimulates several anti-inflammatory pathways and cellular changes that favor this side of the immune system and promote healing, as outlined in Section 3. Among these activities, the promotion of macrophage polarization towards the M2 type may be of particular importance for the shift from pro- to anti-inflammatory behavior, an aspect that has recently received increased attention [137,194,197]. Another potentially decisive action of melatonin concerns the upregulation of SIRT1 in nontumor cells, especially observed in aging animals [3,5,17,18,28,70,395]. Apart from being a relevant factor in aging, SIRT1 displays antioxidant and anti-inflammatory properties (Section 3). As mentioned above, various actions of melatonin are abolished by sirtuin inhibitors or *Sirt1* siRNA. Moreover, some mitochondrial actions of melatonin were shown to be absent in Sirt1$^{-/-}$ mice [396]. The inclusion of SIRT1 and, perhaps, other sirtuins into the spectrum of melatonin's actions represents an important step forward in the understanding of its aging- and inflammation-related properties. However, one cannot expect that all SIRT1 actions mediate melatonergic regulation. SIRT1 is also controlled by various other factors, including accessory components of circadian oscillators that regulate NAMPT expression and NAD$^+$ levels, hormones such as triiodothyronine and glucocorticoids, oncogenes, lncRNAs such as *HOTAIR*, and various miRNAs not regulated by melatonin. The incoherence of melatonin effects on miRNAs and their targeting of typically otherwise melatonin-controlled transcription factors, such as Nrf2 and NF-κB, is evident from Table 1. Moreover, several miRNAs up- or downregulated by melatonin do not cause a rise in SIRT1. However, in the latter case, one has to remain aware that melatonin downregulates SIRT1 in cancer cells, and that several of the miRNAs have been studied in tumors. The selection of miRNAs in Table 1 was restricted to those with demonstrated functions in the control of inflammation. More extensive studies on melatonin, SIRT1, and miRNAs will presumably reveal additional cases that are related to the immune system and also to aging and age-related diseases. As examples, the associated roles of SIRT1 and miRNAs in SASP and in Aβ toxicity shall be briefly mentioned [125,397]. MicroRNAs and other noncoding RNAs have brought about a new, considerably expanded level of complexity into the relationships between melatonin, inflammation, and aging. There is considerable difficulty that arises from multiple mRNAs targeted by a single miRNA species. A further level of complexity in the regulatory networks can be expected as soon as the intercellular communication, via exosomal RNAs, is more profoundly understood in its details and its variations according to diseases and aging.

References

1. Bubenik, G.A.; Konturek, S.J. Melatonin and aging: Prospects for human treatment. *J. Physiol. Pharmacol.* **2011**, *62*, 13–19. [PubMed]
2. Hardeland, R. Melatonin in aging and disease—Multiple consequences of reduced secretion, options and limits of treatment. *Aging Dis.* **2012**, *3*, 194–225. [PubMed]
3. Hardeland, R. Brain inflammaging: Roles of melatonin, circadian clocks and sirtuins. *J. Clin. Cell. Immunol.* **2018**, *9*, 543. [CrossRef]
4. Yamazaki, S.; Straume, M.; Tei, H.; Sakaki, Y.; Menaker, M.; Block, G.D. Effects of aging on central and peripheral mammalian clocks. *Proc. Natl. Acad. Sci. USA* **2002**, *99*, 10801–10806. [CrossRef] [PubMed]
5. Hardeland, R. Melatonin and the pathologies of weakened or dysregulated circadian oscillators. *J. Pineal Res.* **2017**, *62*, e12377. [CrossRef] [PubMed]
6. Ginaldi, L.; De Martinis, M.; D'Ostilio, A.; Marini, L.; Loreto, M.F.; Quaglino, D. Immunological changes in the elderly. *Aging* **1999**, *11*, 281–286. [CrossRef] [PubMed]
7. DelaRosa, O.; Pawelec, G.; Peralbo, E.; Wikby, A.; Mariani, E.; Mocchegiani, E.; Tarazona, R.; Solana, R. Immunological biomarkers of ageing in man: Changes in both innate and adaptive immunity are associated with health and longevity. *Biogerontology* **2006**, *7*, 471–481. [CrossRef] [PubMed]
8. Dewan, S.K.; Zheng, S.B.; Xia, S.J.; Bill, K. Senescent remodeling of the immune system and its contribution to the predisposition of the elderly to infections. *Chin. Med. J.* **2012**, *125*, 3325–3331. [PubMed]
9. Cardinali, D.P.; Esquifino, A.I.; Srinivasan, V.; Pandi-Perumal, S.R. Melatonin and the immune system in aging. *Neuroimmunomodulation* **2008**, *15*, 272–278. [CrossRef] [PubMed]
10. Hardeland, R. Melatonin and the theories of aging: A critical appraisal of melatonin's role in antiaging mechanisms. *J. Pineal Res.* **2013**, *55*, 325–356. [CrossRef] [PubMed]
11. Hardeland, R.; Cardinali, D.P.; Srinivasan, V.; Spence, D.W.; Brown, G.M.; Pandi-Perumal, S.R. Melatonin—A pleiotropic, orchestrating regulator molecule. *Prog. Neurobiol.* **2011**, *93*, 350–384. [CrossRef] [PubMed]
12. Gachon, F.; Nagoshi, E.; Brown, S.A.; Ripperger, J.; Schibler, U. The mammalian circadian timing system: From gene expression to physiology. *Chromosoma* **2004**, *113*, 103–112. [CrossRef] [PubMed]
13. Buijs, R.M.; Scheer, F.A.; Kreier, F.; Yi, C.; Bos, N.; Goncharuk, V.D.; Kalsbeek, A. Organization of circadian functions: Interaction with the body. *Prog. Brain Res.* **2006**, *153*, 341–360. [PubMed]
14. Hardeland, R. Melatonin and circadian oscillators in aging—A dynamic approach to the multiply connected players. *Interdiscip. Top. Gerontol.* **2015**, *40*, 128–140. [PubMed]
15. Carrillo-Vico, A.; Lardone, P.J.; Álvarez-Sánchez, N.; Rodríguez-Rodríguez, A.; Guerrero, J.M. Melatonin: Buffering the immune system. *Int. J. Mol. Sci.* **2013**, *14*, 8638–8683. [CrossRef] [PubMed]
16. Hardeland, R. Opposite effects of melatonin in different systems and under different conditions. *Curr. Top. Biochem. Res.* **2016**, *17*, 57–69.

17. Hardeland, R. Melatonin and inflammation—Story of a double-edged blade. *J. Pineal Res.* **2018**, *65*, e12525. [CrossRef] [PubMed]
18. Hardeland, R. Melatonin and retinoid orphan receptors: Demand for new interpretations after their exclusion as nuclear melatonin receptors. *Melatonin Res.* **2018**, *1*, 77–92. [CrossRef]
19. Nakahata, Y.; Sahar, S.; Astarita, G.; Kaluzova, M.; Sassone-Corsi, P. Circadian control of the NAD^+ salvage pathway by CLOCK-SIRT1. *Science* **2009**, *324*, 654–657. [CrossRef] [PubMed]
20. Bellet, M.M.; Orozco-Solis, R.; Sahar, S.; Eckel-Mahan, K.; Sassone-Corsi, P. The time of metabolism: NAD^+, SIRT1, and the circadian clock. *Cold Spring Harb. Symp. Quant. Biol.* **2011**, *76*, 31–38. [CrossRef] [PubMed]
21. Sahar, S.; Sassone-Corsi, P. The epigenetic language of circadian clocks. *Handb. Exp. Pharmacol.* **2013**, *217*, 29–44.
22. Masri, S. Sirtuin-dependent clock control: New advances in metabolism, aging and cancer. *Curr. Opin. Clin. Nutr. Metab. Care* **2015**, *18*, 521–527. [CrossRef] [PubMed]
23. Li, D.; Bi, F.F.; Chen, N.N.; Cao, J.M.; Sun, W.P.; Zhou, Y.M.; Li, C.Y.; Yang, Q. A novel crosstalk between BRCA1 and sirtuin 1 in ovarian cancer. *Sci. Rep.* **2014**, *4*, 6666. [CrossRef] [PubMed]
24. Ramsey, K.M.; Mills, K.F.; Satoh, A.; Imai, S. Age-associated loss of sirt1-mediated enhancement of glucose-stimulated insulin secretion in beta cell-specific sirt1-overexpressing (besto) mice. *Aging Cell* **2008**, *7*, 78–88. [CrossRef] [PubMed]
25. Elibol, B.; Kilic, U. High levels of SIRT1 expression as a protective mechanism against disease-related conditions. *Front Endocrinol.* **2018**, *9*, 614. [CrossRef] [PubMed]
26. Gutierrez-Cuesta, J.; Tajes, M.; Jiménez, A.; Coto-Montes, A.; Camins, A.; Pallàs, M. Evaluation of potential pro-survival pathways regulated by melatonin in a murine senescence model. *J. Pineal Res.* **2008**, *45*, 497–505. [CrossRef] [PubMed]
27. Tajes, M.; Gutierrez-Cuesta, J.; Ortuño-Sahagun, D.; Camins, A.; Pallàs, M. Anti-aging properties of melatonin in an in vitro murine senescence model: Involvement of the sirtuin 1 pathway. *J. Pineal Res.* **2009**, *47*, 228–237. [CrossRef] [PubMed]
28. Cristòfol, R.; Porquet, D.; Corpas, R.; Coto-Montes, A.; Serret, J.; Camins, A.; Pallàs, M.; Sanfeliu, C. Neurons from senescence-accelerated SAMP8 mice are protected against frailty by the sirtuin 1 promoting agents melatonin and resveratrol. *J. Pineal Res.* **2012**, *52*, 271–281. [CrossRef] [PubMed]
29. Guo, P.; Pi, H.; Xu, S.; Zhang, L.; Li, Y.; Li, M.; Cao, Z.; Tian, L.; Xie, J.; Li, R.; et al. Melatonin Improves mitochondrial function by promoting MT1/SIRT1/PGC-1 alpha-dependent mitochondrial biogenesis in cadmium-induced hepatotoxicity in vitro. *Toxicol. Sci.* **2014**, *142*, 182–195. [CrossRef] [PubMed]
30. Yu, L.; Sun, Y.; Cheng, L.; Jin, Z.; Yang, Y.; Zhai, M.; Pei, H.; Wang, X.; Zhang, H.; Meng, Q.; et al. Melatonin receptor-mediated protection against myocardial ischemia/reperfusion injury: Role of SIRT1. *J. Pineal Res.* **2014**, *57*, 228–238. [CrossRef] [PubMed]
31. Yu, L.; Liang, H.; Dong, X.; Zhao, G.; Jin, Z.; Zhai, M.; Yang, Y.; Chen, W.; Liu, J.; Yi, W.; et al. Reduced silent information regulator 1 signaling exacerbates myocardial ischemia-reperfusion injury in type 2 diabetic rats and the protective effect of melatonin. *J. Pineal Res.* **2015**, *59*, 376–390. [CrossRef] [PubMed]
32. Zhao, L.; An, R.; Yang, Y.; Yang, X.; Liu, H.; Yue, L.; Li, X.; Lin, Y.; Reiter, R.J.; Qu, Y. Melatonin alleviates brain injury in mice subjected to cecal ligation and puncture via attenuating inflammation, apoptosis, and oxidative stress: The role of SIRT1 signaling. *J. Pineal Res.* **2015**, *59*, 230–239. [CrossRef] [PubMed]
33. Zhou, L.; Chen, X.; Liu, T.; Gong, Y.; Chen, S.; Pan, G.; Cui, W.; Luo, Z.P.; Pei, M.; Yang, H.; et al. Melatonin reverses H_2O_2-induced premature senescence in mesenchymal stem cells via the SIRT1-dependent pathway. *J. Pineal Res.* **2015**, *59*, 190–205. [CrossRef] [PubMed]
34. Yang, Y.; Jiang, S.; Dong, Y.; Fan, C.; Zhao, L.; Yang, X.; Li, J.; Di, S.; Yue, L.; Liang, G.; et al. Melatonin prevents cell death and mitochondrial dysfunction via a SIRT1-dependent mechanism during ischemic-stroke in mice. *J. Pineal Res.* **2015**, *58*, 61–70. [CrossRef] [PubMed]
35. Lee, J.H.; Moon, J.H.; Nazim, U.M.; Lee, Y.J.; Seol, J.W.; Eo, S.K.; Lee, J.H.; Park, S.Y. Melatonin protects skin keratinocyte from hydrogen peroxide-mediated cell death via the SIRT1 pathway. *Oncotarget* **2016**, *7*, 12075–12088. [CrossRef] [PubMed]
36. Bai, X.Z.; He, T.; Gao, J.X.; Liu, Y.; Liu, J.Q.; Han, S.C.; Li, Y.; Shi, J.H.; Han, J.T.; Tao, K.; et al. Melatonin prevents acute kidney injury in severely burned rats via the activation of SIRT1. *Sci. Rep.* **2016**, *6*, 32199. [CrossRef] [PubMed]

37. Shah, S.A.; Khan, M.; Jo, M.H.; Jo, M.G.; Amin, F.U.; Kim, M.O. Melatonin stimulates the SIRT1/Nrf2 signaling pathway counteracting lipopolysaccharide (LPS)-induced oxidative stress to rescue postnatal rat brain. *CNS Neurosci. Ther.* **2017**, *23*, 33–44. [CrossRef] [PubMed]
38. Yang, W.; Kang, X.; Qin, N.; Li, F.; Jin, X.; Ma, Z.; Qian, Z.; Wu, S. Melatonin protects chondrocytes from impairment induced by glucocorticoids via NAD^+-dependent SIRT1. *Steroids* **2017**, *126*, 24–29. [CrossRef] [PubMed]
39. Peng, Z.; Zhang, W.; Qiao, J.; He, B. Melatonin attenuates airway inflammation via SIRT1 dependent inhibition of NLRP3 inflammasome and IL-1β in rats with COPD. *Int. Immunopharmacol.* **2018**, *62*, 23–28. [CrossRef] [PubMed]
40. Hardeland, R.; Madrid, J.A.; Tan, D.X.; Reiter, R.J. Melatonin, the circadian multioscillator system and health: The need for detailed analyses of peripheral melatonin signaling. *J. Pineal Res.* **2012**, *52*, 139–166. [CrossRef] [PubMed]
41. Chang, H.C.; Guarente, L. SIRT1 mediates central circadian control in the SCN by a mechanism that decays with aging. *Cell* **2013**, *153*, 1448–1460. [CrossRef] [PubMed]
42. Hardeland, R. Extended signaling by melatonin. *Cell Cell. Life Sci. J.* **2018**, *3*, 000123.
43. Guerrero, J.M.; Reiter, R.J. Melatonin-immune system relationships. Curr. *Top. Med. Chem.* **2002**, *2*, 167–179. [CrossRef]
44. Carrillo-Vico, A.; Guerrero, J.M.; Lardone, P.J.; Reiter, R.J. A review of the multiple actions of melatonin on the immune system. *Endocrine* **2005**, *27*, 189–200. [CrossRef]
45. Carrillo-Vico, A.; Reiter, R.J.; Lardone, P.J.; Herrera, J.L.; Fernández-Montesinos, R.; Guerrero, J.M.; Pozo, D. The modulatory role of melatonin on immune responsiveness. *Curr. Opin. Investig. Drugs* **2006**, *7*, 423–431. [PubMed]
46. Miller, S.C.; Pandi-Perumal, S.R.; Esquifino, A.I.; Cardinali, D.P.; Maestroni, G.J.M. The role of melatonin in immuno-enhancement: potential application in cancer. *Int. J. Exp. Pathol.* **2006**, *87*, 81–87. [CrossRef] [PubMed]
47. Pandi-Perumal, S.R.; Srinivasan, V.; Maestroni, G.J.M.; Cardinali, D.P.; Poeggeler, B.; Hardeland, R. Melatonin: Nature's most versatile biological signal? *FEBS J.* **2006**, *273*, 2813–2838. [CrossRef] [PubMed]
48. Carrillo-Vico, A.; Calvo, J.R.; Abreu, P.; Lardone, P.J.; García-Mauriño, S.; Reiter, R.J.; Guerrero, J.M. Evidence of melatonin synthesis by human lymphocytes and its physiological significance: Possible role as intracrine, autocrine, and/or paracrine substance. *FASEB J.* **2004**, *18*, 537–539. [CrossRef] [PubMed]
49. Carrillo-Vico, A.; Lardone, P.J.; Fernandez-Santos, J.M.; Martín-Lacave, I.; Calvo, J.R.; Karasek, M.; Guerrero, J.M. Human lymphocyte-synthesized melatonin is involved in the regulation of the interleukin-2/interleukin-2 receptor system. *J. Clin. Endocrinol. MeTable* **2005**, *90*, 992–1000. [CrossRef] [PubMed]
50. Maestroni, G.J.M.; Cardinali, D.P.; Esquifino, A.I.; Pandi-Perumal, S.R. Does melatonin play a disease-promoting role in rheumatoid arthritis? *J. Neuroimmunol.* **2005**, *158*, 106–111. [CrossRef] [PubMed]
51. Cutolo, M.; Maestroni, G.J.M. The melatonin-cytokine connection in rheumatoid arthritis. *Ann. Rheum. Dis.* **2005**, *64*, 1109–1111. [CrossRef] [PubMed]
52. Maestroni, G.J.M.; Otsa, K.; Cutolo, M. Melatonin treatment does not improve rheumatoid arthritis. *Br. J. Clin. Pharmacol.* **2008**, *65*, 797–798. [CrossRef] [PubMed]
53. Ghareghani, M.; Dokoohaki, S.; Ghanbari, A.; Farhadi, N.; Zibara, K.; Khodadoust, S.; Parishani, M.; Ghavamizadeh, M.; Sadeghi, H. Melatonin exacerbates acute experimental autoimmune encephalomyelitis by enhancing the serum levels of lactate: A potential biomarker of multiple sclerosis progression. *Clin. Exp. Pharmacol. Physiol.* **2017**, *44*, 52–61. [CrossRef] [PubMed]
54. Carrillo-Vico, A.; García-Mauriño, S.; Calvo, J.R.; Guerrero, J.M. Melatonin counteracts the inhibitory effect of PGE2 on IL-2 production in human lymphocytes via its mt1 membrane receptor. *FASEB J.* **2003**, *17*, 755–757. [CrossRef] [PubMed]
55. Morrey, K.M.; McLachlan, J.A.; Serkin, C.D.; Bakouche, O. Activation of human monocytes by the pineal hormone melatonin. *J. Immunol.* **1994**, *153*, 2671–2680. [PubMed]
56. Kuklina, E.M.; Glebezdina, N.S.; Nekrasova, I.V. Role of melatonin in the regulation of differentiation of T cells producing interleukin-17 (Th17). *Bull. Exp. Biol. Med.* **2016**, *160*, 656–658. [CrossRef] [PubMed]

57. Jovanovic, D.V.; Di Battista, J.A.; Martel-Pelletier, J.; Jolicoeur, F.C.; He, Y.; Zhang, M.; Mineau, F.; Pelletier, J.P. IL-17 stimulates the production and expression of proinflammatory cytokines, IL-beta and TNF-alpha, by human macrophages. *J. Immunol.* **1998**, *160*, 3513–3521. [PubMed]
58. Shalom-Barak, T.; Quach, J.; Lotz, M. Interleukin-17-induced gene expression in articular chondrocytes is associated with activation of mitogen-activated protein kinases and NF-κB. *J. Biol. Chem.* **1998**, *273*, 27467–27473. [CrossRef] [PubMed]
59. Kawaguchi, M.; Kokubu, F.; Kuga, H.; Matsukura, S.; Hoshino, H.; Ieki, K.; Imai, T.; Adachi, M.; Huang, S.K. Modulation of bronchial epithelial cells by IL-17. *J. Allergy Clin. Immunol.* **2001**, *108*, 804–809. [CrossRef] [PubMed]
60. Molet, S.; Hamid, Q.; Davoine, F.; Nutku, E.; Taha, R.; Page, R.N.; Olivenstein, R.; Elias, J.; Chakir, J. IL-17 is increased in asthmatic airways and induces human bronchial fibroblasts to produce cytokines. *J. Allergy Clin. Immunol.* **2001**, *108*, 430–438. [CrossRef] [PubMed]
61. Paradowska, A.; Maśliñiski, W.; Grzybowska-Kowalczyk, A.; Łacki, J. The function of interleukin 17 in the pathogenesis of rheumatoid arthritis. *Arch. Immunol. Ther. Exp.* **2007**, *55*, 329–334. [CrossRef]
62. Ishigame, H.; Kakuta, S.; Nagai, T.; Kadoki, M.; Nambu, A.; Komiyama, Y.; Fujikado, N.; Tanahashi, Y.; Akitsu, A.; Kotaki, H.; et al. Differential roles of interleukin-17A and -17F in host defense against mucoepithelial bacterial infection and allergic responses. *Immunity* **2009**, *30*, 108–119. [CrossRef] [PubMed]
63. Zhang, Y.; Huang, D.; Gao, W.; Yan, J.; Zhou, W.; Hou, X.; Liu, M.; Ren, C.; Wang, S.; Shen, J. Lack of IL-17 signaling decreases liver fibrosis in murine schistosomiasis japonica. *Int. Immunol.* **2015**, *27*, 317–325. [CrossRef] [PubMed]
64. Shabgah, A.G.; Fattahi, E.; Shahneh, F.Z. Interleukin-17 in human inflammatory diseases. *Postepy Dermatol. Alergol.* **2014**, *31*, 256–261. [CrossRef] [PubMed]
65. Yang, Z.Y.; Yuan, C.X. IL-17A promotes the neuroinflammation and cognitive function in sevoflurane anesthetized aged rats via activation of NF-κB signaling pathway. *BMC Anesthesiol.* **2018**, *18*, 147. [CrossRef] [PubMed]
66. Liu, F.; Ng, T.B.; Fung, M.C. Pineal indoles stimulate the gene expression of immunomodulating cytokines. *J. Neural Transm.* **2001**, *108*, 397–405. [CrossRef] [PubMed]
67. Maestroni, G.J.M. The immunoneuroendocrine role of melatonin. *J. Pineal Res.* **1993**, *14*, 1–10. [CrossRef] [PubMed]
68. Maestroni, G.J.M.; Hertens, E.; Galli, P.; Conti, A.; Pedrinis, E. Melatonin-induced T-helper cell hematopoietic cytokines resembling both interleukin-4 and dynorphin. *J. Pineal Res.* **1996**, *21*, 131–139. [CrossRef] [PubMed]
69. Maestroni, G.J.M. κ-Opioid receptors in marrow stroma mediate the hematopoietic effects of melatonin-induced opioid cytokines. *Ann. N. Y. Acad. Sci.* **1998**, *840*, 411–419. [CrossRef] [PubMed]
70. Hardeland, R.; Cardinali, D.P.; Brown, G.M.; Pandi-Perumal, S.R. Melatonin and brain inflammaging. *Prog. Neurobiol.* **2015**, *127–128*, 46–63. [CrossRef] [PubMed]
71. Strindhall, J.; Nilsson, B.O.; Löfgren, S.; Ernerudh, J.; Pawelec, G.; Johansson, B.; Wikby, A. No Immune Risk Profile among individuals who reach 100 years of age: Findings from the Swedish NONA immune longitudinal study. *Exp. Gerontol.* **2007**, *42*, 753–761. [CrossRef] [PubMed]
72. Candore, G.; Caruso, C.; Colonna-Romano, G. Inflammation, genetic background and longevity. *Biogerontology* **2010**, *11*, 565–573. [CrossRef] [PubMed]
73. Ponnappan, S.; Ponnappan, U. Aging and immune function: Molecular mechanisms to interventions. *Antioxid. Redox Signal.* **2011**, *14*, 1551–1585. [CrossRef] [PubMed]
74. Hardeland, R.; Coto-Montes, A. New vistas on oxidative damage and aging. *Open Biol. J.* **2010**, *3*, 39–52. [CrossRef]
75. Hardeland, R. Melatonin and its metabolites as anti-nitrosating and anti-nitrating agents. *J. Exp. Integr. Med.* **2011**, *1*, 67–81. [CrossRef]
76. Hardeland, R. Neuroprotection by radical avoidance: Search for suitable agents. *Molecules* **2009**, *14*, 5054–5102. [CrossRef] [PubMed]
77. Hardeland, R. Melatonin and the electron transport chain. *Cell. Mol. Life Sci.* **2017**, *74*, 3883–3896. [CrossRef] [PubMed]
78. Reiter, R.J.; Rosales-Corral, S.; Tan, D.X.; Jou, M.J.; Galano, A.; Xu, B. Melatonin as a mitochondria-targeted antioxidant: One of evolution's best ideas. *Cell. Mol. Life Sci.* **2017**, *74*, 3863–3881. [CrossRef] [PubMed]

79. Paradies, G.; Paradies, V.; Ruggiero, F.M.; Petrosillo, G. Mitochondrial bioenergetics decay in aging: Beneficial effect of melatonin. *Cell. Mol. Life Sci.* **2017**, *74*, 3897–3911. [CrossRef] [PubMed]
80. Slominski, A.T.; Zmijewski, M.A.; Semak, I.; Kim, T.K.; Janjetovic, Z.; Slominski, R.M.; Zmijewski, J.W. Melatonin, mitochondria, and the skin. *Cell. Mol. Life Sci.* **2017**, *74*, 3913–3925. [CrossRef] [PubMed]
81. Cardinali, D.P.; Vigo, D.E. Melatonin, mitochondria, and the metabolic syndrome. *Cell. Mol. Life Sci.* **2017**, *74*, 3941–3954. [CrossRef] [PubMed]
82. Acuña-Castroviejo, D.; Rahim, I.; Acuña-Fernández, C.; Fernández-Ortiz, M.; Solera-Marín, J.; Sayed, R.K.A.; Díaz-Casado, M.E.; Rusanova, I.; López, L.C.; Escames, G. Melatonin, clock genes and mitochondria in sepsis. *Cell. Mol. Life Sci.* **2017**, *74*, 3965–3987. [CrossRef] [PubMed]
83. Wongprayoon, P.; Govitrapong, P. Melatonin as a mitochondrial protector in neurodegenerative diseases. *Cell. Mol. Life Sci.* **2017**, *74*, 3999–4014. [CrossRef] [PubMed]
84. Tan, B.; Choi, R.H.; Chin, T.J.; Kaur, C.; Ling, E.A. Manipulation of microglial activity as a therapy for Alzheimer's disease. *Front. Biosci. (Schol. Ed.)* **2012**, *4*, 1402–1412. [PubMed]
85. McLarnon, J.G. Correlated inflammatory responses and neurodegeneration in peptide-injected animal models of Alzheimer's disease. *Biomed. Res. Int.* **2014**, *2014*, 923670. [CrossRef] [PubMed]
86. Narayan, P.; Holmström, K.M.; Kim, D.H.; Whitcomb, D.J.; Wilson, M.R.; St George-Hyslop, P.; Wood, N.W.; Dobson, C.M.; Cho, K.; Abramov, A.Y.; et al. Rare individual amyloid-β oligomers act on astrocytes to initiate neuronal damage. *Biochemistry* **2014**, *53*, 2442–2453. [CrossRef] [PubMed]
87. Hanzel, C.E.; Pichet-Binette, A.; Pomentel, L.S.; Iulita, M.F.; Allard, S.; Ducatenzeiler, A.; Do Carmo, S.; Cuello, A.C. Neuronal driven pre-plaque inflammation in a transgenic rat model of Alzheimer's disease. *Neurobiol. Aging* **2014**, *35*, 2249–2262. [CrossRef] [PubMed]
88. Iliff, J.J.; Wang, M.; Liao, Y.; Plogg, B.A.; Peng, W.; Gundersen, G.A.; Benveniste, H.; Vates, G.E.; Deane, R.; Goldman, S.A.; et al. A paravascular pathway facilitates CSF flow through the brain parenchyma and the clearance of interstitial solutes, including amyloid β. *Sci. Transl. Med.* **2012**, *4*, 147ra111. [CrossRef] [PubMed]
89. Mendelsohn, A.R.; Larrick, J.W. Sleep facilitates clearance of metabolites from the brain: Glymphatic function in aging and neurodegenerative diseases. *Rejuvenation Res.* **2013**, *16*, 518–523. [CrossRef] [PubMed]
90. Plog, B.A.; Nedergaard, M. The glymphatic system in central nervous system health and disease: Past, present, and future. *Annu. Rev. Pathol.* **2018**, *13*, 379–394. [CrossRef] [PubMed]
91. Boespflug, E.L.; Iliff, J.J. The emerging relationship between interstitial fluid-cerebrospinal fluid exchange, amyloid-β, and sleep. *Biol. Psychiatry* **2018**, *83*, 328–336. [CrossRef] [PubMed]
92. Yulug, B.; Hanoglu, L.; Kilic, E. Does sleep disturbance affect the amyloid clearance mechanisms in Alzheimer's disease? *Psychiatry Clin. Neurosci.* **2017**, *71*, 673–677. [CrossRef] [PubMed]
93. Pappolla, M.A.; Matsubara, E.; Vidal, R.; Pacheco-Quinto, J.; Poeggeler, B.; Zagorski, M.; Sambamurti, K. Melatonin treatment enhances Aβ lymphatic clearance in a transgenic mouse model of amyloidosis. *Curr. Alzheimer Res.* **2018**, *15*, 637–642. [CrossRef] [PubMed]
94. Spinedi, E.; Cardinali, D.P. Neuroendocrine-metabolic dysfunction and sleep disturbances in neurodegenerative disorders: Focus on Alzheimer's Disease and melatonin. *Neuroendocrinology* **2018**. [CrossRef] [PubMed]
95. Pappolla, M.A.; Chyan, Y.; Poeggeler, B.; Frangione, B.; Wilson, G.; Ghiso, J.; Reiter, R.J. An assessment of the antioxidant and the antiamyloidogenic properties of melatonin: Implications for Alzheimer's disease. *J. Neural Transm.* **2000**, *107*, 203–231. [CrossRef] [PubMed]
96. Srinivasan, V.; Pandi-Perumal, S.R.; Cardinali, D.P.; Poeggeler, B.; Hardeland, R. Melatonin in Alzheimer's disease and other neurodegenerative disorders. *Behav. Brain Funct.* **2006**, *2*, 15. [CrossRef] [PubMed]
97. Rosales-Corral, S.A.; Acuña-Castroviejo, D.; Coto-Montes, A.; Boga, J.A.; Manchester, L.C.; Fuentes-Broto, L.; Korkmaz, A.; Ma, S.; Tan, D.X.; Reiter, R.J. Alzheimer's disease: Pathological mechanisms and the beneficial role of melatonin. *J. Pineal Res.* **2012**, *52*, 167–202. [CrossRef] [PubMed]
98. Lin, L.; Huang, Q.X.; Yang, S.S.; Chu, J.; Wang, J.Z.; Tian, Q. Melatonin in Alzheimer's disease. *Int. J. Mol. Sci.* **2013**, *14*, 14575–14593. [CrossRef] [PubMed]
99. Song, W.; Lahiri, D.K. Melatonin alters the metabolism of the β-amyloid precursor protein in the neuroendocrine cell line PC12. *J. Mol. Neurosci.* **1997**, *9*, 75–92. [CrossRef] [PubMed]

100. Panmanee, J.; Nopparat, C.; Chavanich, N.; Shukla, M.; Mukda, S.; Song, W.; Vincent, B.; Govitrapong, P. Melatonin regulates the transcription of βAPP-cleaving secretases mediated through melatonin receptors in human neuroblastoma SH-SY5Y cells. *J. Pineal Res.* **2015**, *58*, 151–165. [CrossRef] [PubMed]
101. Shukla, M.; Htoo, H.H.; Wintachai, P.; Hernandez, J.F.; Dubois, C.; Postina, R.; Xu, H.; Checler, F.; Smith, D.R.; Govitrapong, P.; et al. Melatonin stimulates the nonamyloidogenic processing of βAPP through the positive transcriptional regulation of ADAM10 and ADAM17. *J. Pineal Res.* **2015**, *58*, 151–165. [CrossRef] [PubMed]
102. Mukda, S.; Panmanee, J.; Boontem, P.; Govitrapong, P. Melatonin administration reverses the alteration of amyloid precursor protein-cleaving secretases expression in aged mouse hippocampus. *Neurosci. Lett.* **2016**, *621*, 39–46. [CrossRef] [PubMed]
103. Shukla, M.; Govitrapong, P.; Boontem, P.; Reiter, R.J.; Satayavivad, J. Mechanisms of melatonin in alleviating Alzheimer's disease. *Curr. Neuropharmacol.* **2017**, *15*, 1010–1031. [CrossRef] [PubMed]
104. Matsubara, E.; Bryant-Thomas, T.; Pacheco Quinto, J.; Henry, T.L.; Poeggeler, B.; Herbert, D.; Cruz-Sanchez, F.; Chyan, Y.J.; Smith, M.A.; Perry, G.; et al. Melatonin increases survival and inhibits oxidative and amyloid pathology in a transgenic model of Alzheimer's disease. *J. Neurochem.* **2003**, *85*, 1101–1108. [CrossRef] [PubMed]
105. Olcese, J.M.; Cao, C.; Mori, T.; Mamcarz, M.B.; Maxwell, A.; Runfeldt, M.J.; Wang, L.; Zhang, C.; Lin, X.; Zhang, G.; et al. Protection against cognitive deficits and markers of neurodegeneration by long-term oral administrations of melatonin in a transgenic model of Alzheimer disease. *J. Pineal Res.* **2009**, *47*, 82–96. [CrossRef] [PubMed]
106. Quinn, J.; Kulhanek, D.; Nowlin, J.; Jones, R.; Praticò, D.; Rokach, J.; Stackman, R. Chronic melatonin therapy fails to alter amyloid burden or oxidative damage in old Tg2576 mice: Implications for clinical trials. *Brain Res.* **2005**, *1037*, 209–213. [CrossRef] [PubMed]
107. Clark, I.A.; Vissel, B. Treatment implications of the altered cytokine-insulin axis in neurodegenerative disease. *Biochem. Pharmacol.* **2013**, *86*, 862–871. [CrossRef] [PubMed]
108. Jiang, T.; Yu, J.T.; Zhu, X.C.; Tan, L. TREM2 in Alzheimer's disease. *Mol. Neurobiol.* **2013**, *48*, 180–185. [CrossRef] [PubMed]
109. Ferreira, L.S.S.; Fernandes, C.S.; Vieira, M.N.N.; De Felice, F.G. Insulin resistance in Alzheimer's disease. *Front. Neurosci.* **2018**, *12*, 830. [CrossRef] [PubMed]
110. Hotamisligil, G.S.; Erbay, E. Nutrient sensing and inflammation in metabolic diseases. *Nat. Rev. Immunol.* **2008**, *8*, 923–934. [CrossRef] [PubMed]
111. Hotamisligil, G.S. Inflammation, metaflammation and immunometabolic disorders. *Nature* **2017**, *542*, 177–185. [CrossRef] [PubMed]
112. Franceschi, C.; Garagnani, P.; Parini, P.; Giuliani, C.; Santoro, A. Inflammaging: A new immune-metabolic viewpoint for age-related diseases. *Nat. Rev. Endocrinol.* **2018**, *14*, 576–590. [CrossRef] [PubMed]
113. Cardinali, D.P.; Hardeland, R. Inflammaging, metabolic syndrome and melatonin: A call for treatment studies. *Neuroendocrinology* **2017**, *104*, 382–397. [CrossRef] [PubMed]
114. Coppé, J.P.; Patil, C.K.; Rodier, F.; Sun, Y.; Muñoz, D.P.; Goldstein, J.; Nelson, P.S.; Desprez, P.Y.; Campisi, J. Senescence-associated secretory phenotypes reveal cell-nonautonomous functions of oncogenic RAS and p53 tumor suppressor. *PLoS Biol.* **2008**, *6*, 2853–2868. [CrossRef] [PubMed]
115. Young, A.R.J.; Narita, M. SASP reflects senescence. *EMBO Rep.* **2009**, *10*, 228–230. [CrossRef] [PubMed]
116. Fumagalli, M.; d'Adda di Fagagna, F. SASPense and DDRama in cancer and ageing. *Nat. Cell Biol.* **2009**, *11*, 921–923. [CrossRef] [PubMed]
117. Coppé, J.P.; Desprez, P.Y.; Krtolica, A.; Campisi, J. The senescence-associated secretory phenotype: The dark side of tumor suppression. *Annu. Rev. Pathol.* **2010**, *5*, 99–118. [CrossRef] [PubMed]
118. Pantsulaia, I.; Ciszewski, W.M.; Niewiarowska, J. Senescent endothelial cells: Potential modulators of immunosenescence and ageing. *Ageing Res. Rev.* **2016**, *29*, 13–25. [CrossRef] [PubMed]
119. Salminen, A.; Ojala, J.; Kaamiranta, K.; Haapasalo, A.; Hiltunen, M.; Soininen, H. Astrocytes in the aging brain express characteristics of senescence-associated secretory phenotype. *Eur. J. Neurosci.* **2011**, *34*, 3–11. [CrossRef] [PubMed]
120. Maciel-Barón, L.Á.; Morales-Rosales, S.L.; Silva-Palacios, A.; Rodríguez-Barrera, R.H.; García-Álvarez, J.A.; Luna-López, A.; Pérez, V.I.; Torres, C.; Königsberg, M. The secretory phenotype of senescent astrocytes isolated from Wistar newborn rats changes with anti-inflammatory drugs, but does not have a short-term effect on neuronal mitochondrial potential. *Biogerontology* **2018**, *19*, 415–433. [CrossRef] [PubMed]

121. Carroll, J.E.; Cole, S.W.; Seeman, T.E.; Breen, E.C.; Witarama, T.; Arevalo, J.M.; Ma, J.; Irwin, M.R. Partial sleep deprivation activates the DNA damage response (DDR) and the senescence-associated secretory phenotype (SASP) in aged adult humans. *Brain Behav. Immun.* **2016**, *51*, 223–229. [CrossRef] [PubMed]
122. Yu, S.; Wang, X.; Geng, P.; Tang, X.; Xiang, L.; Lu, X.; Li, J.; Ruan, Z.; Chen, J.; Xie, G.; et al. Melatonin regulates PARP1 to control the senescence-associated secretory phenotype (SASP) in human fetal lung fibroblast cells. *J. Pineal Res.* **2017**, *63*, e12405. [CrossRef] [PubMed]
123. Bae, W.J.; Park, J.S.; Kang, S.K.; Kwon, I.K.; Kim, E.C. Effects of melatonin and its underlying mechanism on ethanol-stimulated senescence and osteoclastic differentiation in human periodontal ligament cells and cementoblasts. *Int. J. Mol. Sci.* **2018**, *19*, 1742. [CrossRef] [PubMed]
124. Fang, J.; Yan, Y.; Teng, X.; Wen, X.; Li, N.; Peng, S.; Liu, W.; Donadeu, F.X.; Zhao, S.; Hua, J. Melatonin prevents senescence of canine adipose-derived mesenchymal stem cells through activating NRF2 and inhibiting ER stress. *Aging* **2018**, *10*, 2954–2972. [CrossRef] [PubMed]
125. Hekmatimoghaddam, S.; Dehghani Firoozabadi, A.; Zare-Khormizi, M.R.; Pourrajab, F. Sirt1 and Parp1 as epigenome safeguards and microRNAs as SASP-associated signals, in cellular senescence and aging. *Ageing Res. Rev.* **2017**, *40*, 120–141. [CrossRef] [PubMed]
126. Korkmaz, A.; Rosales-Corral, S.; Reiter, R.J. Gene regulation by melatonin linked to epigenetic phenomena. *Gene* **2012**, *503*, 1–11. [CrossRef] [PubMed]
127. Franceschi, C.; Garagnani, P.; Vitale, G.; Capri, M.; Salvioli, S. Inflammaging and 'garb-aging'. *Trends Endocrinol. MeTable* **2017**, *28*, 199–212. [CrossRef] [PubMed]
128. Gilthorpe, J.D.; Oozeer, F.; Nash, J.; Calvo, M.; Bennett, D.L.; Lumsden, A.; Pini, A. Extracellular histone H1 is neurotoxic and drives a pro-inflammatory response in microglia. *F1000Resarch* **2013**, *2*, 148. [CrossRef] [PubMed]
129. Shimada, K.; Crother, T.R.; Karlin, J.; Dagvadorj, J.; Chiba, N.; Chen, S.; Ramanujan, V.K.; Wolf, A.J.; Vergnes, L.; Ojcius, D.M.; et al. Oxidized mitochondrial DNA activates the NLRP3 inflammasome during apoptosis. *Immunity* **2012**, *36*, 401–414. [CrossRef] [PubMed]
130. Fang, C.; Wei, X.; Wei, Y. Mitochondrial DNA in the regulation of innate immune responses. *Protein Cell* **2016**, *7*, 11–16. [CrossRef] [PubMed]
131. Glück, S.; Ablasser, A. Innate immunosensing of DNA in cellular senescence. *Curr. Opin. Immunol.* **2018**, *56*, 31–36. [CrossRef] [PubMed]
132. Rongvaux, A. Innate immunity and tolerance toward mitochondria. *Mitochondrion* **2018**, *41*, 14–20. [CrossRef] [PubMed]
133. Escames, G.; López, L.C.; García, J.A.; García-Corzo, L.; Ortiz, F.; Acuña-Castroviejo, D. Mitochondrial DNA and inflammatory diseases. *Hum. Genet.* **2012**, *131*, 161–173. [CrossRef] [PubMed]
134. Rahim, I.; Djerdjouri, B.; Sayed, R.K.; Fernández-Ortiz, M.; Fernández-Gil, B.; Hidalgo-Gutiérrez, A.; López, L.C.; Escames, G.; Reiter, R.J.; Acuña-Castroviejo, D. Melatonin administration to wild-type mice and nontreated NLRP3 mutant mice share similar inhibition of the inflammatory response during sepsis. *J. Pineal Res.* **2017**, *63*, e12410. [CrossRef] [PubMed]
135. Glück, S.; Guey, B.; Gulen, M.F.; Wolter, K.; Kang, T.W.; Schmacke, N.A.; Bridgeman, A.; Rehwinkel, J.; Zender, L.; Ablasser, A. Innate immune sensing of cytosolic chromatin fragments through cGAS promotes senescence. *Nat. Cell Biol.* **2017**, *19*, 1061–1070. [CrossRef] [PubMed]
136. Hamann, L.; Ruiz-Moreno, J.S.; Szwed, M.; Mossakowska, M.; Lundvall, L.; Schumann, R.R.; Opitz, B.; Puzianowska-Kuznicka, M. STING SNP R293Q is associated with a decreased risk of aging-related diseases. *Gerontology* **2018**, *26*, 1–10. [CrossRef] [PubMed]
137. Liu, Z.; Gan, L.; Xu, Y.; Luo, D.; Ren, Q.; Wu, S.; Sun, C. Melatonin alleviates inflammasome-induced pyroptosis through inhibiting NF-κB/GSDMD signal in mice adipose tissue. *J. Pineal Res.* **2017**, *63*, e12414. [CrossRef] [PubMed]
138. Deng, W.G.; Tang, S.T.; Tseng, H.P.; Wu, K.K. Melatonin suppresses macrophage cyclooxygenase-2 and inducible nitric oxide synthase expression by inhibiting p52 acetylation and binding. *Blood* **2006**, *108*, 518–524. [CrossRef] [PubMed]
139. Negi, G.; Kumar, A.; Sharma, S.S. Melatonin modulates neuroinflammation and oxidative stress in experimental diabetic neuropathy: Effects on NF-κB and Nrf2 cascades. *J. Pineal Res.* **2011**, *50*, 124–131. [CrossRef] [PubMed]

140. Murakami, Y.; Yuhara, K.; Takada, N.; Arai, T.; Tsuda, S.; Takamatsu, S.; Machino, M.; Fujisawa, S. Effect of melatonin on cyclooxygenase-2 expression and nuclear factor-kappa B activation in RAW264. *7 macrophage-like cells stimulated with fimbriae of Porphyromonas gingivalis. In Vivo* **2011**, *25*, 641–647. [PubMed]
141. Shi, D.; Xiao, X.; Wang, J.; Liu, L.; Chen, W.; Fu, L.; Xie, F.; Huang, W.; Deng, W. Melatonin suppresses proinflammatory mediators in lipopolysaccharide-stimulated CRL1999 cells via targeting MAPK, NF-κB, c/EBPβ, and p300 signaling. *J. Pineal Res.* **2012**, *53*, 154–165. [CrossRef] [PubMed]
142. Chinchalongporn, V.; Shukla, M.; Govitrapong, P. Melatonin ameliorates Aβ42 -induced alteration of βAPP-processing secretases via the melatonin receptor through the Pin1/GSK3β/NF-κB pathway in SH-SY5Y cells. *J. Pineal Res.* **2018**, *64*, e12470. [CrossRef] [PubMed]
143. Xia, M.Z.; Liang, Y.L.; Wang, H.; Chen, X.; Huang, Y.Y.; Zhang, Z.H.; Chen, Y.H.; Zhang, C.; Zhao, M.; Xu, D.X.; et al. Melatonin modulates TLR4-mediated inflammatory genes through MyD88- and TRIF-dependent signaling pathways in lipopolysaccharide-stimulated RAW264.7 cells. *J. Pineal Res.* **2012**, *53*, 325–334. [CrossRef] [PubMed]
144. Chuffa, L.G.; Fioruci-Fontanelli, B.A.; Mendes, L.O.; Ferreira Seiva, F.R.; Martinez, M.; Fávaro, W.J.; Domeniconi, R.F.; Pinheiro, P.F.; Delazari Dos Santos, L.; Martinez, F.E. Melatonin attenuates the TLR4-mediated inflammatory response through MyD88- and TRIF-dependent signaling pathways in an in vivo model of ovarian cancer. *BMC Cancer* **2015**, *15*, 34. [CrossRef] [PubMed]
145. Kang, J.W.; Koh, E.J.; Lee, S.M. Melatonin protects liver against ischemia and reperfusion injury through inhibition of toll-like receptor signaling pathway. *J. Pineal Res.* **2011**, *50*, 403–411. [CrossRef] [PubMed]
146. Huang, S.H.; Cao, X.J.; Wei, W. Melatonin decreases TLR3-mediated inflammatory factor expression via inhibition of NF-κB activation in respiratory syncytial virus-infected RAW264.7 macrophages. *J. Pineal Res.* **2008**, *45*, 93–100. [CrossRef] [PubMed]
147. Ding, K.; Wang, H.; Xu, J.; Lu, X.; Zhang, L.; Zhu, L. Melatonin reduced microglial activation and alleviated neuroinflammation induced neuron degeneration in experimental traumatic brain injury: Possible involvement of mTOR pathway. *Neurochem. Int.* **2014**, *76*, 23–31. [CrossRef] [PubMed]
148. Jumnongprakhon, P.; Govitrapong, P.; Tocharus, C.; Pinkaew, D.; Tocharus, J. Melatonin protects methamphetamine-induced neuroinflammation through NF-κB and Nrf2 pathways in glioma cell line. *Neurochem. Res.* **2015**, *40*, 1448–1456. [CrossRef] [PubMed]
149. Ismail, I.A.; El-Bakry, H.A.; Soliman, S.S. Melatonin and tumeric ameliorate aging-induced changes: Implication of immunoglobulins, cytokines, DJ-1/NRF2 and apoptosis regulation. *Int. J. Physiol. Pathophysiol. Pharmacol.* **2018**, *10*, 70–82. [PubMed]
150. El-Bakry, H.A.; Ismail, I.A.; Soliman, S.S. Immunosenescence-like state is accelerated by constant light exposure and counteracted by melatonin or turmeric administration through DJ-1/Nrf2 and P53/Bax pathways. *J. Photochem. Photobiol. B* **2018**, *186*, 69–80. [CrossRef] [PubMed]
151. Wang, J.; Jiang, C.; Zhang, K.; Lan, X.; Chen, X.; Zang, W.; Wang, Z.; Guan, F.; Zhu, C.; Yang, X.; et al. Melatonin receptor activation provides cerebral protection after traumatic brain injury by mitigating oxidative stress and inflammation via the Nrf2 signaling pathway. *Free Radic. Biol. Med.* **2019**, *131*, 345–355. [CrossRef] [PubMed]
152. Ariga, H.; Takahashi-Niki, K.; Kato, I.; Maita, H.; Niki, T.; Iguchi-Ariga, S.M. Neuroprotective function of DJ-1 in Parkinson's disease. *Oxid. Med. Cell. Longev.* **2013**, *2013*, 683920. [CrossRef] [PubMed]
153. Poulose, N.; Raju, R. Sirtuin regulation in aging and injury. *Biochim. Biophys. Acta* **2015**, *1852*, 2442–2455. [CrossRef] [PubMed]
154. Zhang, W.; Huang, Q.; Zeng, Z.; Wu, J.; Zhang, Y.; Chen, Z. Sirt1 inhibits oxidative stress in vascular endothelial cells. *Oxid. Med. Cell. Longev.* **2017**, *2017*, 7543973. [CrossRef] [PubMed]
155. Karbasforooshan, H.; Karimi, G. The role of SIRT1 in diabetic cardiomyopathy. *Biomed. Pharmacother.* **2017**, *90*, 386–392. [CrossRef] [PubMed]
156. Mendes, K.L.; Lelis, D.F.; Santos, S.H.S. Nuclear sirtuins and inflammatory signaling pathways. *Cytokine Growth Factor Rev.* **2017**, *38*, 98–105. [CrossRef] [PubMed]
157. Chai, D.; Zhang, L.; Xi, S.; Cheng, Y.; Jiang, H.; Hu, R. Nrf2 activation induced by Sirt1 ameliorates acute lung injury after intestinal ischemia/reperfusion through NOX4-mediated gene regulation. *Cell. Physiol. Biochem.* **2018**, *46*, 781–792. [CrossRef] [PubMed]

158. Han, J.; Liu, X.; Li, Y.; Zhang, J.; Yu, H. Sirt1/Nrf2 signalling pathway prevents cognitive impairment in diabetic rats through anti-oxidative stress induced by miRNA-23b-3p expression. *Mol. Med. Rep.* **2018**, *17*, 8414–8422. [CrossRef] [PubMed]
159. Huang, K.; Li, R.; Wei, W. Sirt1 activation prevents anti-Thy 1.1 mesangial proliferative glomerulonephritis in the rat through the Nrf2/ARE pathway. *Eur. J. Pharmacol.* **2018**, *832*, 138–144. [CrossRef] [PubMed]
160. Yang, B.; Xu, B.; Zhao, H.; Wang, Y.B.; Zhang, J.; Li, C.W.; Wu, Q.; Cao, Y.K.; Li, Y.; Cao, F. Dioscin protects against coronary heart disease by reducing oxidative stress and inflammation via Sirt1/Nrf2 and p38 MAPK pathways. *Mol. Med. Rep.* **2018**, *18*, 973–980. [CrossRef] [PubMed]
161. Wang, X.; Yuan, B.; Cheng, B.; Liu, Y.; Zhang, B.; Wang, X.; Lin, X.; Yang, B.; Gong, G. Crocin alleviates myocardial ischemia/reperfusion-induced endoplasmic reticulum stress via regulation of miR-34a/Sirt1/Nrf2 pathway. *Shock* **2019**, *51*, 123–130. [CrossRef] [PubMed]
162. Li, Y.; Yang, G.; Yang, X.; Wang, W.; Zhang, J.; He, Y.; Zhang, W.; Jing, T.; Lin, R. Nicotinic acid inhibits NLRP3 inflammasome activation via SIRT1 in vascular endothelial cells. *Int. Immunopharmacol.* **2016**, *40*, 211–218. [CrossRef] [PubMed]
163. Li, Y.; Yang, X.; He, Y.; Wang, W.; Zhang, J.; Zhang, W.; Jing, T.; Wang, B.; Lin, R. Negative regulation of NLRP3 inflammasome by SIRT1 in vascular endothelial cells. *Immunobiology* **2017**, *222*, 552–561. [CrossRef] [PubMed]
164. Zhang, S.; Jiang, L.; Che, F.; Lu, Y.; Xie, Z.; Wang, H. Arctigenin attenuates ischemic stroke via SIRT1-dependent inhibition of NLRP3 inflammasome. *Biochem. Biophys. Res. Commun.* **2017**, *493*, 821–826. [CrossRef] [PubMed]
165. Zou, P.; Liu, X.; Li, G.; Wang, Y. Resveratrol pretreatment attenuates traumatic brain injury in rats by suppressing NLRP3 inflammasome activation via SIRT1. *Mol. Med. Rep.* **2018**, *17*, 3212–3217. [CrossRef] [PubMed]
166. Lin, Q.Q.; Geng, Y.W.; Jiang, Z.W.; Tian, Z.J. SIRT1 regulates lipopolysaccharide-induced CD40 expression in renal medullary collecting duct cells by suppressing the TLR4-NF-κB signaling pathway. *Life Sci.* **2017**, *170*, 100–107. [CrossRef] [PubMed]
167. Yuan, Y.; Liu, Q.; Zhao, J.; Tang, H.; Sun, J. SIRT1 attenuates murine allergic rhinitis by downregulated HMGB 1/TLR4 pathway. *Scand. J. Immunol.* **2018**, *87*, e12667. [CrossRef] [PubMed]
168. Li, K.; Lv, G.; Pan, L. Sirt1 alleviates LPS induced inflammation of periodontal ligament fibroblasts via downregulation of TLR4. *Int. J. Biol. Macromol.* **2018**, *119*, 249–254. [CrossRef] [PubMed]
169. Rabadi, M.M.; Xavier, S.; Vasko, R.; Kaur, K.; Goligorksy, M.S.; Ratliff, B.B. High-mobility group box 1 is a novel deacetylation target of Sirtuin1. *Kidney Int.* **2015**, *87*, 95–108. [CrossRef] [PubMed]
170. Hwang, J.S.; Choi, H.S.; Ham, S.A.; Yoo, T.; Lee, W.J.; Paek, K.S.; Seo, H.G. Deacetylation-mediated interaction of SIRT1-HMGB1 improves survival in a mouse model of endotoxemia. *Sci. Rep.* **2015**, *5*, 15971. [CrossRef] [PubMed]
171. Rickenbacher, A.; Jang, J.H.; Limani, P.; Ungethüm, U.; Lehmann, K.; Oberkofler, C.E.; Weber, A.; Graf, R.; Humar, B.; Clavien, P.A. Fasting protects liver from ischemic injury through Sirt1-mediated downregulation of circulating HMGB1 in mice. *J. Hepatol.* **2014**, *61*, 301–308. [CrossRef] [PubMed]
172. Xu, W.; Lu, Y.; Yao, J.; Li, Z.; Chen, Z.; Wang, G.; Jing, H.; Zhang, X.; Li, M.; Peng, J.; Tian, X. Novel role of resveratrol: Suppression of high-mobility group protein box 1 nucleocytoplasmic translocation by the upregulation of sirtuin 1 in sepsis-induced liver injury. *Shock* **2014**, *42*, 440–447. [CrossRef] [PubMed]
173. Hwang, J.S.; Lee, W.J.; Kang, E.S.; Ham, S.A.; Yoo, T.; Paek, K.S.; Lim, D.S.; Do, J.T.; Seo, H.G. Ligand-activated peroxisome proliferator-activated receptor-δ and -γ inhibit lipopolysaccharide-primed release of high mobility group box 1 through upregulation of SIRT1. *Cell Death Dis.* **2014**, *5*, e1432. [CrossRef] [PubMed]
174. Yin, Y.; Feng, Y.; Zhao, H.; Zhao, Z.; Yua, H.; Xu, J.; Che, H. SIRT1 inhibits releases of HMGB1 and HSP70 from human umbilical vein endothelial cells caused by IL-6 and the serum from a preeclampsia patient and protects the cells from death. *Biomed. Pharmacother.* **2017**, *88*, 449–458. [CrossRef] [PubMed]
175. Chen, X.; Wu, S.; Chen, C.; Wu, S.; Yang, F.; Fang, Z.; Fu, H.; Li, Y. Omega-3 polyunsaturated fatty acid supplementation attenuates microglial-induced inflammation by inhibiting the HMGB1/TLR4/NF-κB pathway following experimental traumatic brain injury. *J. Neuroinflamm.* **2017**, *14*, 143. [CrossRef] [PubMed]
176. Hwang, J.S.; Kang, E.S.; Han, S.G.; Lim, D.S.; Paek, K.S.; Lee, C.H.; Seo, H.G. Formononetin inhibits lipopolysaccharide-induced release of high mobility group box 1 by upregulating SIRT1 in a PPARδ-dependent manner. *Peer J.* **2018**, *6*, e4208. [CrossRef] [PubMed]

177. Su, Z.; Zhang, P.; Yu, Y.; Lu, H.; Liu, Y.; Ni, P.; Su, X.; Wang, D.; Liu, Y.; Wang, J.; et al. HMGB1 facilitated macrophage reprogramming towards a proinflammatory M1-like phenotype in experimental autoimmune myocarditis development. *Sci. Rep.* **2016**, *6*, 21884. [CrossRef] [PubMed]
178. Karuppagounder, V.; Giridharan, V.V.; Arumugam, S.; Sreedhar, R.; Palaniyandi, S.S.; Krishnamurthy, P.; Quevedo, J.; Watanabe, K.; Konishi, T.; Thandavarayan, R.A. Modulation of macrophage polarization and HMGB1-TLR2/TLR4 cascade plays a crucial role for cardiac remodeling in senescence-accelerated prone mice. *PLoS ONE* **2016**, *11*, e0152922. [CrossRef] [PubMed]
179. Son, M.; Porat, A.; He, M.; Suurmond, J.; Santiago-Schwarz, F.; Andersson, U.; Coleman, T.R.; Volpe, B.T.; Tracey, K.J.; Al-Abed, Y.; et al. C1q and HMGB1 reciprocally regulate human macrophage polarization. *Blood* **2016**, *128*, 2218–2228. [CrossRef] [PubMed]
180. Jiang, Y.; Chen, R.; Shao, X.; Ji, X.; Lu, H.; Zhou, S.; Zong, G.; Xu, H.; Su, Z. HMGB1 silencing in macrophages prevented their functional skewing and ameliorated EAM development: Nuclear HMGB1 may be a checkpoint molecule of macrophage reprogramming. *Int. Immunopharmacol.* **2018**, *56*, 277–284. [CrossRef] [PubMed]
181. Gao, T.; Chen, Z.; Chen, H.; Yuan, H.; Wang, Y.; Peng, X.; Wei, C.; Yang, J.; Xu, C. Inhibition of HMGB1 mediates neuroprotection of traumatic brain injury by modulating the microglia/macrophage polarization. *Biochem. Biophys. Res. Commun.* **2018**, *497*, 430–436. [CrossRef] [PubMed]
182. Prieto-Domínguez, N.; Méndez-Blanco, C.; Carbajo-Pescador, S.; Fondevila, F.; García-Palomo, A.; González-Gallego, J.; Mauriz, J.L. Melatonin enhances sorafenib actions in human hepatocarcinoma cells by inhibiting mTORC1/p70S6K/HIF-1α and hypoxia-mediated mitophagy. *Oncotarget* **2017**, *8*, 91402–91414. [CrossRef] [PubMed]
183. Fan, T.; Pi, H.; Li, M.; Ren, Z.; He, Z.; Zhu, F.; Tian, L.; Tu, M.; Xie, J.; Liu, M.; et al. Inhibiting MT2-TFE3-dependent autophagy enhances melatonin-induced apoptosis in tongue squamous cell carcinoma. *J. Pineal Res.* **2018**, *64*, e12457. [CrossRef] [PubMed]
184. Yun, S.M.; Woo, S.H.; Oh, S.T.; Hong, S.E.; Choe, T.B.; Ye, S.K.; Kim, E.K.; Seong, M.K.; Kim, H.A.; Noh, W.C.; et al. Melatonin enhances arsenic trioxide-induced cell death via sustained upregulation of Redd1 expression in breast cancer cells. *Mol. Cell. Endocrinol.* **2016**, *422*, 64–73. [CrossRef] [PubMed]
185. Liu, Z.; Gan, L.; Liu, G.; Chen, Y.; Wu, T.; Feng, F.; Sun, C. Sirt1 decreased adipose inflammation by interacting with Akt2 and inhibiting mTOR/S6K1 pathway in mice. *J. Lipid Res.* **2016**, *57*, 1373–1381. [CrossRef] [PubMed]
186. Chen, H.; Shen, F.; Sherban, A.; Nocon, A.; Li, Y.; Wang, H.; Xu, M.J.; Rui, X.; Han, J.; Jiang, B.; et al. DEP domain-containing mTOR-interacting protein suppresses lipogenesis and ameliorates hepatic steatosis and acute-on-chronic liver injury in alcoholic liver disease. *Hepatology* **2018**, *68*, 496–514. [CrossRef] [PubMed]
187. Guarani, V.; Deflorian, G.; Franco, C.A.; Krüger, M.; Phng, L.K.; Bentley, K.; Toussaint, L.; Dequiedt, F.; Mostoslavsky, R.; Schmidt, M.H.H.; et al. Acetylation-dependent regulation of endothelial Notch signalling by the SIRT1 deacetylase. *Nature* **2011**, *473*, 234–238. [CrossRef] [PubMed]
188. Bai, X.; He, T.; Liu, Y.; Li, X.; Shi, J.; Wang, K.; Han, F.; Zhang, W.; Zhang, Y.; Cai, W.; et al. Acetylation-dependent regulation of Notch signaling in macrophages by SIRT1 affects sepsis development. *Front. Immunol.* **2018**, *9*, 762. [CrossRef] [PubMed]
189. Yang, J.J.; Tao, H.; Liu, L.P.; Hu, W.; Deng, Z.Y.; Li, J. miR-200a controls hepatic stellate cell activation and fibrosis via SIRT1/Notch1 signal pathway. *Inflamm. Res.* **2017**, *66*, 341–352. [CrossRef] [PubMed]
190. Yu, L.; Liang, H.; Lu, Z.; Zhao, G.; Zhai, M.; Yang, Y.; Yang, J.; Yi, D.; Chen, W.; Wang, X.; et al. Membrane receptor-dependent Notch1/Hes1 activation by melatonin protects against myocardial ischemia-reperfusion injury: In vivo and in vitro studies. *J. Pineal Res.* **2015**, *59*, 420–433. [CrossRef] [PubMed]
191. Zhang, S.; Wang, P.; Ren, L.; Hu, C.; Bi, J. Protective effect of melatonin on soluble A$\beta_{1\text{-}42}$-induced memory impairment, astrogliosis, and synaptic dysfunction via the Musashi1/Notch1/Hes1 signaling pathway in the rat hippocampus. *Alzheimers Res. Ther.* **2016**, *8*, 40. [CrossRef] [PubMed]
192. Yu, L.; Fan, C.; Li, Z.; Zhang, J.; Xue, X.; Xu, Y.; Zhao, G.; Yang, Y.; Wang, H. Melatonin rescues cardiac thioredoxin system during ischemia-reperfusion injury in acute hyperglycemic state by restoring Notch1/Hes1/Akt signaling in a membrane receptor-dependent manner. *J. Pineal Res.* **2017**, *62*, e12375. [CrossRef] [PubMed]

193. Jia, Y.; Li, Z.; Cai, W.; Xiao, D.; Han, S.; Han, F.; Bai, X.; Wang, K.; Liu, Y.; Li, X.; et al. SIRT1 regulates inflammation response of macrophages in sepsis mediated by long noncoding RNA. *Biochim. Biophys. Acta* **2018**, *1864*, 784–792. [CrossRef] [PubMed]
194. Xia, Y.; Chen, S.; Zeng, S.; Zhao, Y.; Zhu, C.; Deng, B.; Zhu, G.; Yin, Y.; Wang, W.; Hardeland, R.; et al. Melatonin in macrophage biology: Current understanding and future perspectives. *J. Pineal Res.* **2018**, *66*, e12547. [CrossRef] [PubMed]
195. Lau, W.W.; Ng, J.K.; Lee, M.M.; Chan, A.S.; Wong, Y.H. Interleukin-6 autocrine signaling mediates melatonin $MT_{1/2}$ receptor-induced STAT3 Tyr_{705} phosphorylation. *J. Pineal Res.* **2012**, *52*, 477–489. [CrossRef] [PubMed]
196. Yang, Y.; Duan, W.; Jin, Z.; Yi, W.; Yan, J.; Zhang, S.; Wang, N.; Liang, Z.; Li, Y.; Chen, W.; et al. JAK2/STAT3 activation by melatonin attenuates the mitochondrial oxidative damage induced by myocardial ischemia/reperfusion injury. *J. Pineal Res.* **2013**, *55*, 275–286. [CrossRef] [PubMed]
197. Yi, W.J.; Kim, T.S. Melatonin protects mice against stress-induced inflammation through enhancement of M2 macrophage polarization. *Int. Immunopharmacol.* **2017**, *48*, 146–158. [CrossRef] [PubMed]
198. Ryo, A.; Suizu, F.; Yoshida, Y.; Perrem, K.; Liou, Y.C.; Wulf, G.; Rottapel, R.; Yamaoka, S.; Lu, K.P. Regulation of NF-κB signaling by Pin1-dependent prolyl isomerization and ubiquitin-mediated proteolysis of p65/RelA. *Mol. Cell* **2003**, *12*, 1413–1426. [CrossRef]
199. Strebovsky, J.; Walker, P.; Lang, R.; Dalpke, A.H. Suppressor of cytokine signaling 1 (SOCS1) limits NFκB signaling by decreasing p65 stability within the cell nucleus. *FASEB J.* **2011**, *25*, 863–874. [CrossRef] [PubMed]
200. Liu, Y.; Liu, X.; Hua, W.; Wei, Q.; Fang, X.; Zhao, Z.; Ge, C.; Liu, C.; Chen, C.; Tao, Y.; et al. Berberine inhibits macrophage M1 polarization via AKT1/SOCS1/NF-κB signaling pathway to protect against DSS-induced colitis. *Int. Immunopharmacol.* **2018**, *57*, 121–131. [CrossRef] [PubMed]
201. García, J.A.; Volt, H.; Venegas, C.; Doerrier, C.; Escames, G.; López, L.C.; Acuña-Castroviejo, D. Disruption of the NF-κB/NLRP3 connection by melatonin requires retinoid-related orphan receptor-α and blocks the septic response in mice. *FASEB J.* **2015**, *29*, 3863–3875. [CrossRef] [PubMed]
202. Nejati Moharrami, N.; Bjørkøy Tande, E.; Ryan, L.; Espevik, T.; Boyartchuk, V. RORα controls inflammatory state of human macrophages. *PLoS ONE* **2018**, *13*, e0207374. [CrossRef] [PubMed]
203. Slominski, A.T.; Kim, T.K.; Takeda, Y.; Janjetovic, Z.; Brozyna, A.A.; Skobowiat, C.; Wang, J.; Postlethwaite, A.; Li, W.; Tuckey, R.C.; et al. RORα and RORγ are expressed in human skin and serve as receptors for endogenously produced noncalcemic 20-hydroxy- and 20,23-dihydroxyvitamin D. *FASEB J.* **2014**, *28*, 2775–2789. [CrossRef] [PubMed]
204. Slominski, A.T.; Zmijewski, M.A.; Jetten, A.M. RORα is not a receptor for melatonin (response to DOI 10.1002/bies.201600018). *BioEssays* **2016**, *38*, 1193–1194. [CrossRef] [PubMed]
205. Zhang, S.; Gao, L.; Liu, X.; Lu, T.; Xie, C.; Jia, J. Resveratrol attenuates microglial activation via SIRT1-SOCS1 pathway. *Evid. Based Complement. Alternat. Med.* **2017**, *2017*, 8791832. [CrossRef] [PubMed]
206. Warren, K.J.; Fang, X.; Gowda, N.M.; Thompson, J.J.; Heller, N.M. The TORC1-activated proteins, p70S6K and GRB10, regulate IL-4 signaling and M2 macrophage polarization by modulating phosphorylation of insulin receptor substrate-2. *J. Biol. Chem.* **2016**, *291*, 24922–24930. [CrossRef] [PubMed]
207. Klinge, C.M. Non-coding RNAs in breast cancer: Intracellular and intercellular communication. *Noncoding RNA* **2018**, *4*, 40. [CrossRef] [PubMed]
208. Kufel, J.; Grzechnik, P. Small nucleolar RNAs tell a different tale. *Trends Genet.* **2019**, *35*, 104–117. [CrossRef] [PubMed]
209. Hardeland, R. On the relationships between lncRNAs and other orchestrating regulators: Role of the circadian system. *Epigenomes* **2018**, *2*, 9. [CrossRef]
210. Czech, B.; Munafò, M.; Ciabrelli, F.; Eastwood, E.L.; Fabry, M.H.; Kneuss, E.; Hannon, G.J. piRNA-guided genome defense: From biogenesis to silencing. *Annu. Rev. Genet.* **2018**, *52*, 131–157. [CrossRef] [PubMed]
211. Hardeland, R. Intercellular communication via exosomal and ectosomal microRNAs: Facing a jungle of countless microRNAs and targets. In *Mini-Reviews in Recent Melatonin Research*; Hardeland, R., Ed.; Cuvillier: Göttingen, Germany, 2017; pp. 109–122, ISBN 978-3-7369-9677-9.
212. Hardeland, R. Exosomal and ectosomal noncoding RNAs in cancer—More than diagnostic and prognostic markers. *Open Acc. J. Oncol. Med.* **2018**, *2*, 000144.
213. Hardeland, R. Melatonin, noncoding RNAs, messenger RNA stability and epigenetics—Evidence, hints, gaps and perspectives. *Int. J. Mol. Sci.* **2014**, *15*, 18221–18252. [CrossRef] [PubMed]
214. Hardeland, R. Interactions of melatonin and microRNAs. *Biochem. Mol. Biol. J.* **2018**, *4*, 7. [CrossRef]

215. Hardeland, R. Melatonin and chromatin. *Melatonin Res.* **2019**, *2*, 67–93. [CrossRef]
216. Mann, M.; Mehta, A.; Zhao, J.L.; Lee, K.; Marinov, G.K.; Garcia-Flores, Y.; Lu, L.F.; Rudensky, A.Y.; Baltimore, D. An NF-κB-microRNA regulatory network tunes macrophage inflammatory responses. *Nat. Commun.* **2017**, *8*, 851. [CrossRef] [PubMed]
217. Yang, Y.; Liu, D.; Xi, Y.; Li, J.; Liu, B.; Li, J. Upregulation of miRNA-140-5p inhibits inflammatory cytokines in acute lung injury through the MyD88/NF-κB signaling pathway by targeting TLR4. *Exp. Ther. Med.* **2018**, *16*, 3913–3920. [CrossRef] [PubMed]
218. Zhao, G.; Zhang, T.; Wu, H.; Jiang, K.; Qiu, C.; Deng, G. MicroRNA let-7c improves LPS-induced outcomes of endometritis by suppressing NF-κB signaling. *Inflammation* **2018**. [CrossRef] [PubMed]
219. Zheng, D.; Zang, Y.; Xu, H.; Wang, Y.; Cao, X.; Wang, T.; Pan, M.; Shi, J.; Li, X. MicroRNA-214 promotes the calcification of human aortic valve interstitial cells through the acceleration of inflammatory reactions with activated MyD88/NF-κB signaling. *Clin. Res. Cardiol.* **2018**. [CrossRef] [PubMed]
220. Garavelli, S.; De Rosa, V.; de Candia, P. The multifaceted interface between cytokines and microRNAs: An ancient mechanism to regulate the good and the bad of inflammation. *Front. Immunol.* **2018**, *9*, 3012. [CrossRef] [PubMed]
221. Lee, S.E.; Kim, S.J.; Youn, J.P.; Hwang, S.Y.; Park, C.S.; Park, Y.S. MicroRNA and gene expression analysis of melatonin-exposed breast cancer cell lines indicating involvement of the anticancer effect. *J. Pineal Res.* **2011**, *51*, 345–352. [CrossRef] [PubMed]
222. Hardeland, R. Melatonin and microRNAs: An emerging field. In *Mini-Reviews in Recent Melatonin Research*; Hardeland, R., Ed.; Cuvillier: Göttingen, Germany, 2017; pp. 105–108, ISBN 978-3-7369-9677-9.
223. Koltai, E.; Bori, Z.; Osvath, P.; Ihasz, F.; Peter, S.; Toth, G.; Degens, H.; Rittweger, J.; Boldogh, I.; Radak, Z. Master athletes have higher miR-7, SIRT3 and SOD2 expression in skeletal muscle than age-matched sedentary controls. *Redox Biol.* **2018**, *19*, 46–51. [CrossRef] [PubMed]
224. Kabaria, S.; Choi, D.C.; Chaudhuri, A.D.; Jain, M.R.; Li, H.; Junn, E. MicroRNA-7 activates Nrf2 pathway by targeting Keap1 expression. *Free Radic. Biol. Med.* **2015**, *89*, 548–556. [CrossRef] [PubMed]
225. Choi, D.C.; Chae, Y.J.; Kabaria, S.; Chaudhuri, A.D.; Jain, M.R.; Li, H.; Mouradian, M.M.; Junn, E. MicroRNA-7 protects against 1-methyl-4-phenylpyridinium-induced cell death by targeting RelA. *J. Neurosci.* **2014**, *34*, 12725–12737. [CrossRef] [PubMed]
226. Zhao, X.D.; Lu, Y.Y.; Guo, H.; Xie, H.H.; He, L.J.; Shen, G.F.; Zhou, J.F.; Li, T.; Hu, S.J.; Zhou, L.; et al. MicroRNA-7/NF-κB signaling regulatory feedback circuit regulates gastric carcinogenesis. *J. Cell Biol.* **2015**, *210*, 613–627. [CrossRef] [PubMed]
227. Giles, K.M.; Brown, R.A.; Ganda, C.; Podgorny, M.J.; Candy, P.A.; Wintle, L.C.; Richardson, K.L.; Kalinowski, F.C.; Stuart, L.M.; Epis, M.R.; et al. microRNA-7-5p inhibits melanoma cell proliferation and metastasis by suppressing RelA/NF-κB. *Oncotarget* **2016**, *7*, 31663–31680. [CrossRef] [PubMed]
228. Saunders, L.R.; Sharma, A.D.; Tawney, J.; Nakagawa, M.; Okita, K.; Yamanaka, S.; Willenbring, H.; Verdin, E. miRNAs regulate SIRT1 expression during mouse embryonic stem cell differentiation and in adult mouse tissues. *Aging* **2010**, *2*, 415–431. [CrossRef] [PubMed]
229. Ramachandran, D.; Roy, U.; Garg, S.; Ghosh, S.; Pathak, S.; Kolthur-Seetharam, U. Sirt1 and mir-9 expression is regulated during glucose-stimulated insulin secretion in pancreatic β-islets. *FEBS J.* **2011**, *278*, 1167–1174. [CrossRef] [PubMed]
230. Schonrock, N.; Humphreys, D.T.; Preiss, T.; Götz, J. Target gene repression mediated by miRNAs miR-181c and miR-9 both of which are down-regulated by amyloid-β. *J. Mol. Neurosci.* **2012**, *46*, 324–335. [CrossRef] [PubMed]
231. Ao, R.; Wang, Y.; Tong, J.; Wang, B.F. Altered microRNA-9 expression level is directly correlated with pathogenesis of nonalcoholic fatty liver disease by targeting Onecut2 and SIRT1. *Med. Sci. Monit.* **2016**, *22*, 3804–3819. [CrossRef] [PubMed]
232. D'Adamo, S.; Cetrullo, S.; Guidotti, S.; Borzì, R.M.; Flamigni, F. Hydroxytyrosol modulates the levels of microRNA-9 and its target sirtuin-1 thereby counteracting oxidative stress-induced chondrocyte death. *Osteoarthritis Cartilage* **2017**, *25*, 600–610. [CrossRef] [PubMed]
233. Zhou, L.; Fu, L.; Lv, N.; Chen, X.S.; Liu, J.; Li, Y.; Xu, Q.Y.; Huang, S.; Zhang, X.D.; Dou, L.P.; et al. A minicircuitry comprised of microRNA-9 and SIRT1 contributes to leukemogenesis in t(8;21) acute myeloid leukemia. *Eur. Rev. Med. Pharmacol. Sci.* **2017**, *21*, 786–794. [PubMed]

234. Owczarz, M.; Budzinska, M.; Domaszewska-Szostek, A.; Borkowska, J.; Polosak, J.; Gewartowska, M.; Slusarczyk, P.; Puzianowska-Kuznicka, M. miR-34a and miR-9 are overexpressed and SIRT genes are downregulated in peripheral blood mononuclear cells of aging humans. *Exp. Biol. Med.* **2017**, *242*, 1453–1461. [CrossRef] [PubMed]
235. Bu, P.; Luo, C.; He, Q.; Yang, P.; Li, X.; Xu, D. MicroRNA-9 inhibits the proliferation and migration of malignant melanoma cells via targeting sirtuin 1. *Exp. Ther. Med.* **2017**, *14*, 931–938. [CrossRef] [PubMed]
236. Khosravi, A.; Alizadeh, S.; Jalili, A.; Shirzad, R.; Saki, N. The impact of Mir-9 regulation in normal and malignant hematopoiesis. *Oncol. Rev.* **2018**, *12*, e348. [CrossRef] [PubMed]
237. Rushworth, S.A.; Murray, M.Y.; Barrera, L.N.; Heasman, S.A.; Zaitseva, L.; MacEwan, D.J. Understanding the role of miRNA in regulating NF-κB in blood cancer. *Am. J. Cancer Res.* **2012**, *2*, 65–74. [PubMed]
238. Wang, L.Q.; Kwong, Y.L.; Kho, C.S.; Wong, K.F.; Wong, K.Y.; Ferracin, M.; Calin, G.A.; Chim, C.S. Epigenetic inactivation of miR-9 family microRNAs in chronic lymphocytic leukemia—Implications on constitutive activation of NFκB pathway. *Mol. Cancer* **2013**, *12*, 173. [CrossRef] [PubMed]
239. Zhang, Z.X.; Liu, Z.Q.; Jiang, B.; Lu, X.Y.; Ning, X.F.; Yuan, C.T.; Wang, A.L. BRAF activated non-coding RNA (BANCR) promoting gastric cancer cells proliferation via regulation of NF-κB1. *Biochem. Biophys. Res. Commun.* **2015**, *465*, 225–231. [CrossRef] [PubMed]
240. Chakraborty, S.; Zawieja, D.C.; Davis, M.J.; Muthuchamy, M. MicroRNA signature of inflamed lymphatic endothelium and role of miR-9 in lymphangiogenesis and inflammation. *Am. J. Physiol. Cell Physiol.* **2015**, *309*, C680–C692. [CrossRef] [PubMed]
241. Gu, R.; Liu, N.; Luo, S.; Huang, W.; Zha, Z.; Yang, J. MicroRNA-9 regulates the development of knee osteoarthritis through the NF-kappaB1 pathway in chondrocytes. *Medicine* **2016**, *95*, e4315. [CrossRef] [PubMed]
242. Qian, D.; Wei, G.; Xu, C.; He, Z.; Hua, J.; Li, J.; Hu, Q.; Lin, S.; Gong, J.; Meng, H.; et al. Bone marrow-derived mesenchymal stem cells (BMSCs) repair acute necrotized pancreatitis by secreting microRNA-9 to target the NF-κB1/p50 gene in rats. *Sci. Rep.* **2017**, *7*, 581. [CrossRef] [PubMed]
243. Yao, H.; Ma, R.; Yang, L.; Hu, G.; Chen, X.; Duan, M.; Kook, Y.; Niu, F.; Liao, K.; Fu, M.; et al. MiR-9 promotes microglial activation by targeting MCPIP1. *Nat. Commun.* **2014**, *5*, 4386. [CrossRef] [PubMed]
244. Huang, G.; Liu, X.; Zhao, X.; Zhao, J.; Hao, J.; Ren, J.; Chen, Y. MiR-9 promotes multiple myeloma progression by regulating TRIM56/NF-κB pathway. *Cell Biol. Int.* **2019**. [CrossRef] [PubMed]
245. Zhu, M.; Zhou, X.; Du, Y.; Huang, Z.; Zhu, J.; Xu, J.; Cheng, G.; Shu, Y.; Liu, P.; Zhu, W.; et al. miR-20a induces cisplatin resistance of a human gastric cancer cell line via targeting CYLD. *Mol. Med. Rep.* **2016**, *14*, 1742–1750. [CrossRef] [PubMed]
246. Liu, Z.; Yu, H.; Guo, Q. MicroRNA-20a promotes inflammation via the nuclear factor-κB signaling pathway in pediatric pneumonia. *Mol. Med. Rep.* **2018**, *17*, 612–617. [CrossRef] [PubMed]
247. Lin, Q.; Geng, Y.; Zhao, M.; Lin, S.; Zhu, Q.; Tian, Z. MiR-21 regulates TNF-α-induced CD40 expression via the SIRT1-NF-κB pathway in renal inner medullary collecting duct cells. *Cell. Physiol. Biochem.* **2017**, *41*, 124–136. [CrossRef] [PubMed]
248. Kim, S.J.; Kang, H.S.; Lee, J.H.; Park, J.H.; Jung, C.H.; Bae, J.H.; Oh, B.C.; Song, D.K.; Baek, W.K.; Im, S.S. Melatonin ameliorates ER stress-mediated hepatic steatosis through miR-23a in the liver. *Biochem. Biophys. Res. Commun.* **2015**, *458*, 462–469. [CrossRef] [PubMed]
249. Weinberg, R.B.; Mufson, E.J.; Counts, S.E. Evidence for a neuroprotective microRNA pathway in amnestic mild cognitive impairment. *Front. Neurosci.* **2015**, *9*, 430. [CrossRef] [PubMed]
250. Sruthi, T.V.; Edatt, L.; Raji, G.R.; Kunhiraman, H.; Shankar, S.S.; Shankar, V.; Ramachandran, V.; Poyyakkara, A.; Kumar, S.V.B. Horizontal transfer of miR-23a from hypoxic tumor cell colonies can induce angiogenesis. *J. Cell. Physiol.* **2018**, *233*, 3498–3514. [CrossRef] [PubMed]
251. Luo, H.; Han, Y.; Liu, J.; Zhang, Y. Identification of microRNAs in granulosa cells from patients with different levels of ovarian reserve function and the potential regulatory function of miR-23a in granulosa cell apoptosis. *Gene* **2019**, *686*, 250–260. [CrossRef] [PubMed]
252. Khan, A.U.H.; Rathore, M.G.; Allende-Vega, N.; Vo, D.N.; Belkhala, S.; Orecchioni, S.; Talarico, G.; Bertolini, F.; Cartron, G.; Lecellier, C.H.; et al. Human leukemic cells performing oxidative phosphorylation (OXPHOS) generate an antioxidant response independently of reactive oxygen species (ROS) production. *EBioMedicine* **2015**, *3*, 43–53. [CrossRef] [PubMed]

253. Zhang, D.; Qiu, X.; Li, J.; Zheng, S.; Li, L.; Zhao, H. MiR-23a-3p-regulated abnormal acetylation of FOXP3 induces regulatory T cell function defect in Graves' disease. *Biol. Chem.* **2018**. [CrossRef] [PubMed]
254. Zhao, S.; Li, T.; Li, J.; Lu, Q.; Han, C.; Wang, N.; Qiu, Q.; Cao, H.; Xu, X.; Chen, H.; et al. miR-23b-3p induces the cellular metabolic memory of high glucose in diabetic retinopathy through a SIRT1-dependent signalling pathway. *Diabetologia* **2016**, *59*, 644–654. [CrossRef] [PubMed]
255. Mori, F.; Ferraiuolo, M.; Santoro, R.; Sacconi, A.; Goeman, F.; Pallocca, M.; Pulito, C.; Korita, E.; Fanciulli, M.; Muti, P.; et al. Multitargeting activity of miR-24 inhibits long-term melatonin anticancer effects. *Oncotarget* **2016**, *7*, 20532–20548. [CrossRef] [PubMed]
256. Tong, X.; Wang, X.; Wang, C.; Li, L. Elevated levels of serum MiR-152 and miR-24 in uterine sarcoma: Potential for inducing autophagy via SIRT1 and deacetylated LC3. *Br. J. Biomed. Sci.* **2018**, *75*, 7–12. [CrossRef] [PubMed]
257. Xiao, X.; Lu, Z.; Lin, V.; May, A.; Shaw, D.H.; Wang, Z.; Che, B.; Tran, K.; Du, H.; Shaw, P.X. MicroRNA miR-24-3p reduces apoptosis and regulates Keap1-Nrf2 pathway in mouse cardiomyocytes responding to ischemia/reperfusion injury. *Oxid. Med. Cell. Longev.* **2018**, *2018*, 7042105. [CrossRef] [PubMed]
258. Xie, Q.; Wei, M.; Kang, X.; Liu, D.; Quan, Y.; Pan, X.; Liu, X.; Liao, D.; Liu, J.; Zhang, B. Reciprocal inhibition between miR-26a and NF-κB regulates obesity-related chronic inflammation in chondrocytes. *Biosci. Rep.* **2015**, *35*, e00204. [CrossRef] [PubMed]
259. Thulasingam, S.; Massilamany, C.; Gangaplara, A.; Dai, H.; Yarbaeva, S.; Subramaniam, S.; Riethoven, J.J.; Eudy, J.; Lou, M.; Reddy, J. miR-27b*, an oxidative stress-responsive microRNA modulates nuclear factor-κB pathway in RAW 264.7 cells. *Mol. Cell. Biochem.* **2011**, *352*, 181–188. [CrossRef] [PubMed]
260. Kurtz, C.L.; Fannin, E.E.; Toth, C.L.; Pearson, D.S.; Vickers, K.C.; Sethupathy, P. Inhibition of miR-29 has a significant lipid-lowering benefit through suppression of lipogenic programs in liver. *Sci. Rep.* **2015**, *5*, 12911. [CrossRef] [PubMed]
261. Zhou, L.; Xu, D.Y.; Sha, W.G.; Shen, L.; Lu, G.Y.; Yin, X.; Wang, M.J. High glucose induces renal tubular epithelial injury via Sirt1/NF-kappaB/microR-29/Keap1 signal pathway. *J. Transl. Med.* **2015**, *13*, 352. [CrossRef] [PubMed]
262. Wei, R.; Zhang, R.; Li, H.; Li, H.; Zhang, S.; Xie, Y.; Shen, L.; Chen, F. MiR-29 Targets PUMA to suppress oxygen and glucose deprivation/reperfusion (OGD/R)-induced cell death in hippocampal neurons. *Curr. Neurovasc. Res.* **2018**, *15*, 47–54. [CrossRef] [PubMed]
263. Egan Benova, T.; Viczenczova, C.; Szeiffova Bacova, B.; Knezl, V.; Dosenko, V.; Rauchova, H.; Zeman, M.; Reiter, R.J.; Tribulova, N. Obesity-associated alterations in cardiac connexin-43 and PKC signaling are attenuated by melatonin and omega-3 fatty acids in female rats. *Mol. Cell. Biochem.* **2018**. [CrossRef] [PubMed]
264. Guan, Y.; Rao, Z.; Chen, C. miR-30a suppresses lung cancer progression by targeting SIRT1. *Oncotarget* **2017**, *9*, 4924–4934. [CrossRef] [PubMed]
265. Wan, Q.; Zhou, Z.; Ding, S.; He, J. The miR-30a negatively regulates IL-17-mediated signal transduction by targeting Traf3ip2. *J. Interferon Cytokine Res.* **2015**, *35*, 917–923. [CrossRef] [PubMed]
266. Volkmann, I.; Kumarswamy, R.; Pfaff, N.; Fiedler, J.; Dangwal, S.; Holzmann, A.; Batkai, S.; Geffers, R.; Lother, A.; Hein, L.; et al. MicroRNA-mediated epigenetic silencing of sirtuin1 contributes to impaired angiogenic responses. *Circ. Res.* **2013**, *113*, 997–1003. [CrossRef] [PubMed]
267. Kumarswamy, R.; Volkmann, I.; Beermann, J.; Napp, L.C.; Jabs, O.; Bhayadia, R.; Melk, A.; Ucar, A.; Chowdhury, K.; Lorenzen, J.M.; et al. Vascular importance of the miR-212/132 cluster. *Eur. Heart J.* **2014**, *35*, 3224–3231. [CrossRef] [PubMed]
268. Meng, F.; Dai, E.; Yu, X.; Zhang, Y.; Chen, X.; Liu, X.; Wang, S.; Wang, L.; Jiang, W. Constructing and characterizing a bioactive small molecule and microRNA association network for Alzheimer's disease. *J. R. Soc. Interface* **2013**, *11*, 20131057. [CrossRef] [PubMed]
269. Rajbhandari, R.; McFarland, B.C.; Patel, A.; Gerigk, M.; Gray, G.K.; Fehling, S.C.; Bredel, M.; Berbari, N.F.; Kim, H.; Marks, M.P.; et al. Loss of tumor suppressive microRNA-31 enhances TRADD/NF-κB signaling in glioblastoma. *Oncotarget* **2015**, *6*, 17805–17816. [CrossRef] [PubMed]
270. Carloni, S.; Favrais, G.; Saliba, E.; Albertini, M.C.; Chalon, S.; Longini, M.; Gressens, P.; Buonocore, G.; Balduini, W. Melatonin modulates neonatal brain inflammation through endoplasmic reticulum stress, autophagy, and miR-34a/silent information regulator 1 pathway. *J. Pineal Res.* **2016**, *61*, 370–830. [CrossRef] [PubMed]

271. Pogribny, I.P.; Muskhelishvili, L.; Tryndyak, V.P.; Beland, F.A. The tumor-promoting activity of 2-acetylaminofluorene is associated with disruption of the p53 signaling pathway and the balance between apoptosis and cell proliferation. *Toxicol. Appl. Pharmacol.* **2009**, *235*, 305–311. [CrossRef] [PubMed]
272. Tabuchi, T.; Satoh, M.; Itoh, T.; Nakamura, M. MicroRNA-34a regulates the longevity-associated protein SIRT1 in coronary artery disease: Effect of statins on SIRT1 and microRNA-34a expression. *Clin. Sci.* **2012**, *123*, 161–171. [CrossRef] [PubMed]
273. Roy, A.; Zhang, M.; Saad, Y.; Kolattukudy, P.E. Antidicer RNAse activity of monocyte chemotactic protein-induced protein-1 is critical for inducing angiogenesis. *Am. J. Physiol. Cell Physiol.* **2013**, *305*, C1021–C1032. [CrossRef] [PubMed]
274. Khee, S.G.; Yusof, Y.A.; Makpol, S. Expression of senescence-associated microRNAs and target genes in cellular aging and modulation by tocotrienol-rich fraction. *Oxid. Med. Cell. Longev.* **2014**, *2014*, 725929. [PubMed]
275. Karbasforooshan, H.; Karimi, G. The role of SIRT1 in diabetic retinopathy. *Biomed. Pharmacother.* **2018**, *97*, 190–194. [CrossRef] [PubMed]
276. Rossi, S.; Di Filippo, C.; Gesualdo, C.; Testa, F.; Trotta, M.C.; Maisto, R.; Ferraro, B.; Ferraraccio, F.; Accardo, M.; Simonelli, F.; et al. Interplay between intravitreal RvD1 and local endogenous sirtuin-1 in the protection from endotoxin-induced uveitis in rats. *Mediat. Inflamm.* **2015**, *2015*, 126408. [CrossRef] [PubMed]
277. Gao, A.M.; Zhang, X.Y.; Ke, Z.P. Apigenin sensitizes BEL-7402/ADM cells to doxorubicin through inhibiting miR-101/Nrf2 pathway. *Oncotarget* **2017**, *8*, 82085–82091. [CrossRef] [PubMed]
278. Raji, G.R.; Sruthi, T.V.; Edatt, L.; Haritha, K.; Sharath Shankar, S.; Sameer Kumar, V.B. Horizontal transfer of miR-106a/b from cisplatin resistant hepatocarcinoma cells can alter the sensitivity of cervical cancer cells to cisplatin. *Cell. Signal.* **2017**, *38*, 146–158. [CrossRef] [PubMed]
279. Heyn, J.; Luchting, B.; Hinske, L.C.; Hübner, M.; Azad, S.C.; Kreth, S. miR-124a and miR-155 enhance differentiation of regulatory T cells in patients with neuropathic pain. *J. Neuroinflamm.* **2016**, *13*, 248. [CrossRef] [PubMed]
280. Kim, S.W.; Ramasamy, K.; Bouamar, H.; Lin, A.P.; Jiang, D.; Aguiar, R.C. MicroRNAs miR-125a and miR-125b constitutively activate the NF-κB pathway by targeting the tumor necrosis factor alpha-induced protein 3 (TNFAIP3, A20). *Proc. Natl. Acad. Sci. USA* **2012**, *109*, 7865–7870. [CrossRef] [PubMed]
281. Haemmig, S.; Baumgartner, U.; Glück, A.; Zbinden, S.; Tschan, M.P.; Kappeler, A.; Mariani, L.; Vajtai, I.; Vassella, E. miR-125b controls apoptosis and temozolomide resistance by targeting TNFAIP3 and NKIRAS2 in glioblastomas. *Cell Death Dis.* **2014**, *5*, e1279. [CrossRef] [PubMed]
282. Parisi, C.; Napoli, G.; Amadio, S.; Spalloni, A.; Apolloni, S.; Longone, P.; Volonté, C. MicroRNA-125b regulates microglia activation and motor neuron death in ALS. *Cell Death Differ.* **2016**, *23*, 531–541. [CrossRef] [PubMed]
283. Zheng, Z.; Qu, J.Q.; Yi, H.M.; Ye, X.; Huang, W.; Xiao, T.; Li, J.Y.; Wang, Y.Y.; Feng, J.; Zhu, J.F.; et al. MiR-125b regulates proliferation and apoptosis of nasopharyngeal carcinoma by targeting A20/NF-κB signaling pathway. *Cell Death Dis.* **2017**, *8*, e2855. [CrossRef] [PubMed]
284. Xue, N.; Qi, L.; Zhang, G.; Zhang, Y. miRNA-125b regulates osteogenic differentiation of periodontal ligament cells through NKIRAS2/NF-κB pathway. *Cell. Physiol. Biochem.* **2018**, *48*, 1771–1781. [CrossRef] [PubMed]
285. Wang, D.; Cao, L.; Xu, Z.; Fang, L.; Zhong, Y.; Chen, Q.; Luo, R.; Chen, H.; Li, K.; Xiao, S. MiR-125b reduces porcine reproductive and respiratory syndrome virus replication by negatively regulating the NF-κB pathway. *PLoS ONE* **2013**, *8*, e55838. [CrossRef] [PubMed]
286. Wang, X.; Ha, T.; Zou, J.; Ren, D.; Liu, L.; Zhang, X.; Kalbfleisch, J.; Gao, X.; Williams, D.; Li, C. MicroRNA-125b protects against myocardial ischaemia/reperfusion injury via targeting p53-mediated apoptotic signalling and TRAF6. *Cardiovasc. Res.* **2014**, *102*, 385–395. [CrossRef] [PubMed]
287. Ma, H.; Wang, X.; Ha, T.; Gao, M.; Liu, L.; Wang, R.; Yu, K.; Kalbfleisch, J.H.; Kao, R.L.; Williams, D.L.; et al. MicroRNA-125b prevents cardiac dysfunction in polymicrobial sepsis by targeting TRAF6-mediated nuclear factor κB activation and p53-mediated apoptotic signaling. *J. Infect. Dis.* **2016**, *214*, 1773–1783. [CrossRef] [PubMed]
288. Wang, Y.; Tang, P.; Chen, Y.; Chen, J.; Ma, R.; Sun, L. Overexpression of microRNA-125b inhibits human acute myeloid leukemia cells invasion, proliferation and promotes cells apoptosis by targeting NF-κB signaling pathway. *Biochem. Biophys. Res. Commun.* **2017**, *488*, 60–66. [CrossRef] [PubMed]

289. Jia, J.; Wang, J.; Zhang, J.; Cui, M.; Sun, X.; Li, Q.; Zhao, B. MiR-125b inhibits LPS-induced inflammatory injury via targeting MIP-1α in chondrogenic cell ATDC5. *Cell. Physiol. Biochem.* **2018**, *45*, 2305–2316. [CrossRef] [PubMed]
290. Togliatto, G.; Trombetta, A.; Dentelli, P.; Gallo, S.; Rosso, A.; Cotogni, P.; Granata, R.; Falcioni, R.; Delale, T.; Ghigo, E.; et al. Unacylated ghrelin induces oxidative stress resistance in a glucose intolerance and peripheral artery disease mouse model by restoring endothelial cell miR-126 expression. *Diabetes* **2015**, *64*, 1370–1382. [CrossRef] [PubMed]
291. Oglesby, I.K.; Bray, I.M.; Chotirmall, S.H.; Stallings, R.L.; O'Neill, S.J.; McElvaney, N.G.; Greene, C.M. miR-126 is downregulated in cystic fibrosis airway epithelial cells and regulates TOM1 expression. *J. Immunol.* **2010**, *184*, 1702–1709. [CrossRef] [PubMed]
292. Feng, X.; Wang, H.; Ye, S.; Guan, J.; Tan, W.; Cheng, S.; Wei, G.; Wu, W.; Wu, F.; Zhou, Y. Up-regulation of microRNA-126 may contribute to pathogenesis of ulcerative colitis via regulating NF-kappaB inhibitor IκBα. *PLoS ONE* **2012**, *7*, e52782. [CrossRef] [PubMed]
293. Feng, X.; Tan, W.; Cheng, S.; Wang, H.; Ye, S.; Yu, C.; He, Y.; Zeng, J.; Cen, J.; Hu, J.; et al. Upregulation of microRNA-126 in hepatic stellate cells may affect pathogenesis of liver fibrosis through the NF-κB pathway. *DNA Cell Biol.* **2015**, *34*, 470–480. [CrossRef] [PubMed]
294. Adlakha, Y.K.; Saini, N. miR-128 exerts pro-apoptotic effect in a p53 transcription-dependent and -independent manner via PUMA-Bak axis. *Cell Death Dis.* **2013**, *4*, e542. [CrossRef] [PubMed]
295. Lian, B.; Yang, D.; Liu, Y.; Shi, G.; Li, J.; Yan, X.; Jin, K.; Liu, X.; Zhao, J.; Shang, W.; et al. miR-128 targets the SIRT1/ROS/DR5 pathway to sensitize colorectal cancer to TRAIL-induced apoptosis. *Cell. Physiol. Biochem.* **2018**, *49*, 2151–2162. [CrossRef] [PubMed]
296. Pan, S.; Cui, Y.; Fu, Z.; Zhang, L.; Xing, H. MicroRNA-128 is involved in dexamethasone-induced lipid accumulation via repressing SIRT1 expression in cultured pig preadipocytes. *J. Steroid Biochem. Mol. Biol.* **2019**, *186*, 185–195. [CrossRef] [PubMed]
297. Xia, Z.; Meng, F.; Liu, Y.; Fang, Y.; Wu, X.; Zhang, C.; Liu, D.; Li, G. Decreased MiR-128-3p alleviates the progression of rheumatoid arthritis by up-regulating the expression of TNFAIP3. *Biosci. Rep.* **2018**, *38*, BSR20180540. [CrossRef] [PubMed]
298. Geng, L.; Zhang, T.; Liu, W.; Chen, Y. Inhibition of miR-128 abates Aβ-mediated cytotoxicity by targeting PPAR-γ via NF-κB inactivation in primary mouse cortical neurons and Neuro2a cells. *Yonsei Med. J.* **2018**, *59*, 1096–1106. [CrossRef] [PubMed]
299. Ali, T.; Mushtaq, I.; Maryam, S.; Farhan, A.; Saba, K.; Jan, M.I.; Sultan, A.; Anees, M.; Duygu, B.; Hamera, S.; et al. Interplay of N-acetyl cysteine and melatonin in regulating oxidative stress-induced cardiac hypertrophic factors and microRNAs. *Arch. Biochem. Biophys.* **2019**, *661*, 56–65. [CrossRef] [PubMed]
300. Liu, L.; Sun, T.; Liu, Z.; Chen, X.; Zhao, L.; Qu, G.; Li, Q. Traumatic brain injury dysregulates microRNAs to modulate cell signaling in rat hippocampus. *PLoS ONE* **2014**, *9*, e103948. [CrossRef] [PubMed]
301. Smith, E.J.; Shay, K.P.; Thomas, N.O.; Butler, J.A.; Finlay, L.F.; Hagen, T.M. Age-related loss of hepatic Nrf2 protein homeostasis: Potential role for heightened expression of miR-146a. *Free Radic. Biol. Med.* **2015**, *89*, 1184–1191. [CrossRef] [PubMed]
302. Kamali, K.; Korjan, E.S.; Eftekhar, E.; Malekzadeh, K.; Soufi, F.G. The role of miR-146a on NF-κB expression level in human umbilical vein endothelial cells under hyperglycemic condition. *Bratisl. Lek. Listy* **2016**, *117*, 376–380. [CrossRef] [PubMed]
303. Loubaki, L.; Chabot, D.; Paré, I.; Drouin, M.; Bazin, R. MiR-146a potentially promotes IVIg-mediated inhibition of TLR4 signaling in LPS-activated human monocytes. *Immunol. Lett.* **2017**, *185*, 64–73. [CrossRef] [PubMed]
304. An, R.; Feng, J.; Xi, C.; Xu, J.; Sun, L. miR-146a attenuates sepsis-induced myocardial dysfunction by suppressing IRAK1 and TRAF6 via targeting ErbB4 expression. *Oxid. Med. Cell. Longev.* **2018**, *2018*, 7163057. [CrossRef] [PubMed]
305. Lindeløv Vestergaard, A.; Heiner Bang-Berthelsen, C.; Fløyel, T.; Lucien Stahl, J.; Christen, L.; Taheri Sotudeh, F.; de Hemmer Horskjær, P.; Stensgaard Frederiksen, K.; Greek Kofod, F.; Bruun, C.; et al. MicroRNAs and histone deacetylase inhibition-mediated protection against inflammatory β-cell damage. *PLoS ONE* **2018**, *13*, e0203713. [CrossRef] [PubMed]

306. Sang, W.; Wang, Y.; Zhang, C.; Zhang, D.; Sun, C.; Niu, M.; Zhang, Z.; Wei, X.; Pan, B.; Chen, W.; et al. MiR-150 impairs inflammatory cytokine production by targeting ARRB-2 after blocking CD28/B7 costimulatory pathway. *Immunol. Lett.* **2016**, *172*, 1–10. [CrossRef] [PubMed]
307. Xue, H.; Li, M.X. MicroRNA-150 protects against cigarette smoke-induced lung inflammation and airway epithelial cell apoptosis through repressing p53: MicroRNA-150 in CS-induced lung inflammation. *Hum. Exp. Toxicol.* **2018**, *37*, 920–928. [CrossRef] [PubMed]
308. Ma, Y.; Liu, Y.; Hou, H.; Yao, Y.; Meng, H. MiR-150 predicts survival in patients with sepsis and inhibits LPS-induced inflammatory factors and apoptosis by targeting NF-κB1 in human umbilical vein endothelial cells. *Biochem. Biophys. Res. Commun.* **2018**, *500*, 828–837. [CrossRef] [PubMed]
309. Luo, X.Y.; Zhu, X.Q.; Li, Y.; Wang, X.B.; Yin, W.; Ge, Y.S.; Ji, W.M. MicroRNA-150 restores endothelial cell function and attenuates vascular remodeling by targeting PTX3 through the NF-κB signaling pathway in mice with acute coronary syndrome. *Cell Biol. Int.* **2018**. [CrossRef] [PubMed]
310. Gu, J.; Lu, Z.; Ji, C.; Chen, Y.; Liu, Y.; Lei, Z.; Wang, L.; Zhang, H.T.; Li, X. Melatonin inhibits proliferation and invasion via repression of miRNA-155 in glioma cells. *Biomed. Pharmacother.* **2017**, *93*, 969–975. [CrossRef]
311. Wang, Y.; Zheng, Z.J.; Jia, Y.J.; Yang, Y.L.; Xue, Y.M. Role of p53/miR-155-5p/sirt1 loop in renal tubular injury of diabetic kidney disease. *J. Transl. Med.* **2018**, *16*, 146. [CrossRef] [PubMed]
312. Wang, X.; Wang, B.; Zhao, J.; Liu, C.; Qu, X.; Li, Y. MiR-155 is involved in major depression disorder and antidepressant treatment via targeting SIRT1. *Biosci. Rep.* **2018**, *38*, 20181139. [CrossRef] [PubMed]
313. Wan, C.; Han, R.; Liu, L.; Zhang, F.; Li, F.; Xiang, M.; Ding, W. Role of miR-155 in fluorooctane sulfonate-induced oxidative hepatic damage via the Nrf2-dependent pathway. *Toxicol. Appl. Pharmacol.* **2016**, *295*, 85–93. [CrossRef] [PubMed]
314. Gu, S.; Lai, Y.; Chen, H.; Liu, Y.; Zhang, Z. miR-155 mediates arsenic trioxide resistance by activating Nrf2 and suppressing apoptosis in lung cancer cells. *Sci. Rep.* **2017**, *7*, 12155. [CrossRef] [PubMed]
315. Rodriguez-Ortiz, C.J.; Baglietto-Vargas, D.; Martinez-Coria, H.; LaFerla, F.M.; Kitazawa, M. Upregulation of miR-181 decreases c-Fos and SIRT-1 in the hippocampus of 3xTg-AD mice. *J. Alzheimers Dis.* **2014**, *42*, 1229–1238. [CrossRef] [PubMed]
316. Chen, X.Y.; Zhang, H.S.; Wu, T.C.; Sang, W.W.; Ruan, Z. Down-regulation of NAMPT expression by miR-182 is involved in Tat-induced HIV-1 long terminal repeat (LTR) transactivation. *Int. J. Biochem. Cell Biol.* **2013**, *45*, 292–298. [CrossRef] [PubMed]
317. Eyler, C.E.; Rich, J.N. Looking in the miR-ror: TGF-β-mediated activation of NF-κB in glioma. *J. Clin. Investig.* **2012**, *122*, 3473–3475. [CrossRef] [PubMed]
318. Song, L.; Liu, L.; Wu, Z.; Li, Y.; Ying, Z.; Lin, C.; Wu, J.; Hu, B.; Cheng, S.Y.; Li, M.; et al. TGF-β induces miR-182 to sustain NF-κB activation in glioma subsets. *J. Clin. Investig.* **2012**, *122*, 3563–3578. [CrossRef] [PubMed]
319. Guo, Y.; Liao, Y.; Jia, C.; Ren, J.; Wang, J.; Li, T. MicroRNA-182 promotes tumor cell growth by targeting transcription elongation factor A-like 7 in endometrial carcinoma. *Cell. Physiol. Biochem.* **2013**, *32*, 581–590. [CrossRef] [PubMed]
320. Ling, T.; Yu, F.; Cao, H. miR-182 controls cell growth in gastrointestinal stromal tumors by negatively regulating CYLD expression. *Oncol. Rep.* **2018**, *40*, 3705–3713. [CrossRef] [PubMed]
321. Liu, Y.; Li, L.N.; Guo, S.; Zhao, X.Y.; Liu, Y.Z.; Liang, C.; Tu, S.; Wang, D.; Li, L.; Dong, J.Z.; et al. Melatonin improves cardiac function in a mouse model of heart failure with preserved ejection fraction. *Redox Biol.* **2018**, *18*, 211–221. [CrossRef] [PubMed]
322. Wang, R.; Zhou, S.; Wu, P.; Li, M.; Ding, X.; Sun, L.; Xu, X.; Zhou, X.; Zhou, L.; Cao, C.; et al. Identifying involvement of H19-miR-675-3p-IGF1R and H19-miR-200a-PDCD4 in treating pulmonary hypertension with melatonin. *Mol. Ther. Nucleic Acids* **2018**, *13*, 44–54. [CrossRef] [PubMed]
323. Eades, G.; Yao, Y.; Yang, M.; Zhang, Y.; Chumsri, S.; Zhou, Q. miR-200a regulates SIRT1 expression and epithelial to mesenchymal transition (EMT)-like transformation in mammary epithelial cells. *J. Biol. Chem.* **2011**, *286*, 25992–26002. [CrossRef] [PubMed]
324. Pan, F.; Qiu, X.F.; Yu, W.; Zhang, Q.P.; Chen, Q.; Zhang, C.Y.; Chen, Y.; Pan, L.J.; Zhang, A.X.; Dai, Y.T. MicroRNA-200a is up-regulated in aged rats with erectile dysfunction and could attenuate endothelial function via SIRT1 inhibition. *Asian J. Androl.* **2016**, *18*, 74–79. [PubMed]

325. Zhang, P.; Xu, L.; Guan, H.; Liu, L.; Liu, J.; Huang, Z.; Cao, X.; Liao, Z.; Xiao, H.; Li, Y. Beraprost sodium, a prostacyclin analogue, reduces fructose-induced hepatocellular steatosis in mice and in vitro via the microRNA-200a and SIRT1 signaling pathway. *Metabolism* **2017**, *73*, 9–21. [CrossRef] [PubMed]
326. Fu, H.; Song, W.; Chen, X.; Guo, T.; Duan, B.; Wang, X.; Tang, Y.; Huang, L.; Zhang, C. MiRNA-200a induce cell apoptosis in renal cell carcinoma by directly targeting SIRT1. *Mol. Cell. Biochem.* **2018**, *437*, 143–152. [CrossRef] [PubMed]
327. Salimian, N.; Peymani, M.; Ghaedi, K.; Nasr Esfahani, M.H. Modulation in miR-200a/SIRT1axis is associated with apoptosis in MPP$^+$-induced SH-SY5Y cells. *Gene* **2018**, *674*, 25–30. [CrossRef] [PubMed]
328. Eades, G.; Yang, M.; Yao, Y.; Zhang, Y.; Zhou, Q. miR-200a regulates Nrf2 activation by targeting Keap1 mRNA in breast cancer cells. *J. Biol. Chem.* **2011**, *286*, 40725–40733. [CrossRef] [PubMed]
329. Murray-Stewart, T.; Hanigan, C.L.; Woster, P.M.; Marton, L.J.; Casero, R.A., Jr. Histone deacetylase inhibition overcomes drug resistance through a miRNA-dependent mechanism. *Mol. Cancer Ther.* **2013**, *12*, 2088–2099. [CrossRef] [PubMed]
330. Wei, J.; Zhang, Y.; Luo, Y.; Wang, Z.; Bi, S.; Song, D.; Dai, Y.; Wang, T.; Qiu, L.; Wen, L.; et al. Aldose reductase regulates miR-200a-3p/141-3p to coordinate Keap1-Nrf2, Tgfβ1/2, and Zeb1/2 signaling in renal mesangial cells and the renal cortex of diabetic mice. *Free Radic. Biol. Med.* **2014**, *67*, 91–102. [CrossRef] [PubMed]
331. Liu, Q.L.; Zhang, J.; Liu, X.; Gao, J.Y. Role of growth hormone in maturation and activation of dendritic cells via miR-200a and the Keap1/Nrf2 pathway. *Cell Prolif.* **2015**, *48*, 573–581. [CrossRef] [PubMed]
332. Liu, M.; Hu, C.; Xu, Q.; Chen, L.; Ma, K.; Xu, N.; Zhu, H. Methylseleninic acid activates Keap1/Nrf2 pathway via up-regulating miR-200a in human oesophageal squamous cell carcinoma cells. *Biosci. Rep.* **2015**, *35*, e00256. [CrossRef] [PubMed]
333. Sun, X.; Zuo, H.; Liu, C.; Yang, Y. Overexpression of miR-200a protects cardiomyocytes against hypoxia-induced apoptosis by modulating the kelch-like ECH-associated protein 1-nuclear factor erythroid 2-related factor 2 signaling axis. *Int. J. Mol. Med.* **2016**, *38*, 1303–1311. [CrossRef] [PubMed]
334. Wu, H.; Kong, L.; Tan, Y.; Epstein, P.N.; Zeng, J.; Gu, J.; Liang, G.; Kong, M.; Chen, X.; Miao, L.; et al. C66 ameliorates diabetic nephropathy in mice by both upregulating NRF2 function via increase in miR-200a and inhibiting miR-21. *Diabetologia* **2016**, *59*, 1558–1568. [CrossRef] [PubMed]
335. Zhao, S.; Mao, L.; Wang, S.G.; Chen, F.L.; Ji, F.; Fe, H.D. MicroRNA-200a activates Nrf2 signaling to protect osteoblasts from dexamethasone. *Oncotarget* **2017**, *8*, 104867–104876. [CrossRef] [PubMed]
336. Zhao, X.J.; Yu, H.W.; Yang, Y.Z.; Wu, W.Y.; Chen, T.Y.; Jia, K.K.; Kang, L.L.; Jiao, R.Q.; Kong, L.D. Polydatin prevents fructose-induced liver inflammation and lipid deposition through increasing miR-200a to regulate Keap1/Nrf2 pathway. *Redox Biol.* **2018**, *18*, 124–137. [CrossRef] [PubMed]
337. Shi, Z.; Hu, Z.; Chen, D.; Huang, J.; Fan, J.; Zhou, S.; Wang, X.; Hu, J.; Huang, F. MicroRNA-200a mediates nasopharyngeal carcinoma cell proliferation through the activation of nuclear factor-κB. *Mol. Med. Rep.* **2016**, *13*, 1732–1738. [CrossRef] [PubMed]
338. Zhang, Q.S.; Liu, W.; Lu, G.X. miR-200a-3p promotes β-Amyloid-induced neuronal apoptosis through down-regulation of SIRT1 in Alzheimer's disease. *J. Biosci.* **2017**, *42*, 397–404. [CrossRef] [PubMed]
339. Li, L.; Wang, Q.; Yuan, Z.; Chen, A.; Liu, Z.; Li, H.; Wang, Z. Long non-coding RNA H19 contributes to hypoxia-induced CPC injury by suppressing Sirt1 through miR-200a-3p. *Acta Biochim. Biophys. Sin.* **2018**, *50*, 950–959. [CrossRef] [PubMed]
340. Qi, J.; Qiao, Y.; Wang, P.; Li, S.; Zhao, W.; Gao, C. microRNA-210 negatively regulates LPS-induced production of proinflammatory cytokines by targeting NF-κB1 in murine macrophages. *FEBS Lett.* **2012**, *586*, 1201–1207. [CrossRef] [PubMed]
341. Zhang, D.; Cao, X.; Li, J.; Zhao, G. MiR-210 inhibits NF-κB signaling pathway by targeting DR6 in osteoarthritis. *Sci. Rep.* **2015**, *5*, 12775. [CrossRef] [PubMed]
342. Ramalinga, M.; Roy, A.; Srivastava, A.; Bhattarai, A.; Harish, V.; Suy, S.; Collins, S.; Kumar, D. MicroRNA-212 negatively regulates starvation induced autophagy in prostate cancer cells by inhibiting SIRT1 and is a modulator of angiogenesis and cellular senescence. *Oncotarget* **2015**, *6*, 34446–34457. [CrossRef] [PubMed]
343. Miao, H.; Zeng, H.; Gong, H. microRNA-212 promotes lipid accumulation and attenuates cholesterol efflux in THP-1 human macrophages by targeting SIRT1. *Gene* **2018**, *643*, 55–60. [CrossRef] [PubMed]
344. Li, D.; Bai, L.; Wang, T.; Xie, Q.; Chen, M.; Fu, Y.; Wen, Q. Function of miR-212 as a tumor suppressor in thyroid cancer by targeting SIRT1. *Oncol. Rep.* **2018**, *39*, 695–702. [CrossRef] [PubMed]

345. Fiorentino, L.; Cavalera, M.; Mavilio, M.; Conserva, F.; Menghini, R.; Gesualdo, L.; Federici, M. Regulation of TIMP3 in diabetic nephropathy: A role for microRNAs. *Acta Diabetol.* **2013**, *50*, 965–969. [CrossRef] [PubMed]
346. Lu, Z.; Li, Y.; Takwi, A.; Li, B.; Zhang, J.; Conklin, D.J.; Young, K.H.; Martin, R.; Li, Y. miR-301a as an NF-κB activator in pancreatic cancer cells. *EMBO J.* **2011**, *30*, 57–67. [CrossRef] [PubMed]
347. Zhou, P.; Jiang, W.; Wu, L.; Chang, R.; Wu, K.; Wang, Z. miR-301a is a candidate oncogene that targets the homeobox gene Gax in human hepatocellular carcinoma. *Dig. Dis. Sci.* **2012**, *57*, 1171–1180. [CrossRef] [PubMed]
348. Huang, L.; Liu, Y.; Wang, L.; Chen, R.; Ge, W.; Lin, Z.; Zhang, Y.; Liu, S.; Shan, Y.; Lin, Q.; et al. Down-regulation of miR-301a suppresses pro-inflammatory cytokines in Toll-like receptor-triggered macrophages. *Immunology* **2013**, *140*, 314–322. [PubMed]
349. Ma, X.; Yan, F.; Deng, Q.; Li, F.; Lu, Z.; Liu, M.; Wang, L.; Conklin, D.J.; McCracken, J.; Srivastava, S.; et al. Modulation of tumorigenesis by the pro-inflammatory microRNA miR-301a in mouse models of lung cancer and colorectal cancer. *Cell Discov.* **2015**, *1*, 15005. [CrossRef] [PubMed]
350. Tavakolpour, V.; Shokri, G.; Naser Moghadasi, A.; Mozafari Nahavandi, P.; Hashemi, M.; Kouhkan, F. Increased expression of mir-301a in PBMCs of patients with relapsing-remitting multiple sclerosis is associated with reduced NKRF and PIAS3 expression levels and disease activity. *J. Neuroimmunol.* **2018**, *325*, 79–86. [CrossRef] [PubMed]
351. Wu, C.T.; Huang, Y.; Pei, Z.Y.; Xi, X.; Zhu, G.F. MicroRNA-326 aggravates acute lung injury in septic shock by mediating the NF-κB signaling pathway. *Int. J. Biochem. Cell Biol.* **2018**, *101*, 1–11. [CrossRef] [PubMed]
352. Shi, L.; Chen, Z.G.; Wu, L.L.; Zheng, J.J.; Yang, J.R.; Chen, X.F.; Chen, Z.Q.; Liu, C.L.; Chi, S.Y.; Zheng, J.Y.; et al. miR-340 reverses cisplatin resistance of hepatocellular carcinoma cell lines by targeting Nrf2-dependent antioxidant pathway. *Asian Pac. J. Cancer Prev.* **2014**, *15*, 10439–10444. [CrossRef] [PubMed]
353. Wu, L.L.; Cai, W.P.; Lei, X.; Shi, Q.; Lin, X.Y.; Shi, L. NRAL mediates cisplatin resistance in hepatocellular carcinoma via miR-340-5p/Nrf2 axis. *J. Cell. Commun. Signal.* **2018**. [CrossRef] [PubMed]
354. Prins, S.A.; Przybycien-Szymanska, M.M.; Rao, Y.S.; Pak, T.R. Long-term effects of peripubertal binge EtOH exposure on hippocampal microRNA expression in the rat. *PLoS ONE* **2014**, *9*, e83166. [CrossRef] [PubMed]
355. Cai, B.; Ma, W.; Bi, C.; Yang, F.; Zhang, L.; Han, Z.; Huang, Q.; Ding, F.; Li, Y.; Yan, G.; et al. Long noncoding RNA H19 mediates melatonin inhibition of premature senescence of c-kit$^+$ cardiac progenitor cells by promoting miR-675. *J. Pineal Res.* **2016**, *61*, 82–95. [CrossRef] [PubMed]
356. Liu, J.; Zhu, L.; Xie, G.L.; Bao, J.F.; Yu, Q. Let-7 miRNAs modulate the activation of NF-κB by targeting TNFAIP3 and are involved in the pathogenesis of lupus nephritis. *PLoS ONE* **2015**, *10*, e0121256. [CrossRef] [PubMed]
357. Yang, S.; Tang, W.; He, Y.; Wen, L.; Sun, B.; Li, S. Long non-coding RNA and microRNA-675/let-7a mediates the protective effect of melatonin against early brain injury after subarachnoid hemorrhage via targeting TP53 and neural growth factor. *Cell Death Dis.* **2018**, *9*, 99. [CrossRef] [PubMed]
358. Lin, Z.; Ge, J.; Wang, Z.; Ren, J.; Wang, X.; Xiong, H.; Gao, J.; Zhang, Y.; Zhang, Q. Let-7e modulates the inflammatory response in vascular endothelial cells through ceRNA crosstalk. *Sci. Rep.* **2017**, *7*, 42498. [CrossRef] [PubMed]
359. Kumar, M.; Sahu, S.K.; Kumar, R.; Subuddhi, A.; Maji, R.K.; Jana, K.; Gupta, P.; Raffetseder, J.; Lerm, M.; Ghosh, Z.; et al. MicroRNA let-7 modulates the immune response to *Mycobacterium tuberculosis* infection via control of A20, an inhibitor of the NF-κB pathway. *Cell Host Microbe* **2015**, *17*, 345–356. [CrossRef] [PubMed]
360. Wang, Y.S.; His, E.; Cheng, H.Y.; Hsu, S.H.; Liao, Y.C.; Juo, S.H. Let-7g suppresses both canonical and non-canonical NF-κB pathways in macrophages leading to anti-atherosclerosis. *Oncotarget* **2017**, *8*, 101026–101041. [PubMed]
361. Xie, H.; Lei, N.; Gong, A.Y.; Chen, X.M.; Hu, G. *Cryptosporidium parvum* induces SIRT1 expression in host epithelial cells through downregulating let-7i. *Hum. Immunol.* **2014**, *75*, 760–765. [CrossRef] [PubMed]
362. Sarver, A.L.; Sarver, A.E.; Yuan, C.; Subramanian, S. OMCD: OncomiR Cancer Database. *BMC Cancer* **2018**, *18*, 1223. [CrossRef] [PubMed]
363. Ushio, N.; Rahman, M.M.; Maemura, T.; Lai, Y.C.; Iwanaga, T.; Kawaguchi, H.; Miyoshi, N.; Momoi, Y.; Miura, N. Identification of dysregulated microRNAs in canine malignant melanoma. *Oncol. Lett.* **2019**, *17*, 1080–1088. [CrossRef] [PubMed]

364. Zargar, S.; Tomar, V.; Shyamsundar, V.; Vijayalakshmi, R.; Somasundaram, K.; Karunagaran, D. A feedback loop between miRNA-155, Programmed cell death 4 and Activation Protein-1 modulates the expression of miR-155 and tumorigenesis in tongue cancer. *Mol. Cell. Biol.* **2019**. [CrossRef] [PubMed]
365. Jung-Hynes, B.; Schmit, T.L.; Reagan-Shaw, S.R.; Siddiqui, I.A.; Mukhtar, H.; Ahmad, N. Melatonin, a novel Sirt1 inhibitor, imparts proliferative effects against prostate cancer cells in vitro culture and in vivo in TRAMP model. *J. Pineal Res.* **2011**, *50*, 140–149. [PubMed]
366. Zhang, Y.; Liu, X.; Bai, X.; Lin, Y.; Li, Z.; Fu, J.; Li, M.; Zhao, T.; Yang, H.; Xu, R.; et al. Melatonin prevents endothelial cell pyroptosis via regulation of long noncoding RNA MEG3/miR-223/NLRP3 axis. *J. Pineal Res.* **2018**, *64*, e12449. [CrossRef] [PubMed]
367. Jin, M.; Cao, M.; Cao, Q.; Piao, J.; Zhao, F.; Piao, J. Long noncoding RNA and gene expression analysis of melatonin-exposed Liaoning cashmere goat fibroblasts indicating cashmere growth. *Naturwissenschaften* **2018**, *105*, 60. [CrossRef] [PubMed]
368. Wang, T.H.; Wu, C.H.; Yeh, C.T.; Su, S.C.; Hsia, S.M.; Liang, K.H.; Chen, C.C.; Hsueh, C.; Chen, C.Y. Melatonin suppresses hepatocellular carcinoma progression via lncRNA-CPS1-IT-mediated HIF-1α inactivation. *Oncotarget* **2017**, *8*, 82280–82293. [PubMed]
369. Chen, C.C.; Chen, C.Y.; Wang, S.H.; Yeh, C.T.; Su, S.C.; Ueng, S.H.; Chuang, W.Y.; Hsueh, C.; Wang, T.H. Melatonin sensitizes hepatocellular carcinoma cells to chemotherapy through long non-coding RNA RAD51-AS1-mediated suppression of DNA repair. *Cancers* **2018**, *10*, 320. [CrossRef] [PubMed]
370. Su, S.C.; Reiter, R.J.; Hsiao, H.Y.; Chung, W.H.; Yang, S.F. Functional interaction between melatonin signaling and noncoding RNAs. *Trends Endocrinol. MeTable* **2018**, *29*, 435–445. [CrossRef] [PubMed]
371. Fan, Z.; Zhao, M.; Joshi, P.D.; Li, P.; Zhang, Y.; Guo, W.; Xu, Y.; Wang, H.; Zhao, Z.; Yan, J. A class of circadian long non-coding RNAs mark enhancers modulating long-range circadian gene regulation. *Nucleic Acids Res.* **2017**, *45*, 5720–5738. [CrossRef] [PubMed]
372. Pereira Fernandes, D.; Bitar, M.; Jacobs, F.M.J.; Barry, G. Long non-coding RNAs in neuronal aging. *Noncoding RNA* **2018**, *4*, 12. [CrossRef] [PubMed]
373. Gomez-Verjan, J.C.; Vazquez-Martinez, E.R.; Rivero-Segura, N.A.; Medina-Campos, R.H. The RNA world of human ageing. *Hum. Genet.* **2018**, *137*, 865–879. [CrossRef] [PubMed]
374. Heward, J.A.; Lindsay, M.A. Long non-coding RNAs in the regulation of the immune response. *Trends Immunol.* **2014**, *35*, 408–419. [CrossRef] [PubMed]
375. Elling, R.; Chan, J.; Fitzgerald, K.A. Emerging role of long noncoding RNAs as regulators of innate immune cell development and inflammatory gene expression. *Eur. J. Immunol.* **2016**, *46*, 504–512. [CrossRef] [PubMed]
376. Murphy, M.B.; Medvedev, A.E. Long noncoding RNAs as regulators of Toll-like receptor signaling and innate immunity. *J. Leukoc. Biol.* **2016**, *99*, 839–850. [CrossRef] [PubMed]
377. Panda, A.C.; Abdelmohsen, K.; Gorospe, M. SASP regulation by noncoding RNA. *Mech. Ageing Dev.* **2017**, *168*, 37–43. [CrossRef] [PubMed]
378. Carpenter, S.; Fitzgerald, K.A. Cytokines and long noncoding RNAs. *Cold Spring Harb. Perspect. Biol.* **2018**, *10*, a028589. [CrossRef] [PubMed]
379. Wang, Z.; Zheng, Y. lncRNAs regulate innate immune responses and their roles in macrophage polarization. *Mediat. Inflamm.* **2018**, *2018*, 8050956. [CrossRef] [PubMed]
380. Yarani, R.; Mirza, A.H.; Kaur, S.; Pociot, F. The emerging role of lncRNAs in inflammatory bowel disease. *Exp. Mol. Med.* **2018**, *50*, 161. [CrossRef] [PubMed]
381. Memczak, S.; Jens, M.; Elefsinioti, A.; Torti, F.; Krueger, J.; Rybak, A.; Maier, L.; Mackowiak, S.D.; Gregersen, L.H.; Munschauer, M.; et al. Circular RNAs are a large class of animal RNAs with regulatory potency. *Nature* **2013**, *495*, 333–338. [CrossRef] [PubMed]
382. Hansen, T.B.; Jensen, T.I.; Clausen, B.H.; Bramsen, J.B.; Finsen, B.; Damgaard, C.K.; Kjems, J. Natural RNA circles function as efficient microRNA sponges. *Nature* **2013**, *495*, 384–388. [CrossRef] [PubMed]
383. Ebbesen, K.K.; Hansen, T.B.; Kjems, J. Insights into circular RNA biology. *RNA Biol.* **2017**, *14*, 1035–1045. [CrossRef] [PubMed]
384. Shi, Z.; Chen, T.; Yao, Q.; Zheng, L.; Zhang, Z.; Wang, J.; Hu, Z.; Cui, H.; Han, Y.; Han, X.; et al. The circular RNA ciRS-7 promotes APP and BACE1 degradation in an NF-κB-dependent manner. *FEBS J.* **2017**, *284*, 1096–1109. [CrossRef] [PubMed]

385. Su, C.; Han, Y.; Zhang, H.; Li, Y.; Yi, L.; Wang, X.; Zhou, S.; Yu, D.; Song, X.; Xiao, N.; et al. CiRS-7 targeting miR-7 modulates the progression of non-small cell lung cancer in a manner dependent on NF-κB signalling. *J. Cell. Mol. Med.* **2018**, *22*, 3097–3107. [CrossRef] [PubMed]
386. Huang, H.; Wei, L.; Qin, T.; Yang, N.; Li, Z.; Xu, Z. Circular RNA ciRS-7 triggers the migration and invasion of esophageal squamous cell carcinoma via miR-7/KLF4 and NF-κB signals. *Cancer Biol. Ther.* **2019**, *20*, 73–80. [CrossRef] [PubMed]
387. Piwecka, M.; Glažar, P.; Hernandez-Miranda, L.R.; Memczak, S.; Wolf, S.A.; Rybak-Wolf, A.; Filipchyk, A.; Klironomos, F.; Cerda Jara, C.A.; Fenske, P.; et al. Loss of a mammalian circular RNA locus causes miRNA deregulation and affects brain function. *Science* **2017**, *357*, eaam8526. [CrossRef] [PubMed]
388. Srinivasan, V.; Cardinali, D.P.; Srinivasan, U.S.; Kaur, C.; Brown, G.M.; Spence, D.W.; Hardeland, R.; Pandi-Perumal, S.R. Therapeutic potential of melatonin and its analogs in Parkinson's disease: Focus on sleep and neuroprotection. *Ther. Adv. Neurol. Disord.* **2011**, *4*, 297–317. [CrossRef] [PubMed]
389. Willis, G.L. Parkinson's disease as a neuroendocrine disorder of circadian function: Dopamine-melatonin imbalance and the visual system in the genesis and progression of the degenerative process. *Rev. Neurosci.* **2008**, *19*, 245–316. [CrossRef] [PubMed]
390. Willis, G.L. The role of ML-23 and other melatonin analogues in the treatment and management of Parkinson's disease. *Drug News Perspect.* **2005**, *18*, 437–444. [CrossRef] [PubMed]
391. Hardeland, R. Melatonin and synthetic melatoninergic agonists in psychiatric and age-associated disorders: Successful and unsuccessful approaches. *Curr. Pharm. Des.* **2016**, *22*, 1086–1101. [CrossRef] [PubMed]
392. Rodella, L.F.; Favero, G.; Rossini, C.; Foglio, E.; Bonomini, F.; Reiter, R.J.; Rezzani, R. Aging and vascular dysfunction: Beneficial melatonin effects. *Age* **2013**, *35*, 103–115. [CrossRef] [PubMed]
393. Favero, G.; Franceschetti, L.; Buffoli, B.; Moghadasian, M.H.; Reiter, R.J.; Rodella, L.F.; Rezzani, R. Melatonin: Protection against age-related cardiac pathology. *Ageing Res. Rev.* **2017**, *35*, 336–349. [CrossRef] [PubMed]
394. Majidinia, M.; Reiter, R.J.; Shakouri, S.K.; Yousefi, B. The role of melatonin, a multitasking molecule, in retarding the processes of ageing. *Ageing Res. Rev.* **2018**, *47*, 198–213. [CrossRef] [PubMed]
395. Kireev, R.A.; Vara, E.; Viña, J.; Tresguerres, J.A.F. Melatonin and oestrogen treatments were able to improve neuroinflammation and apoptotic processes in dentate gyrus of old ovariectomized female rats. *Age* **2014**, *36*, 9707. [CrossRef] [PubMed]
396. Ding, M.; Feng, N.; Tang, D.; Feng, J.; Li, Z.; Jia, M.; Liu, Z.; Gu, X.; Wang, Y.; Fu, F.; et al. Melatonin prevents Drp1-mediated mitochondrial fission in diabetic hearts through SIRT1-PGC1α pathway. *J. Pineal Res.* **2018**, *65*, e12491. [CrossRef] [PubMed]
397. Hadar, A.; Milanesi, E.; Walczak, M.; Puzianowska-Kuźnicka, M.; Kuźnicki, J.; Squassina, A.; Niola, P.; Chillotti, C.; Attems, J.; Gozes, I.; et al. SIRT1, miR-132 and miR-212 link human longevity to Alzheimer's Disease. *Sci. Rep.* **2018**, *8*, 8465. [CrossRef] [PubMed]

9

Network-Driven Proteogenomics Unveils an Aging-Related Imbalance in the Olfactory IκBα-NFκB p65 Complex Functionality in Tg2576 Alzheimer's Disease Mouse Model

Maialen Palomino-Alonso [1], Mercedes Lachén-Montes [1,2,3], Andrea González-Morales [1,2,3], Karina Ausín [2,3], Alberto Pérez-Mediavilla [3,4], Joaquín Fernández-Irigoyen [1,2,3,†] and Enrique Santamaría [1,2,3,*,†]

1 Clinical Neuroproteomics Group, Navarrabiomed, Departamento de Salud, Universidad Pública de Navarra, 31008 Pamplona, Spain; mpalomino@alumni.unav.es (M.P.-A); mercedes.lachen.montes@navarra.es (M.L.-M.); andrea.gonzalez.morales@navarra.es (A.G.-M.); jokfer@gmail.com (J.F.-I.)

2 Proteored-ISCIII, Proteomics Unit, Navarrabiomed, Departamento de Salud, Universidad Pública de Navarra, 31008 Pamplona, Spain; karina.ausin.perez@navarra.es

3 Instituto de Investigación Sanitaria de Navarra (IdiSNA), Navarra Institute for Health Research, 31008 Pamplona, Spain; lamediav@unav.es

4 Neurobiology of Alzheimer's Disease, Neurosciences Division, Center for Applied Medical Research (CIMA), Department of Biochemistry, University of Navarra, 31008 Pamplona, Spain

* Correspondence: esantamma@navarra.es

† These authors contributed equally to this work.

Abstract: Olfaction is often deregulated in Alzheimer's disease (AD) patients, and is also impaired in transgenic Tg2576 AD mice, which overexpress the Swedish mutated form of human amyloid precursor protein (APP). However, little is known about the molecular mechanisms that accompany the neurodegeneration of olfactory structures in aged Tg2576 mice. For that, we have applied proteome- and transcriptome-wide approaches to probe molecular disturbances in the olfactory bulb (OB) dissected from aged Tg2576 mice (18 months of age) as compared to those of age matched wild-type (WT) littermates. Some over-represented biological functions were directly relevant to neuronal homeostasis and processes of learning, cognition, and behavior. In addition to the modulation of CAMP responsive element binding protein 1 (CREB1) and APP interactomes, an imbalance in the functionality of the IκBα-NFκB p65 complex was observed during the aging process in the OB of Tg2576 mice. At two months of age, the phosphorylated isoforms of olfactory IκBα and NFκB p65 were inversely regulated in transgenic mice. However, both phosphorylated proteins were increased at 6 months of age, while a specific drop in IκBα levels was detected in 18-month-old Tg2576 mice, suggesting a transient activation of NFκB in the OB of Tg2576 mice. Taken together, our data provide a metabolic map of olfactory alterations in aged Tg2576 mice, reflecting the progressive effect of APP overproduction and β-amyloid (Aβ) accumulation on the OB homeostasis in aged stages.

Keywords: Tg2576 mice; olfactory bulb; proteogenomics; mass-spectrometry

1. Introduction

Olfactory dysfunction has been related to aging and Alzheimer's disease (AD) [1,2]. The smell impairment is considered an early event of AD, preceding the appearance of dementia symptoms. The Tg2576 transgenic mice express the hAPPSw via the hamster prion promoter, an isoform of the human amyloid precursor protein (APP) with double mutation K670N, M671L [3]. These mice displayed an increase of APP production with consequent overproduction of β-amyloid (Aβ) 40 and Aβ42 and plaques formation in the frontal, temporal, and entorhinal cortices, hippocampus, presubiculum, and cerebellum at about 11–13 months of age [4]. There is strong evidence that accumulation of Aβ peptide is responsible for age-related memory decline in these mice [5–7]. Other than the increase in Aβ production, these mice can also display hyperphosphorylated tau at old age. Synaptic deficits, and mitochondrial imbalance have been reported for this late-plaque model [8,9]. Metabolic and posttranslational modification alterations occur long before the onset of behavioral impairment [10–12]. However, Tg2576 mice did not present a profound cognitive impairment, even at old ages [13].

The olfactory bulb (OB) is the first brain structure of the olfactory pathway [14]. APP processing products have been observed in the OB of 1-month-old Tg2576 mice, as has Aβ deposition at 13.5 months of age [15]. Moreover, Tg2576 mice (between ages of 6.5 and 8 months) present a reduced rate of OB neurogenesis, a reduction in the volume of the granular cell layers of the OB [16], and some olfactory memory deficits [16,17]. A detailed analysis of olfaction in Tg2576 mice also revealed behavioral deficits in odor habituation and discrimination [18,19]. Interestingly, the appearance of these behavioral impairments corresponds with a progressive Aβ deposition in specific olfactory structures [18]. In view of these data, an in depth biochemical characterization of the OB is necessary to reveal the missing links in the biochemical understanding of smell impairments in Tg2576 AD mice.

In this study, we used a discovery platform, applying mass-spectrometry based quantitative proteomics and transcriptome-wide analyses, to decipher the pathophysiological mechanisms that are disturbed in the OB from aged Tg2576 mice (18 months of age) as compared to those of age matched background strain control mice. 107 differential genes and 25 differentially expressed proteins were detected, pinpointing specific molecular pathways, protein interactomes, and potential olfactory therapeutic targets.

2. Results and Discussion

OB perturbations are responsible for olfactory dysfunction in neurological syndromes [2], however, few studies have examined this structure using high throughput molecular approaches [20–23]. Focusing on the transgenic Tg2576 mouse AD model, different proteomic and transcriptomic studies were performed to characterize novel molecular mediators associated with AD pathophysiology in brain structures affected during the disease progression [9,24–30]. To our knowledge, this is the first study that characterizes olfactory-associated molecular changes in this late-plaque model using omics technologies.

2.1. Molecular Alterations Detected in the Olfactory Bulb (OB) of 18-Month-Old Tg2576 Mice

Tg2576 transgenic mice suffer from memory deficits accompanied by β-amyloid plaques that increase with disease progression [5–7]. We have applied a dual-omic approach to analyze the molecular imbalance induced by the hAPPSw isoform at the olfactory level, with the final goal to reveal novel information about the OB site-specific molecular signature at late AD stages in 18-month-old Tg2576 mice. To analyze the potential differences in olfactory molecular expression profiles, OB specimens for each experimental group (Tg2576 and WT mice) were subjected to chemical tags (isobaric tag for relative and absolute quantitation, iTRAQ) coupled to tandem mass spectrometry (3 mice/condition) and into RNA microarray platform (3 mice/condition) (Figure 1).

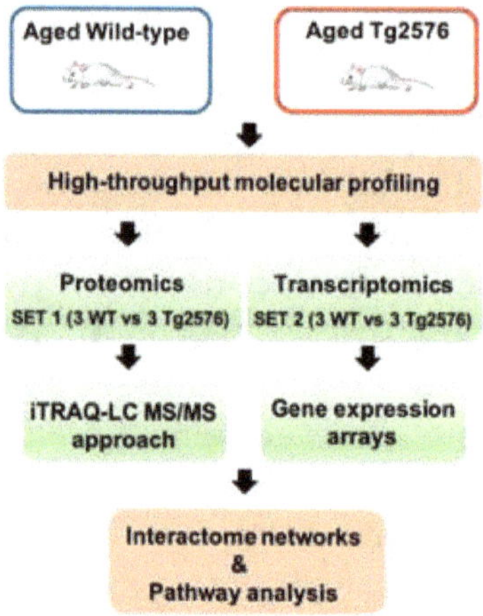

Figure 1. An overview of the workflow used for the molecular characterization of the olfactory bulbs (OBs) derived from aged Tg2576 mice.

Among 2466 quantified proteins (Table S1), differential analysis revealed 25 de-regulated proteins in Tg2576 OBs with respect to wild-type (WT) OBs (11 down- and 14 up-regulated in aged Tg2576 mice) (Figure 2A,B and Table S2). The up-regulation of our intrinsic positive control (APP) was verified by Western-blotting (Figure 2A). According to the STRING Database [31], this subproteome is mainly involved in membrane organization (False discovery rate (FDR): 1.21×10^{-5}; e.g., *SYNE2, NOL3, AP1G1*), protein transport (FDR: 0.047; e.g., *RAB5B, RPL28, SRPR, RPL18, CHMP3, COPE*), and negative regulation of neuron differentiation (FDR: 0.041; e.g., *APP, APOE, GFAP, MT3*). In the transcriptomic phase, 107 protein-coding genes were differentially regulated in the OB of aged Tg2576 mice (16 down- and 91 up-regulated genes with respect to WTs) (Table S3). Gene interactome networks suggested an alteration in the response to cyclic adenosine monophosphate (cAMP) (down regulation of *EGR1, EGR2, NR4A1, JUNB,* and *FOSB* genes) and in the olfactory transduction signaling due to the up-regulation of *ADCY3,* and *GNAL* genes, together with the overexpression of some olfactory receptors (OR) like *OLFR553, OLFR1312,* and *OLFR597* genes (dashed circles in Figure 2C).

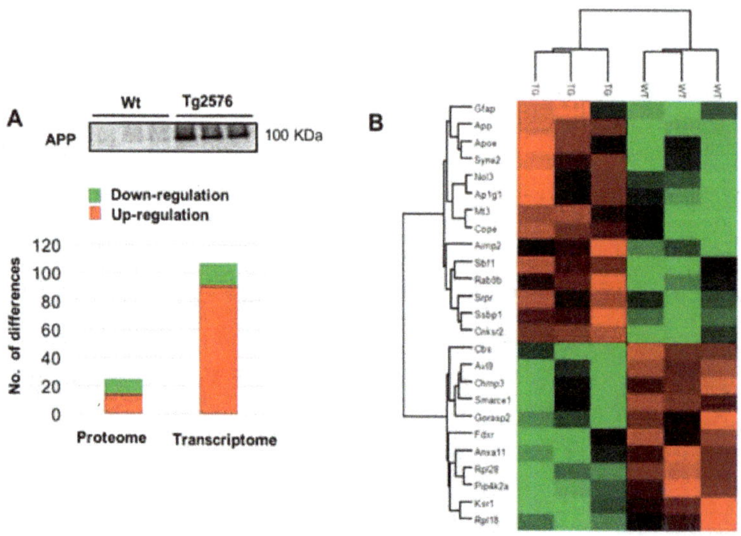

Figure 2. *Cont.*

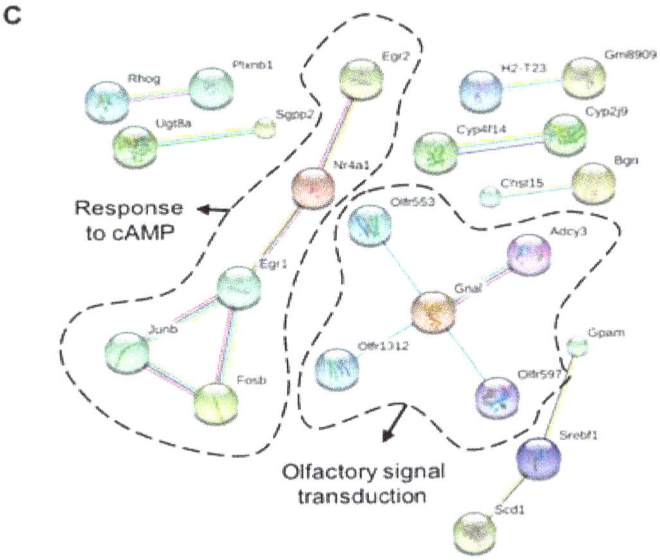

Figure 2. Multi-omic approach to decipher the OB site-specific molecular signature in aged Tg2576 mice. (**A**) Differential molecular profiling detected by the dual-omic approach in Tg2576 OBs. The olfactory protein expression levels of amyloid precursor protein (APP) at late Alzheimer's disease (AD) stages in 18-month-old Tg2576 mice is shown. Equal loading control and quantitation values have been included in Table S5; (**B**) Heat map representing the degree of change for the differentially expressed proteins (Table S2) between 18-month-old wild-type (WT) and Tg2576 mice. Red and green, up- and down-regulated proteins, respectively; (**C**) Gene interactome networks for the differentially expressed genes detected in aged Tg2576 mice. Network analysis was performed submitting the corresponding gene IDs to the STRING software (v. 10.5) (Available online: https://string-db.org/). Only interactions tagged as "high confidence" (>0.7) in STRING database were considered. Dashed circles highlight the potential alteration in the response to cyclic adenosine monophosphate (cAMP) and in the olfactory transduction signaling.

Moreover, *RTP2* (Receptor-transporter-protein 2) was also up-regulated in the OB of Tg2576 mice. RTP2 promotes OR cell-surface expression and activation in response to odorant stimulation [32]. Based on transcriptomic information from the prefrontal cortex, it has been suggested as a cause of the alteration in the smell perception of AD subjects [33]. According to our data, *OR* gene dysregulation has been also demonstrated in the OB, entorhinal, and frontal cortex in human AD subjects [34,35]. On the other hand, there was not an evident RNA-protein correlation derived from the differential datasets obtained from Tg2576 OBs. This may be due to the use of different sets of animals for each technology platform. Moreover, other reasons may also explain the observed discrepancy, such as the spatial and temporal delayed synthesis between mRNA and protein [36], post-transcriptional events, and the different hydrophobicity and solubility of the "missing proteome" during the proteomic phase, hampering its characterization and quantitation by mass-spectrometry (e.g., ORs) [37].

2.2. *Biological Functions and Neuronal-Specific Processes Altered in the OB of Aged Tg2576 Mice*

To obtain a more detailed description of the proteogenomic modulation in the Tg2576 OBs, differential datasets were analyzed for higher-level organization of genes and proteins into common biological pathways. For that, differential proteomic and transcriptomic datasets were merged and functionally analyzed across specific biological functions using the Ingenuity Pathway Analysis (IPA) software (V. 36601845, Release Date: 22 June 2017, Ingenuity Systems®, Redwood City, CA, USA). Some statistically over-represented processes were directly relevant to cell movement (p-value: 0.0003), cell survival (p-value: 0.00015), and cell death (p-value: 1.08×10^{-6}) (Figure 3A and Table S4).

Moreover, molecular clusters involved in learning (p-value: 0.004), cognition (p-value: 0.0007), behavior (p-value: 0.003), and dementia (p-value: 0.003) were also significantly represented (Figure 3B and Table S4).

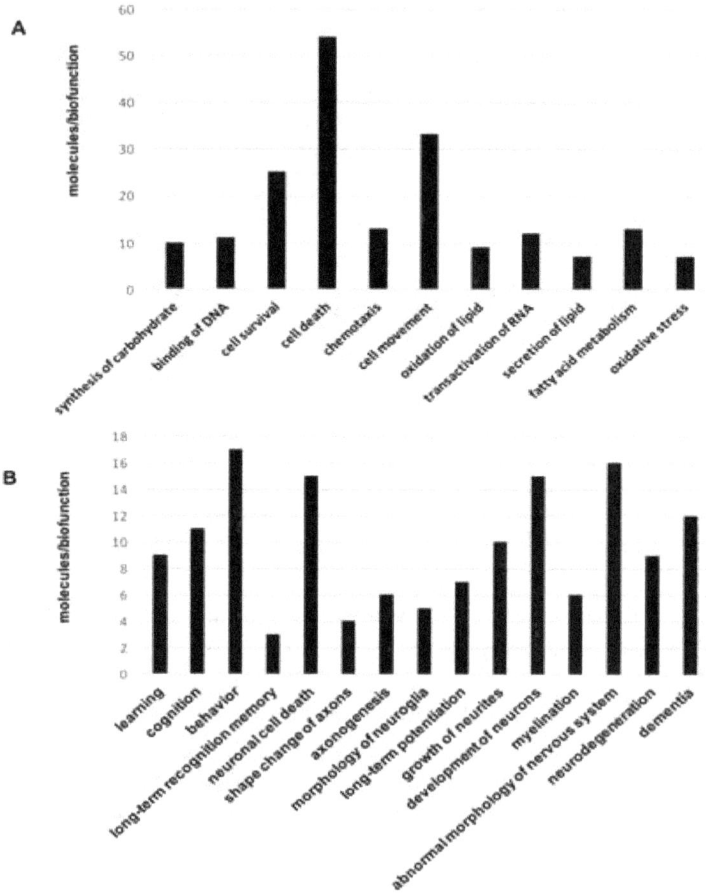

Figure 3. Significantly represented biofunctions in the OB of aged Tg2576 mice. Canonical (**A**) and neuronal-specific (**B**) over-represented biofunctions in omic datasets derived from 18-month-old Tg2576 mice. In (**A**), 45 out of 54 molecules present in cell death category are related to apoptosis (See Table S4).

Although the role of β-amyloid in olfactory deficits detected in Tg2576 mice has been extensively studied [18,19], there is no information about the survival potential of OB neurons in aged Tg2576 mice. To complement our proteogenomic workflow, survival and apoptotic pathways were monitored to analyze the effect of the β-amyloid burden on the viability of the olfactory neurons in aged Tg2576 mice. For that, steady-state levels of survival proteins like Bcl-xL and activated forms of caspase-3, -9, and -12 were measured in protein extracts from Tg2576 OBs at 18 months. The characterization of pro- and anti-apoptotic factors revealed no activation of mitochondrial or endoplasmic reticulum apoptotic routes in aged Tg2576 mice at the level of OB. Subsequent experiments were performed to monitor specific survival pathways at the level of OB. Total and residue-specific phosphorylation of focal adhesion kinase (FAK), protein kinase B (Akt), ERK activator kinase 1 (MEK)/extracellular signal-regulated kinase (ERK), Phosphoinositide-dependent protein kinase 1 (PDK1), protein kinase C (PKC), p38 mitogen-activated protein kinase (p38 MAPK), and mitogen-activated protein kinase kinase 4 (SEK1/MKK4)were measured in Tg2576 and WT OBs. As shown in Figure 4, no changes in the activation state of this survival panel were observed between transgenic and WT mice at 18 months of age, except a slight increase (non-significant) in the activation state of SEK1/MKK4 kinase (Figure 4).

However, deregulation of MAP kinases (MEK, ERK) and the PDK1/PKC axis has been observed in human OB at advanced AD stages [22,23]. These differences may be partially explained by stage, and species-dependent responses [23] and differences in molecular mechanisms associated to β-amyloidogenesis.

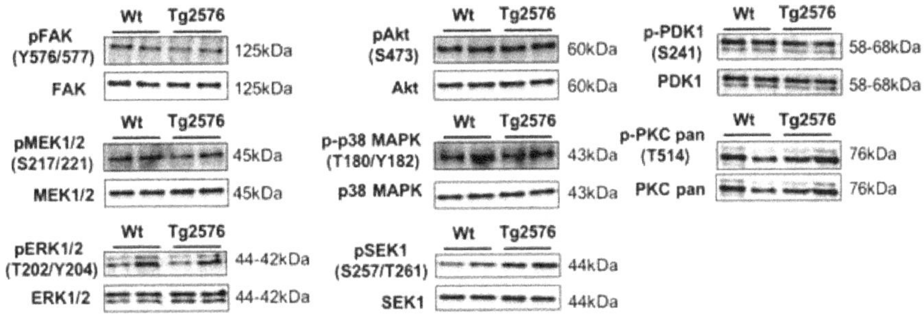

Figure 4. Activation state of specific survival pathways in the OB of aged Tg2576 mice. Levels and residue-specific phosphorylation of focal adhesion kinase (FAK), ERK Activator Kinase 1 (MEK)/extracellular signal-regulated kinase (ERK), protein kinase B (Akt), phosphoinositide-dependent protein kinase 1 (PDK1), protein kinase C (PKC), p38 mitogen-activated protein kinase (p38 MAPK), and mitogen-activated protein kinase kinase 4 (SEK1/MKK4), in the OB of aged Tg2576 mice. Equal loading of the gels was assessed by stain free digitalization. Equal loading control and quantitation values have been included in Table S5.

2.3. Functional Interactome of the hAPPSw Isoform at the Olfactory Level: Characterization of Potential Hubs by Network-Driven Proteogenomics

To explore the cooperative action among differentially expressed OB genes/proteins in aged Tg2576 mice, we performed molecular interaction networks, merging the olfactory targets that tend to be de-regulated in this model. We consider the discovery of unexpected relationships between apparently unrelated proteins and AD-causing neuropathological substrates as a powerful strategy for the characterization of novel AD causative/susceptibility targets with a central role during olfactory neurodegeneration. Functional interactome maps were generated using IPA software (Figures 5 and 6). We explored whether the hAPPSw isoform, highly expressed in Tg2576 mice, may potentially be interconnected with differential molecular targets detected by our dual-omic approach. As shown in Figure 5, differential functional interactors for APP protein were identified in the OB from aged transgenic mice. The functional APP interactome was composed by targets potentially distributed in different cellular compartments: (i) *APOE*, *SERPINH1*, and *BGN* in the extracellular space; (ii) *VAPA* at the plasma membrane level; (iii) *Irgm1*, *GFAP*, *MT3*, *ARC*, *GAB1*, *ZDHHC23*, and *GORASP2* in the cytoplasm; and (iv) *FOSB*, *JUNB*, *ZFP36L1*, *NR4A2*, *HEY2*, *EGR1*, *TP63*, and *Mmp* in the nuclear compartment (Figure 5).

Moreover, integrative network analysis also allowed us to establish a framework to map interactions between differentially expressed targets and network hubs. According to IPA analysis, CREB1, NFKBIA (IκBα), and NFκB were postulated as potential upstream regulators of part of the differential targets detected in our study (Table 1).

Even though changes in their expression were not detected in our system-wide approaches, the alteration of some of their targets may correspond to a dysregulation in their functionality in the OB of aged Tg2576 mice. For that, subsequent experiments were performed to monitor the protein expression of CREB1 as well as the activation state of IκBα-NFκB p65 complex in the OB of aged Tg2576 mice. CREB1 is a pivotal molecule during synaptic strengthening and memory formation processes [38–40]. Protein expression levels of transcription factor CREB1 were significantly reduced in the OB of Tg2576 mice (Figure 6) in parallel with the down-regulation of *FOSB*, *NR4A2*, and *EGR1*, well-known CREB target genes [41] (Figure 6 and Table S3). Our data obtained in aged Tg2576 mice reinforce the direct relationship between a reduction of CREB1 activation and AD pathology [41,42].

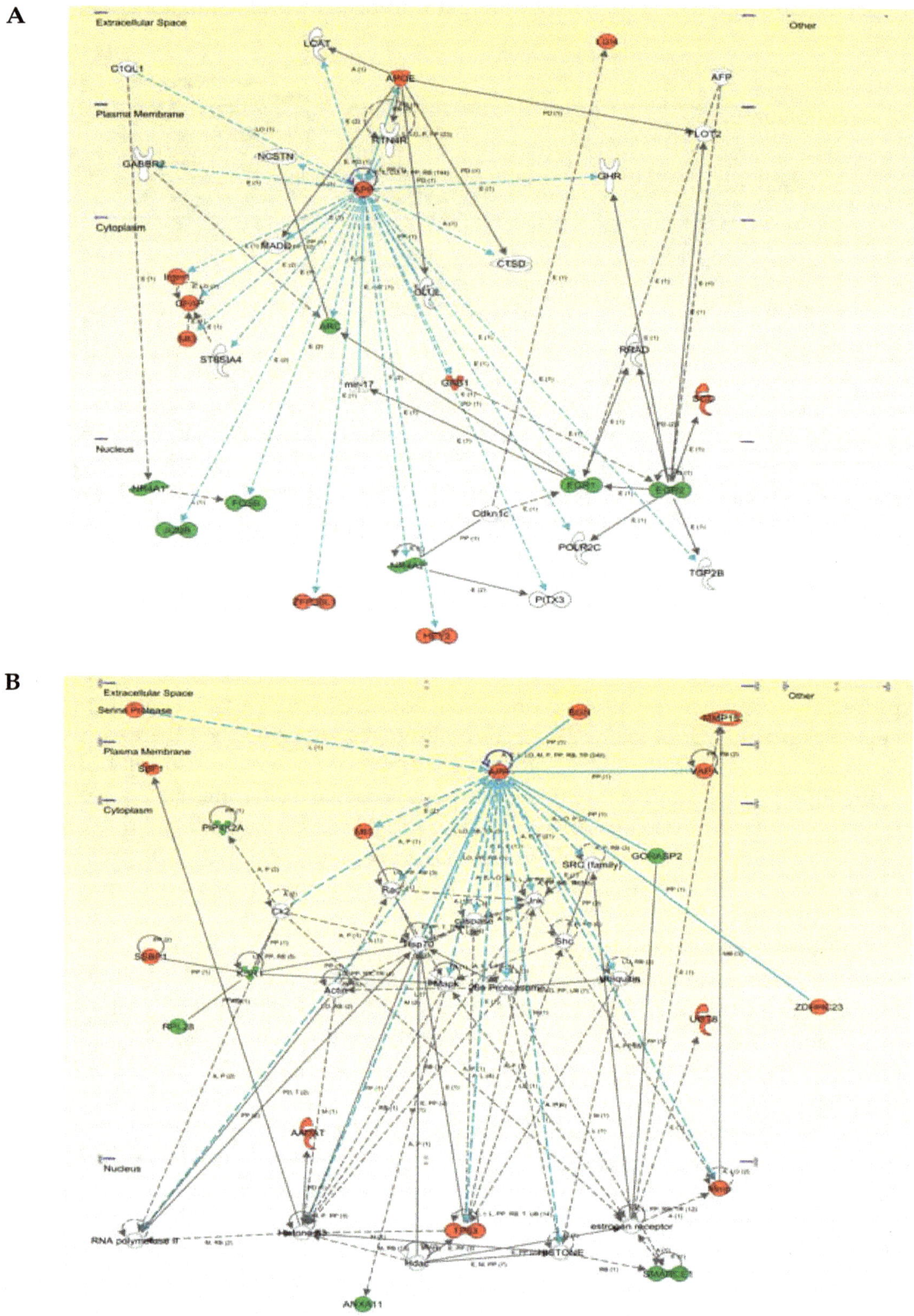

Figure 5. Modulation of APP molecular interaction network in the OB of aged Tg2576 mice. Visual representation of the relationships between differentially expressed genes/proteins and APP functional interactors (blue lines) are shown in both potentially deregulated networks in Tg2576 OBs (**A** and **B**). Continuous lines represent direct interactions, while discontinuous lines correspond to indirect functional interactions. Up-regulated molecules are shown in red, down-regulated molecules in green, and proteins proposed by the software in white. The complete legend of this type of interactomes may be found at http://ingenuity.force.com/ipa/articles/Feature_Description/Legend (accessed on 10 October 2017).

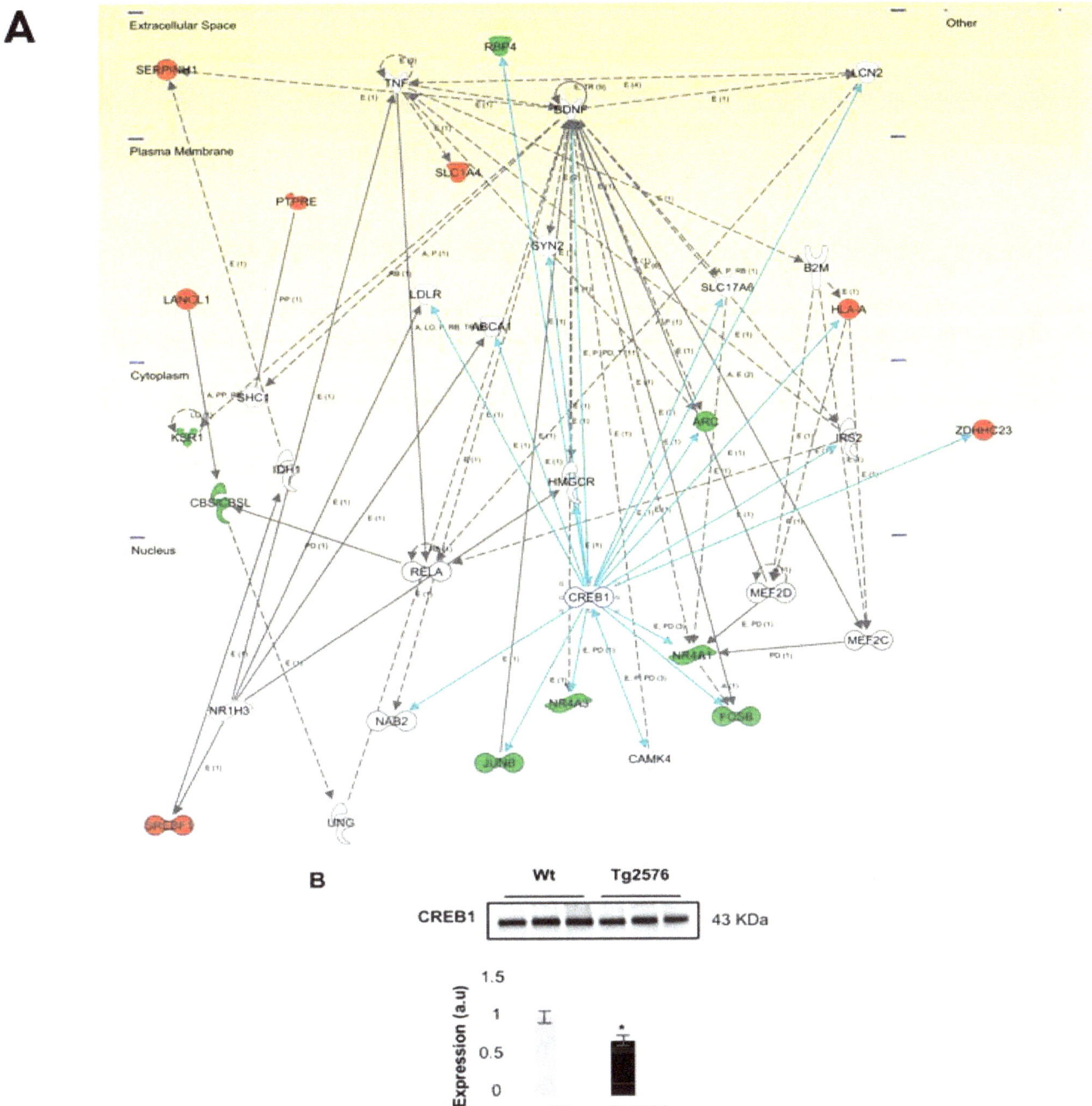

Figure 6. Modulation of CREB1 molecular interactome in the OB of aged Tg2576 mice. Visual representation of the relationships between differential expressed genes/proteins and CREB1 functional interactors (blue lines) are shown in the deregulated network in Tg2576 OBs (**A**); Continuous lines represent direct interactions, while discontinuous lines correspond to indirect functional interactions. Up-regulated molecules are shown in red, down-regulated molecules in green, and molecules proposed by the software in white. The complete legend of this type of interactomes may be found at http://ingenuity.force.com/ipa/articles/Feature_Description/Legend (accessed on 17 October 2017). CREB1 protein levels were down-regulated in the OB of aged Tg2576 mice. * $p < 0.05$ vs. WT group (**B**). Equal loading control and quantitation values have been included in Table S5. a.u., arbitrary units.

Table 1. Potential upstream regulators of differential targets detected in our study.

Upstream Regulator	Molecule Type	*p*-Value	Target Molecules in OB Omics Dataset
CREB1	transcription regulator	0.00000209	*APOE, ARC, EGR1, EGR2, FOSB, GNAL, HLA-A, JUNB, NR4A1, NR4A2, NR4A3, RBP4, SCD, ZDHHC23*
NFKBIA	transcription regulator	0.00916	*BCL2A1, CD82, HLA-A, JUNB, MMP15, NID1, NR4A1*
NFKB1	transcription regulator	0.0000748	*APOE, APP, BCL2A1, CD82, EGR1, HLA-DMB, NR4A1, TBX21*
NFκB (complex)	complex	0.00174	*APOE, APP, BCL2A1, CD82, EGR1, GFAP, HLA-A, HLA-DMB, JUNB, KLF3*

2.4. An Impairment in the Olfactory IκBα-NFκB p65 Complex Functionality during the Progression of Alzheimer's Disease (AD) in Tg2576 Mice

The nuclear factor NFκB controls the transcription of a wide variety of genes including pro-apoptotic and pro-survival genes, proinflammatory cytokines, antioxidant enzymes, pro-oxidant enzymes, and many others [43]. In general, the formation of a complex of NFκB dimer with a typical member of IkB family prevents the nuclear translocation and gene activation function of NFκB [44]. The phosphorylation of serine 32 of IκBα leads to ubiquitination and proteasomal degradation of IκBα, allowing for the phosphorylation of the NFκB p65 subunit and the enhancement of the p65 transactivation potential [44]. In our study, we monitored the functionality of the IκBα-NFκB p65 complex at three stages of AD: long before (2 months of age), immediately before (6 months), and after (18 months) the appearance of Aβ plaques [9]. At two months of age, the phosphorylated isoforms of IκBα and NFκB p65 were inversely regulated in Tg2576 transgenic mice (Figure 7A,B). However, both phosphorylated proteins were increased at 6 months of age, whereas a specific drop in IκBα levels was detected in 18-month-old Tg2576 mice (Figure 7A,B). Based on these data, it may be hypothesized that APP overproduction induces a transient activation of NFκB in the OB of Tg2576 mice compared to that of WT mice. It has been previously observed that there is an increased NFκB activity in different hippocampal and cortical structures in post-mortem AD brains [45–47], probably due to increased oxidative stress, inflammatory reactions, and toxicity of accumulated Aβ peptides [43]. To deepen our understanding of the functional dynamics of the olfactory IκBα-NFκB p65 complexes during the aging process, steady-state levels and phosphorylated isoforms were independently evaluated in WT and Tg2576 mice during aging. For that, protein profiles were quantified in a time-dependent manner. With respect to data obtained at 2 months of age, a specific drop in NFκB p65 protein levels and a progressive decrease in the phosphorylated NFκB p65 subunit were observed in WT mice, whereas an increase in NFκB p65 activity at 6 months was exclusively observed in Tg2576 mice (Figure 7C). In addition, the increase in total and phosphorylated levels of IkB α observed in 18-month-old WT mice, was blocked in aged Tg2576 mice (Figure 7C). Previous reports have shown that NFκB inhibitors prevent Aβ-induced toxicity in vivo and in vitro AD experimental models [48]. To our knowledge, the early impairment in NFκB functionality observed in Tg2576 mice at the level of OB, might open new avenues of targeting the NFκB signaling cascade at the olfactory level, gaining new insight into disease pathogenesis and identifying potential disease modifying agents. However, it is important to note that the phosphoproteome of IκBα-NFκB complexes is highly complicated [44], and many post-translational modifications (PTMs) have been characterized (see http://www.uniprot.org/uniprot/Q04206 (accessed on 10 October 2017), and http://www.uniprot.org/uniprot/P25963 (accessed on 10 October 2017)), but it is still unclear how the tangled crosstalk between all PTMs regulates the ability of NFκB proteins to induce or to repress defined target genes. Due to the early olfactory imbalance detected in the IκBα-NFκB p65 complex in Tg2576 mice, additional studies are necessary to decipher the effects of APP-dependent NFκB dysregulation on the OB molecular landscape at early stages of AD pathology to understand the smell impairment that appears during the AD progression in Tg2576 mice.

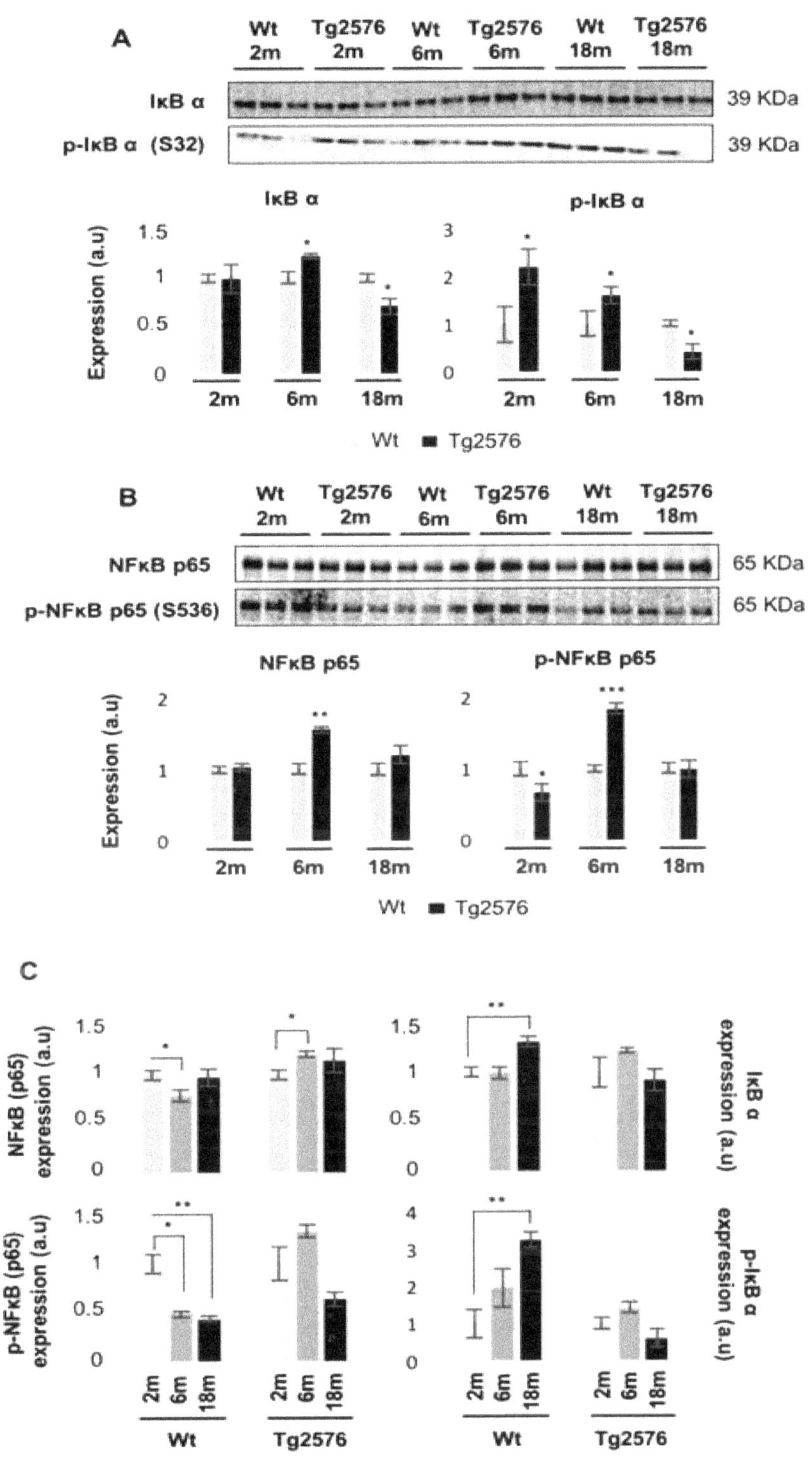

Figure 7. Time-dependent functionality of the OB IκBα-NFκB p65 complex in Tg2576 mice. Levels and residue-specific phosphorylation of the IκBα (**A**); levels and residue-specific phosphorylation of NFκB p65 subunit (**B**); Equal loading of the gels was assessed by stain-free digitalization. Panels show histograms of band densities. Data are presented as mean ± SEM from three independent OB samples per group. * $p < 0.05$ vs. control group; ** $p < 0.01$ vs. control group; *** $p < 0.001$ vs. control group. The expression of the IκBα-NFκB p65 complex was also evaluated during the aging process in WT and Tg2576 mice. * $p < 0.05$ vs. 2-month-old mice; ** $p < 0.01$ vs. 2-month-old mice (**C**). Equal loading control and quantitation values have been included in Table S5. m, month; a.u., arbitrary units.

Although the accumulation of Aβ oligomers in specific OB regions results in impaired neural integrity in specific OB cell layers in Tg2576 mice during AD progression [49], our results indicate that: (i) 1% of the 2.466 quantified proteins are differentially expressed; and (ii) 0.5% of the 20.900 protein-coding genes are differentially modulated in the OB of 18-month-old Tg2576 mice. These data pointed out that AD-related effects on the OB transcriptome and proteome composition at the bulk level are not as massive at RNA and protein levels at they are at old stages. It is important to note that due to technical reasons, only the most abundant OB proteins corresponding to approximately 10% of the mouse proteome were explored. Consequently, alterations other than those reported in this study might also participate in the AD neurodegeneration at the level of the OB in aged Tg2576 mice. Despite the analysis of the OB proteogenome providing a unique window into their biochemistry and dysfunction in aged Tg2576 mice, there are limitations of our study that warrant discussion. The OB is composed by multiple cell types with a tangled connectivity and architecture [50]. In our case, the information about specific-cell types from where proteins and mRNAs originated is lost due to the processing of the bulk OB in our omic strategy. The implementation of novel approaches that allow the exploration of olfactory cell-type specific molecular profiling would complement the output of our nonbiased exploration of the OB transcriptome/proteome, reducing the effect of multiple neuronal populations in the aged Tg2576 OBs.

3. Materials and Methods

3.1. Materials

The following reagents and materials were used. From Cell Signaling technology (Danvers, MA, USA): anti-APP (ref. 2450), anti-FAK (ref. 3285), anti-phospho-FAK (Y576/577) (ref. 3281), anti-Akt (ref. 4685), anti-phospho-Akt (S473) (ref. 4060), anti-PDK1 (ref. 3062), anti-phospho-PDK1 (S241) (ref. 3061), anti-phospho-PKC pan (T514) (ref. 9379), anti-p38 MAPK (ref. 9212), anti-phospho-p38 MAPK (T180/Y182) (ref. 9211), anti-MEK1/2 (ref. 9126), anti-phospho-MEK1/2 (S217/221) (ref. 9154), anti-ERK1/2 (ref. 9102), anti-phospho-ERK1/2 (T202/y204) (ref. 4370), anti-CREB (ref. 9104), anti-IκBα (ref. 4814S), anti-phospho-IκBα (S32) (ref. 2859), anti-NFκB p65 (ref. 8242), anti-phospho-NFκB p65 (ref. 3033S), anti-SEK1 (ref. 9152), and anti-phospho-SEK1 (S257/T261) (Ref. 9156). Anti-PKC-pan was from SigmaAldrich (St Louis, MO, USA) (ref. SAB4502356). Electrophoresis reagents were purchased from Bio-Rad (Hercules, CA, USA) and trypsin from Promega (Madison, WI, USA).

3.2. Animals

Female Tg2576 transgenic mice were used [3]. Animals were housed 4–5 per cage with free access to water and food, and they were maintained in a temperature-controlled environment on a 12 h light–dark cycle. The progressive development of AD signs in our colony has been previously described [51]. Animal care procedures were conducted in accordance with the European Community Council Directive (2010/63/EU, 22 September 2010) and approved by the local ethics committee. Twelve aged animals (6 WT and 6 Tg2576 mice of 18 months of age), divided into two sets, were used for proteomics and transcriptomics analysis (3 mice/group/platform).

3.3. Olfactory Proteomics

OB protein extraction, protein digestion, and peptide iTRAQ labelling was performed as previously described [20–23]. Tryptic digests were labelled according to the manufacturer's instructions with one isobaric amine-reactive tag as follows: Tag113, WT-1; Tag114, WT-2; Tag115, WT-3; Tag116, Tg2576-1; Tag117, Tg2576-2; Tag118, Tg2576-3. After 2 h incubation, the set of labelled samples were pooled and evaporated in a vacuum centrifuge. To increase the proteome coverage, the peptide pool was submitted to cation exchange chromatography using spin Columns (Pierce, Rockford, IL, USA). Twelve fractions were collected (from 10 mM to 150 mM KCl), evaporated under vacuum, and reconstituted into 10 μL of 2% acetonitrile, 0.1% formic acid, and 98% MilliQ-H_2O prior to mass spectrometric analysis. Peptide mixtures were separated by reverse phase chromatography and analyzed by mass-spectrometry as previously described [20–23]. The raw MS/MS spectra search were processed using the MaxQuant software (v. 1.5.8.3) [52]. The parameters used were as follows: initial maximum precursor (25 ppm), fragment mass deviations (40 ppm); variable modification (methionine oxidation and N-terminal acetylation) and fixed modification (MMTS); enzyme (trypsin) with a maximum of one missed cleavage; minimum peptide length (7 amino acids); false discovery rate (FDR) for peptide spectrum match (PSM), and protein identification (1%). The frequently observed laboratory contaminants were removed. Protein identification was considered valid with at least one unique or "razor" peptide. The protein quantification was calculated using at least two razor + unique peptides, and statistical significance was calculated by a two-way Student-t test ($p < 0.05$). A 1.3-fold change cut-off was used. Proteins with iTRAQ ratios below the low range (0.77) were considered to be down-regulated, whereas those above the high range (1.3) were considered to be upregulated. The Perseus software (version 1.5.6.0) [53] was used for statistical analysis and data visualization. Search results files and MS raw data were deposited to the ProteomeXchange Consortium (Available online: http://proteomecentral.proteomexchange.org; accessed on 20 September 2017) via the PRIDE partner repository [54] with the identifier PXD007795.

3.4. OB Transcriptomics

Maxwell® 16 simplyRNA Kit (Promega) was used to extract the OB mitochondrial RNAs (mRNAs) from aged Tg2576 mice and WT littermates. The sense complementary DNA (cDNA) was fragmented and biotinylated using the Affymetrix Clarion S Pico assay (902932; ThermoFisher Scientific, Waltham, MA, USA). Affymetrix mouse Clarion S chips (ThermoFisher Scientific) were used according to the manufacturer protocols. Hybridization, washing, staining, scanning, and data analysis [55] were performed as previously described [34,35]. As in other transcriptomic studies performed in AD brains [56,57], we worked with a p-value < 0.01 (without using any method for multiple testing correction). Microarray data files were submitted to the GEO (Gene Expression Omnibus) database and are available under accession number GSE103835.

3.5. Bioinformatics

The identification of specifically dysregulated regulatory/metabolic networks was analyzed using QIAGEN's Ingenuity Pathway Analysis (IPA) (Available online: www.qiagen.com/ingenuity; accessed on 10 October 2017) and STRING software [31]. The IPA software considers signaling pathway/biofunctions according to the calculated p-value and reports it hierarchically.

3.6. Immunoblotting Analysis

Equal amounts of OB protein (5 μg) were resolved in 4–15% TGX stain-free gels (Bio-Rad). OB proteins derived from murine samples were electrophoretically transferred onto nitrocellulose membranes using a Trans-blot Turbo transfer system (up to 25 V, 7 min) (Bio-Rad). Equal loading of the gels was assessed by stain free digitalization and by Ponceau staining. Western-blotting was performed as previously described [20–23]. After densitometric analyses (Image Lab Software Version 5.2; Bio-Rad), optical density values were expressed as arbitrary units and normalized to total stain in each gel lane.

4. Conclusions

The largely similar OB proteogenome of aged WT and Tg2576 mice suggests that abnormal protein-protein interactions or post-translational modifications, defective intracellular trafficking, or misfolding of proteins could play a pivotal part in driving the neurodegeneration that occurs at the olfactory level in aged Tg2576 mice. Moreover, omics sciences have partially revealed the potential interactome of the hAPPSw isoform at the olfactory level as well as the disruption of the IκBα-NFκB p65 complex during the neurodegenerative process, providing molecular features that may be used as novel olfactory drug target candidates to treat AD.

Acknowledgments: This work was funded by grants from the Spanish Ministry of Economy and Competitiveness (MINECO) (Ref. SAF2014-59340-R), Department of Economic Development from Government of Navarra (Ref. PC023-24) and Obra Social la Caixa to Enrique Santamaría. Andrea González-Morales and Karina Ausín were supported by PEJ-2014-A-61949 and PEJ-2014-A-72151 (MINECO). Mercedes Lachén-Montes is supported by a predoctoral fellowship from the Public University of Navarra (UPNA). Authors thank all of the proteomics identifications (PRIDE) Team for helping with the mass spectrometric data deposit in ProteomeXChange/PRIDE. The Proteomics Unit of Navarrabiomed is a member of Proteored, PRB2-ISCIII, and is supported by grant PT13/0001, of the PE I + D + I 2013–2016 funded by ISCIII and FEDER. This project is part of the HUPO Brain Proteome Project and these results are lined up with the Spanish Initiative on the Human Proteome Project (SpHPP).

Author Contributions: Joaquín Fernández-Irigoyen and Enrique Santamaría designed and supervised the complete study. Maialen Palomino-Alonso, Mercedes Lachen-Montes, Andrea González-Morales, Karina Ausín, and Alberto Pérez-Mediavilla performed sample selection and sample preparation for proteomic and transcriptomic phases. Maialen Palomino-Alonso performed proteomic analysis. Maialen Palomino-Alonso, Mercedes Lachen-Montes, and Andrea González-Morales performed functional assays. Joaquín Fernández-Irigoyen and Enrique Santamaría performed liquid chromatography-tandem mass spectrometry analysis and data interpretation. Enrique Santamaría wrote the paper.

Abbreviations

AD	Alzheimer's disease
APP	Amyloid precursor protein
Aβ	β-amyloid
ERK	Extracellular signal-regulated kinase
FAK	Focal adhesion kinase
OB	Olfactory bulb
MS/MS	Tandem mass-spectrometry
PDK1	Phosphoinositide-dependent protein kinase 1
PKC	Protein kinase C
p38 MAPK	p38 Mitogen-activated protein kinase
WT	Wild-type

References

1. Bahar-Fuchs, A.; Chetelat, G.; Villemagne, V.L.; Moss, S.; Pike, K.; Masters, C.L.; Rowe, C.; Savage, G. Olfactory deficits and amyloid-β burden in Alzheimer's disease, mild cognitive impairment, and healthy aging: A PIB PET study. *J. Alzheimers Dis.* **2010**, *22*, 1081–1087. [CrossRef] [PubMed]
2. Attems, J.; Walker, L.; Jellinger, K.A. Olfactory bulb involvement in neurodegenerative diseases. *Acta Neuropathol.* **2014**, *127*, 459–475. [CrossRef] [PubMed]
3. Hsiao, K.; Chapman, P.; Nilsen, S.; Eckman, C.; Harigaya, Y.; Younkin, S.; Yang, F.; Cole, G. Correlative memory deficits, Aβ elevation, and amyloid plaques in transgenic mice. *Science* **1996**, *274*, 99–102. [CrossRef] [PubMed]
4. Puzzo, D.; Gulisano, W.; Palmeri, A.; Arancio, O. Rodent models for Alzheimer's disease drug discovery. *Expert Opin. Drug Discov.* **2015**, *10*, 703–711. [CrossRef] [PubMed]
5. Westerman, M.A.; Cooper-Blacketer, D.; Mariash, A.; Kotilinek, L.; Kawarabayashi, T.; Younkin, L.H.; Carlson, G.A.; Younkin, S.G.; Ashe, K.H. The relationship between Aβ and memory in the Tg2576 mouse model of Alzheimer's disease. *J. Neurosci.* **2002**, *22*, 1858–1867. [PubMed]
6. Janus, C.; Pearson, J.; McLaurin, J.; Mathews, P.M.; Jiang, Y.; Schmidt, S.D.; Chishti, M.A.; Horne, P.; Heslin, D.; French, J.; et al. Aβ peptide immunization reduces behavioural impairment and plaques in a model of Alzheimer's disease. *Nature* **2000**, *408*, 979–982. [CrossRef] [PubMed]

7. Chen, G.; Chen, K.S.; Knox, J.; Inglis, J.; Bernard, A.; Martin, S.J.; Justice, A.; McConlogue, L.; Games, D.; Freedman, S.B.; et al. A learning deficit related to age and β-amyloid plaques in a mouse model of Alzheimer's disease. *Nature* **2000**, *408*, 975–979. [CrossRef] [PubMed]
8. Jacobsen, J.S.; Wu, C.C.; Redwine, J.M.; Comery, T.A.; Arias, R.; Bowlby, M.; Martone, R.; Morrison, J.H.; Pangalos, M.N.; Reinhart, P.H.; et al. Early-onset behavioral and synaptic deficits in a mouse model of Alzheimer's disease. *Proc. Natl. Acad. Sci. USA* **2006**, *103*, 5161–5166. [CrossRef] [PubMed]
9. Reddy, P.H.; McWeeney, S.; Park, B.S.; Manczak, M.; Gutala, R.V.; Partovi, D.; Jung, Y.; Yau, V.; Searles, R.; Mori, M.; et al. Gene expression profiles of transcripts in amyloid precursor protein transgenic mice: Up-regulation of mitochondrial metabolism and apoptotic genes is an early cellular change in Alzheimer's disease. *Hum. Mol. Genet.* **2004**, *13*, 1225–1240. [CrossRef] [PubMed]
10. Lalande, J.; Halley, H.; Balayssac, S.; Gilard, V.; Dejean, S.; Martino, R.; Frances, B.; Lassalle, J.M.; Malet-Martino, M. 1H NMR metabolomic signatures in five brain regions of the AβPPswe Tg2576 mouse model of Alzheimer's disease at four ages. *J. Alzheimers Dis.* **2014**, *39*, 121–143. [PubMed]
11. Nistico, R.; Ferraina, C.; Marconi, V.; Blandini, F.; Negri, L.; Egebjerg, J.; Feligioni, M. Age-related changes of protein sumoylation balance in the AβPP Tg2576 mouse model of Alzheimer's disease. *Front. Pharmacol.* **2014**, *5*, 63. [PubMed]
12. Fodero, L.R.; Saez-Valero, J.; McLean, C.A.; Martins, R.N.; Beyreuther, K.; Masters, C.L.; Robertson, T.A.; Small, D.H. Altered glycosylation of acetylcholinesterase in APP (SW) Tg2576 transgenic mice occurs prior to amyloid plaque deposition. *J. Neurochem.* **2002**, *81*, 441–448. [CrossRef] [PubMed]
13. King, D.L.; Arendash, G.W. Behavioral characterization of the Tg2576 transgenic model of Alzheimer's disease through 19 months. *Physiol. Behav.* **2002**, *75*, 627–642. [CrossRef]
14. Doty, R.L. The olfactory vector hypothesis of neurodegenerative disease: Is it viable? *Ann. Neurol.* **2008**, *63*, 7–15. [CrossRef] [PubMed]
15. Lehman, E.J.; Kulnane, L.S.; Lamb, B.T. Alterations in β-amyloid production and deposition in brain regions of two transgenic models. *Neurobiol. Aging* **2003**, *24*, 645–653. [CrossRef]
16. Guerin, D.; Sacquet, J.; Mandairon, N.; Jourdan, F.; Didier, A. Early locus coeruleus degeneration and olfactory dysfunctions in Tg2576 mice. *Neurobiol. Aging* **2009**, *30*, 272–283. [CrossRef] [PubMed]
17. Young, J.W.; Sharkey, J.; Finlayson, K. Progressive impairment in olfactory working memory in a mouse model of mild cognitive impairment. *Neurobiol. Aging* **2009**, *30*, 1430–1443. [CrossRef] [PubMed]
18. Wesson, D.W.; Levy, E.; Nixon, R.A.; Wilson, D.A. Olfactory dysfunction correlates with amyloid-β burden in an Alzheimer's disease mouse model. *J. Neurosci.* **2010**, *30*, 505–514. [CrossRef] [PubMed]
19. Wesson, D.W.; Borkowski, A.H.; Landreth, G.E.; Nixon, R.A.; Levy, E.; Wilson, D.A. Sensory network dysfunction, behavioral impairments, and their reversibility in an Alzheimer's β-amyloidosis mouse model. *J. Neurosci.* **2011**, *31*, 15962–15971. [CrossRef] [PubMed]
20. Fernandez-Irigoyen, J.; Corrales, F.J.; Santamaria, E. Proteomic atlas of the human olfactory bulb. *J. Proteom.* **2012**, *75*, 4005–4016. [CrossRef] [PubMed]
21. Zelaya, M.V.; Perez-Valderrama, E.; de Morentin, X.M.; Tunon, T.; Ferrer, I.; Luquin, M.R.; Fernandez-Irigoyen, J.; Santamaria, E. Olfactory bulb proteome dynamics during the progression of sporadic Alzheimer's disease: Identification of common and distinct olfactory targets across alzheimer-related co-pathologies. *Oncotarget* **2015**, *6*, 39437–39456. [CrossRef] [PubMed]
22. Lachen-Montes, M.; Gonzalez-Morales, A.; Zelaya, M.V.; Perez-Valderrama, E.; Ausin, K.; Ferrer, I.; Fernandez-Irigoyen, J.; Santamaria, E. Olfactory bulb neuroproteomics reveals a chronological perturbation of survival routes and a disruption of prohibitin complex during Alzheimer's disease progression. *Sci. Rep.* **2017**, *7*, 9115. [CrossRef] [PubMed]
23. Lachen-Montes, M.; Gonzalez-Morales, A.; de Morentin, X.M.; Perez-Valderrama, E.; Ausin, K.; Zelaya, M.V.; Serna, A.; Aso, E.; Ferrer, I.; Fernandez-Irigoyen, J.; et al. An early dysregulation of FAK and MEK/ERK signaling pathways precedes the β-amyloid deposition in the olfactory bulb of APP/PS1 mouse model of Alzheimer's disease. *J. Proteom.* **2016**, *148*, 149–158. [CrossRef] [PubMed]
24. Stein, T.D.; Johnson, J.A. Lack of neurodegeneration in transgenic mice overexpressing mutant amyloid precursor protein is associated with increased levels of transthyretin and the activation of cell survival pathways. *J. Neurosci.* **2002**, *22*, 7380–7388. [PubMed]

25. George, A.J.; Gordon, L.; Beissbarth, T.; Koukoulas, I.; Holsinger, R.M.; Perreau, V.; Cappai, R.; Tan, S.S.; Masters, C.L.; Scott, H.S.; et al. A serial analysis of gene expression profile of the Alzheimer's disease Tg2576 mouse model. *Neurotox. Res.* **2010**, *17*, 360–379. [CrossRef] [PubMed]
26. Tan, L.; Wang, X.; Ni, Z.F.; Zhu, X.; Wu, W.; Zhu, L.Q.; Liu, D. A systematic analysis of genomic changes in Tg2576 mice. *Mol. Neurobiol.* **2013**, *47*, 883–891. [CrossRef] [PubMed]
27. Shin, S.J.; Lee, S.E.; Boo, J.H.; Kim, M.; Yoon, Y.D.; Kim, S.I.; Mook-Jung, I. Profiling proteins related to amyloid deposited brain of Tg2576 mice. *Proteomics* **2004**, *4*, 3359–3368. [CrossRef] [PubMed]
28. Gillardon, F.; Rist, W.; Kussmaul, L.; Vogel, J.; Berg, M.; Danzer, K.; Kraut, N.; Hengerer, B. Proteomic and functional alterations in brain mitochondria from Tg2576 mice occur before amyloid plaque deposition. *Proteomics* **2007**, *7*, 605–616. [CrossRef] [PubMed]
29. Shevchenko, G.; Wetterhall, M.; Bergquist, J.; Hoglund, K.; Andersson, L.I.; Kultima, K. Longitudinal characterization of the brain proteomes for the Tg2576 amyloid mouse model using shotgun based mass spectrometry. *J. Proteome Res.* **2012**, *11*, 6159–6174. [CrossRef] [PubMed]
30. Cuadrado-Tejedor, M.; Cabodevilla, J.F.; Zamarbide, M.; Gomez-Isla, T.; Franco, R.; Perez-Mediavilla, A. Age-related mitochondrial alterations without neuronal loss in the hippocampus of a transgenic model of Alzheimer's disease. *Curr. Alzheimer Res.* **2013**, *10*, 390–405. [CrossRef] [PubMed]
31. Szklarczyk, D.; Morris, J.H.; Cook, H.; Kuhn, M.; Wyder, S.; Simonovic, M.; Santos, A.; Doncheva, N.T.; Roth, A.; Bork, P.; et al. The string database in 2017: Quality-controlled protein-protein association networks, made broadly accessible. *Nucleic Acids Res.* **2017**, *45*, D362–D368. [CrossRef] [PubMed]
32. Saito, H.; Kubota, M.; Roberts, R.W.; Chi, Q.; Matsunami, H. RTP family members induce functional expression of mammalian odorant receptors. *Cell* **2004**, *119*, 679–691. [CrossRef] [PubMed]
33. Zhang, B.; Gaiteri, C.; Bodea, L.G.; Wang, Z.; McElwee, J.; Podtelezhnikov, A.A.; Zhang, C.; Xie, T.; Tran, L.; Dobrin, R.; et al. Integrated systems approach identifies genetic nodes and networks in late-onset Alzheimer's disease. *Cell* **2013**, *153*, 707–720. [CrossRef] [PubMed]
34. Ansoleaga, B.; Garcia-Esparcia, P.; Llorens, F.; Moreno, J.; Aso, E.; Ferrer, I. Dysregulation of brain olfactory and taste receptors in AD, PSP and CJD, and AD-related model. *Neuroscience* **2013**, *248*, 369–382. [CrossRef] [PubMed]
35. Lachen-Montes, M.; Zelaya, M.; Segura, V.; Fernández-Irigoyen, J.; Santamaría, E. Progressive modulation of the human olfactory bulb transcriptome during Alzheimer's disease evolution: Novel insights into the olfactory signaling across proteinopathies. *Oncotarget* **2017**. [CrossRef] [PubMed]
36. Liu, Y.; Beyer, A.; Aebersold, R. On the dependency of cellular protein levels on mRNA abundance. *Cell* **2016**, *165*, 535–550. [CrossRef] [PubMed]
37. Baker, M.S.; Ahn, S.B.; Mohamedali, A.; Islam, M.T.; Cantor, D.; Verhaert, P.D.; Fanayan, S.; Sharma, S.; Nice, E.C.; Connor, M.; et al. Accelerating the search for the missing proteins in the human proteome. *Nat. Commun.* **2017**, *8*, 14271. [CrossRef] [PubMed]
38. Sakamoto, K.; Karelina, K.; Obrietan, K. CREB: A multifaceted regulator of neuronal plasticity and protection. *J. Neurochem.* **2011**, *116*, 1–9. [CrossRef] [PubMed]
39. Tully, T.; Bourtchouladze, R.; Scott, R.; Tallman, J. Targeting the CREB pathway for memory enhancers. *Nat. Rev. Drug Discov.* **2003**, *2*, 267–277. [CrossRef] [PubMed]
40. Teich, A.F.; Nicholls, R.E.; Puzzo, D.; Fiorito, J.; Purgatorio, R.; Fa, M.; Arancio, O. Synaptic therapy in Alzheimer's disease: A CREB-centric approach. *Neurotherapeutics* **2015**, *12*, 29–41. [CrossRef] [PubMed]
41. Saura, C.A. CREB-regulated transcription coactivator 1-dependent transcription in Alzheimer's disease mice. *Neurodegener. Dis.* **2012**, *10*, 250–252. [CrossRef] [PubMed]
42. Saura, C.A.; Valero, J. The role of CREB signaling in Alzheimer's disease and other cognitive disorders. *Rev. Neurosci.* **2011**, *22*, 153–169. [CrossRef] [PubMed]
43. Kaur, U.; Banerjee, P.; Bir, A.; Sinha, M.; Biswas, A.; Chakrabarti, S. Reactive oxygen species, redox signaling and neuroinflammation in Alzheimer's disease: The NF-κB connection. *Curr. Top. Med. Chem.* **2015**, *15*, 446–457. [CrossRef] [PubMed]
44. Viatour, P.; Merville, M.P.; Bours, V.; Chariot, A. Phosphorylation of NF-κB and IκB proteins: Implications in cancer and inflammation. *Trends Biochem. Sci.* **2005**, *30*, 43–52. [CrossRef] [PubMed]
45. Kaltschmidt, B.; Uherek, M.; Volk, B.; Baeuerle, P.A.; Kaltschmidt, C. Transcription factor NF-κB is activated in primary neurons by amyloid β peptides and in neurons surrounding early plaques from patients with alzheimer disease. *Proc. Natl. Acad. Sci. USA* **1997**, *94*, 2642–2647. [CrossRef] [PubMed]

46. Terai, K.; Matsuo, A.; McGeer, P.L. Enhancement of immunoreactivity for NF-kappa B in the hippocampal formation and cerebral cortex of Alzheimer's disease. *Brain Res.* **1996**, *735*, 159–168. [CrossRef]
47. Ferrer, I.; Marti, E.; Lopez, E.; Tortosa, A. NF-κB immunoreactivity is observed in association with β A4 diffuse plaques in patients with Alzheimer's disease. *Neuropathol. Appl. Neurobiol.* **1998**, *24*, 271–277. [CrossRef] [PubMed]
48. Paris, D.; Patel, N.; Quadros, A.; Linan, M.; Bakshi, P.; Ait-Ghezala, G.; Mullan, M. Inhibition of Aβ production by NF-κB inhibitors. *Neurosci. Lett.* **2007**, *415*, 11–16. [CrossRef] [PubMed]
49. Yoo, S.J.; Lee, J.H.; Kim, S.Y.; Son, G.; Kim, J.Y.; Cho, B.; Yu, S.W.; Chang, K.A.; Suh, Y.H.; Moon, C. Differential spatial expression of peripheral olfactory neuron-derived BACE1 induces olfactory impairment by region-specific accumulation of β-amyloid oligomer. *Cell Death Dis.* **2017**, *8*, e2977. [CrossRef] [PubMed]
50. Nagayama, S.; Homma, R.; Imamura, F. Neuronal organization of olfactory bulb circuits. *Front. Neural Circuits* **2014**, *8*, 98. [CrossRef] [PubMed]
51. Cuadrado-Tejedor, M.; Garcia-Osta, A. Current animal models of Alzheimer's disease: Challenges in translational research. *Front. Neurol.* **2014**, *5*, 182. [CrossRef] [PubMed]
52. Tyanova, S.; Temu, T.; Cox, J. The maxquant computational platform for mass spectrometry-based shotgun proteomics. *Nat. Protoc.* **2016**, *11*, 2301–2319. [CrossRef] [PubMed]
53. Tyanova, S.; Temu, T.; Sinitcyn, P.; Carlson, A.; Hein, M.Y.; Geiger, T.; Mann, M.; Cox, J. The perseus computational platform for comprehensive analysis of (prote)omics data. *Nat. Methods* **2016**, *13*, 731–740. [CrossRef] [PubMed]
54. Vizcaino, J.A.; Deutsch, E.W.; Wang, R.; Csordas, A.; Reisinger, F.; Rios, D.; Dianes, J.A.; Sun, Z.; Farrah, T.; Bandeira, N.; et al. Proteomexchange provides globally coordinated proteomics data submission and dissemination. *Nat. Biotechnol.* **2014**, *32*, 223–226. [CrossRef] [PubMed]
55. Irizarry, R.A.; Bolstad, B.M.; Collin, F.; Cope, L.M.; Hobbs, B.; Speed, T.P. Summaries of Affymetrix GeneChip probe level data. *Nucleic Acids Res.* **2003**, *31*, e15. [CrossRef] [PubMed]
56. Silva, A.R.; Grinberg, L.T.; Farfel, J.M.; Diniz, B.S.; Lima, L.A.; Silva, P.J.; Ferretti, R.E.; Rocha, R.M.; Filho, W.J.; Carraro, D.M.; et al. Transcriptional alterations related to neuropathology and clinical manifestation of Alzheimer's disease. *PLoS ONE* **2012**, *7*, e48751. [CrossRef] [PubMed]
57. Cuadrado-Tejedor, M.; Garcia-Barroso, C.; Sanchez-Arias, J.A.; Rabal, O.; Perez-Gonzalez, M.; Mederos, S.; Ugarte, A.; Franco, R.; Segura, V.; Perea, G.; et al. A first-in-class small-molecule that acts as a dual inhibitor of HDAC and PDE5 and that rescues hippocampal synaptic impairment in Alzheimer's disease mice. *Neuropsychopharmacology* **2016**, *42*, 524–539. [CrossRef] [PubMed]

10

Triple Test Plus Rapid Cognitive Screening Test: A Combination of Clinical Signs and a Tool for Cognitive Assessment in Older Adults

Saadet Koc Okudur [1], Ozge Dokuzlar [2], Derya Kaya [2], Pinar Soysal [3] and Ahmet Turan Isik [2,*]

1 Department of Geriatric Medicine, Manisa State Hospital, Manisa 45040, Turkey
2 Unit for Brain Aging and Dementia, Department of Geriatric Medicine, Faculty of Medicine, Dokuz Eylul University, Izmir 35340, Turkey
3 Department of Geriatric Medicine, Faculty of Medicine, Bezmialem Vakif University, Istanbul 34093, Turkey
* Correspondence: atisik@yahoo.com

Abstract: Less time-consuming, easy-to-apply and more reliable cognitive screening tests are essential for use in primary care. The aim of this study was to investigate the diagnostic value of the Turkish version of the Rapid Cognitive Screen (RCS-T) and Triple Test individually and the combination of RCS-T with each sign and Triple Test to screen elderly patients for cognitive impairment (CI). A total of 357 outpatients aged 60 or older, who underwent comprehensive geriatric assessment, were included in the study. Presence or absence of attended alone sign (AAS), head-turning sign, and applause sign was investigated. The mean age of the patients was 74.29 ± 7.46. Of those, 61 patients (28 men, 33 women) had Alzheimer's disease (AD), 59 patients had mild cognitive impairment (MCI) (29 men, 30 women), and 237 (80 men, 157 women) were cognitively robust. The sensitivity of the combination of RCS-T and negative for AAS for CI, AD and MCI is 0.79, 0.86 and 0.61, respectively; the specificity was 0.92, 0.93 and 0.92, respectively; and the positive and negative predictive values revealed good diagnostic accuracy. The combination of RCS-T and negative for AAS is a simple, effective and rapid way to identify possible CI in older adults.

Keywords: cognitive screening instruments; dementia; mild cognitive impairment; cognitive impairment; Rapid Cognitive Screen; Triple Test

---

1. Introduction

Memory complaints, which should be distinguished from cognitive impairments (CI) related to neurodegenerative diseases such as Alzheimer's disease (AD), are quite prevalent among older adults [1,2]. It is difficult to devote time for detailed neuropsychological tests during a busy clinical day, which is the first approach to determine whether or not a patient requires further clinical evaluation for CI [3]. Therefore, less time-consuming, easy-to-apply and more reliable cognitive screening tests (which are essential to accurately diagnose patients with CI, especially for primary care settings) may help primary care professionals determine whether it is necessary to refer a patient to a tertiary care or a memory center for cognitive diseases [4].

Elaborate medical history, physical examination, and neurocognitive assessment should be performed to identify the etiology of memory loss [5]. The Rapid Cognitive Screen (RCS) is a brief screening tool derived from the Saint Louis University Mental Status (SLUMS) examination for the detection of cognitive dysfunction in primary care settings [6] and the Turkish version of the RCS (RCS-T) is validated in Turkish older adults [7]. Additionally, inclusion of some clinical signs of neurodegenerative diseases leading to dementia, such as the attended alone sign (AAS) [8], head-turning sign (HTS) [9,10] and applause sign (AS) [11] in cognitive assessment, may play a significant role in the diagnostic process [4,12].

The Triple Test consisting of AAS, HTS and AS has been shown to be a simple, rapid and effective screening tool for detecting cognitive impairment, and deterioration of daily living activities in older adults [4,12]. AS is also called the clapping test, three-clap test, or signe d'applause. The evaluation is as follows: The patient is asked to clap three times as quickly as possible after the examiner had performed a demonstration. When the patient claps three times, this is considered negative for AS. When the patient claps more than three times, this is considered positive for AS. Patients clapping less than three times are considered pathologic, and positive for AS, as reported previously [13,14]. In the literature [9,15], HTS is assessed while the patient's caregiver sat silently at a 45° angle, approximately 1 m behind the patient, who is encouraged to speak about their cognitive function history. When the patient turns her/his head away from the collocutor and towards the caregiver(s) for help, the patient is considered positive for HTS. When the patient did not want any help, this is considered negative for HTS. AAS is evaluated based on whether the patient attended the clinic with a family member, caregiver, or friend. When the patient is accompanied, this is considered negative for attended alone sign [15].

Early definitive diagnosis of cognitive impairment may be difficult in busy clinic settings, in which the main purpose of combining tests is to ensure early recognition of patients with cognitive impairment and referral to a higher center.

Nevertheless, it is not known whether the combination of the RCS-T test, a clinical screening tool, and the Triple Test, a test based on clinical symptoms, has positive effects on the management of memory problems. Therefore, in the present study we aimed to investigate the diagnostic value of the RCS-T and Triple Test individually and the combination of RCS-T with each sign and Triple Test to screen elderly patients for CI.

2. Materials and Methods

A total of 357 patients aged over 60 years, who were admitted to the geriatric outpatient clinic with memory complaints between June 2014 and February 2019, and underwent comprehensive geriatric assessment, were included in the study. All the participants, who provided informed consent to participate in the study, were evaluated by comprehensive geriatric assessment, including physical and mental status examination and laboratory evaluation. The ethics committee of Dokuz Eylul University, Turkey, approved the study protocol with decision number 2018/22-19, and the project identification code is 4241-GOA (September 13, 2018). Each participant or a legal guardian provided written, informed consent to participate in the study. We carried out this study in accordance with the provisions of the Declaration of Helsinki.

Major and minor CI was diagnosed according to the Diagnostic and Statistical Manual of Mental Disorders (fifth edition) diagnostic criteria [16] and AD was diagnosed according to National Institute on Aging–Alzheimer's Association workgroup's criteria [17]. The cognitively robust group consisted of patients who had memory complaints despite normal cognitive assessments and those who attended our geriatric outpatient clinic for prevention programs because of other medical issues.

Socio-demographic characteristics of the patients, including gender, age and education, were recorded. All patients were examined to see if they had hearing loss, cataracts, hypertension, diabetes mellitus, coronary artery disease, peripheral vascular disease, hyperlipidemia, cerebrovascular disease, congestive heart failure, depression, dementia, or polypharmacy in their medical history. For each patient, a comprehensive geriatric assessment, including detailed and complete physical and mental examinations, was performed [18]. Patients were evaluated based on the RCS-T [7], Mini-Mental State Examination (MMSE) [19], Geriatric Depression Scale [20], Instrumental Activities of Daily Living [21], Basic Activities of Daily Living Scale [22], Clinical Dementia Rating, and a clock drawing test. For the patients with CI, further evaluations, such as laboratory examination and brain imaging (essential for the differential diagnosis CI) were also performed.

The signs were assessed by two physicians (S.K.O and O.D.), who were blinded to the diagnosis of the patients. High interrater agreements were observed (1.00 for AAS, 0.98 for HTS, and 1.00 for AS). Presence or absence of AS, AAS, and HTS was investigated.

The RCS test includes 3 items: recall of 5 words, a clock drawing test, and the ability to remember a story [6]. Scores ranged from 0 and 10. The RCS-T optimal cut-off scores were ≤ 4 for dementia and ≤ 6 for mild cognitive impairment (MCI) [7].

Patients with unilateral hearing impairment or blindness and deafness, and those considered to be too sick to be questioned, including those in delirium, were excluded. Those who had been taking medications that might influence their thinking or memory, who had previous head trauma resulting in unconsciousness and/or a period of memory impairment, who were unable to provide informed consent to participate in the study, who cannot speak Turkish, or who were illiterate, were excluded. Reversible CI related to vitamin B12 or folic acid deficiency, hypothyroidism, subdural hematoma, hyponatremia, medications (e.g., corticosteroids, antipsychotics, and benzodiazepines), substance abuse problems and the institutionalized older adults were excluded.

The package program, Statistical Package for Social Sciences (SPSS) version 23.0 for Windows (SPSS Inc., Chicago, IL, USA), was used for the statistical analysis. Descriptive statistics are presented as means ± standard deviations or percentages. Nominal variables were evaluated by Pearson's $\chi 2$-test. Kruskal–Wallis test was used to analyze the presence of non-normal distribution, and continuous variables with normal distribution were assessed with one-way ANOVA (shown as the P_1 value in Table 1). Adjustment according to age and gender was carried out by multinomial logistic regression analysis (shown as the P_2 and P_3 value in Table 1). Sensitivity refers to proportion of correct positive classifications, and specificity refers to proportion of correct negative classifications. p-value < 0.05 was considered significant. Sensitivity, specificity, and positive and negative predictive values (PPV, NPV) were calculated for diagnosis of any CI, AD, and MCI. A sample size of 214 participants was calculated as the minimum required size to be within a 5% of the true proportion.

Table 1. Descriptive characteristics of participants (n = 357).

	Control (n = 237)	MCI (n = 59)	AD (n = 61)	P_1	P_2	P_3
Women (%)	66.2	51.7	53.3	0.041	-	-
Age	72.45 ± 7.08	76.37 ± 6.09	78.95 ± 7.63	<0.001	-	-
Education (year)	8.61 ± 3.84	7.98 ± 3.76	8.48 ± 4.09	0.390	-	-
Number of drugs	5.33 ± 3.33	5.65 ± 3.02	5.92 ± 3.07	0.214	-	-
MMSE	28.26 ± 1.71	25.25 ± 3.44	17.92 ± 4.86	<0.001	<0.001	<0.001
SLUMS	25.14 ± 3.19	19.50 ± 4.56	10.88 ± 4.64	<0.001	<0.001	<0.001
RCS-T	8.28 ± 1.52	5.42 ± 2.13	2.15	<0.001	<0.001	<0.001
CDR	0.0 ± 0.1	0.5 ± 0.2	1.5 ± 0.6	<0.001	<0.001	<0.001
CDT	4.7 ± 0.8	4.2 ± 1.2	2.2 ± 1.3	<0.001	<0.001	<0.001
GDS	2.8 ± 3.3	3.1 ± 3.3	3.7 ± 3.3	0.139	-	-
BADL	95.46 ± 5.87	93.15 ± 13.22	83.58 ± 18.28	<0.001	<0.001	0.259
IADL	14.99 ± 3.13	13.58 ± 3.94	8.07 ± 4.95	<0.001	<0.001	0.169

AD, Alzheimer's disease; BADL, Basic Activities of Daily Living; CDR, Clinical Dementia Rating; CDT, clock-drawing; GDS, Geriatric Depression Scale; IADL, Instrumental Activities of Daily Living; MCI, mild cognitive impairment; MMSE, Mini-Mental State Examination; P_1, p-values for comparison of three groups; P_2, p-values for comparison of AD and control group after adjusted for age and gender; P_3, p-values for comparison of MCI and control group after adjusted for age and gender; RCS-T, Turkish version of the Rapid Cognitive Screen test; SLUMS, Saint Louis University Mental Status Examination. Score range for each of the assessments: BADL, 0 (worst)–100 (best); CDR, 0 (best)–3 (worst); CDT, 0 (worst)–5 (best); GDS, 0 (best)–15 (worst); IADL, 0 (worst)–17 (best); MMSE, 0 (worst)–30 (best), RCS-T, 0 (worst)–10 (best); SLUMS, 0 (worst)–30 (best). All data are expressed as means ± standard deviations.

3. Results

A total of 357 outpatients (137 men, 220 women) with a mean age of 74.29 ± 7.46 years were assessed. Of the patients, 61 (28 men, 33 women) were diagnosed with AD, 59 were diagnosed with MCI (29 men, 30 women) and 237 (80 men, 157 women) were cognitively robust (controls). There was a significant difference among AD, MCI and controls in terms of gender and age; there were more female participants in controls ($p < 0.05$) and older patients in AD group ($p < 0.001$). There was no difference in the patients with MCI, AD, and controls with regards to total years of education or educational level of the participants (for each, $p > 0.05$). There was no difference for the number of drugs between the groups ($p > 0.05$). After comprehensive geriatric assessment, when MMSE, SLUMS, RCS-T, clinical dementia rating test, clock-drawing test, Geriatric Depression Scale, Basic Activities of Daily Living Scales and Instrumental Activities of Daily Living were evaluated, there was a significant difference between the groups ($p < 0.001$) except for Geriatric Depression Scale. Descriptive data of the patients are summarized in Table 1. After adjustments for age and gender by multinomial logistic regression analysis MMSE, RCS-T, SLUMS, clock-drawing test (CDT), Clinical Dementia Rating (CDR), Basic Activities of Daily Living (BADL), and Instrumental Activities of Daily Living (IADL) were still significant in the AD group compared to the control group ($p < 0.001$). When MCI and control group were compared, statistical significance was maintained for MMSE, SLUMS, RCS-T, CDR, CDT ($p < 0.001$); but BADL ($p = 0.259$) and IADL ($p = 0.169$) showed no statistical significance.

Patients' neuropsychological profiles were assessed based on the presence or absence of AS, HTS and AAS and the neuropsychological tests (MMSE, SLUMS, RCS-T and clock-drawing test). The sensitivity and specificity, and PPV and NPV values of the tests are shown in Table 2.

Table 2. Assessment of the diagnostic value of the RCS-T and Triple Test individually and the combination of RCS-T with each sign and Triple Test.

	Each Test		**Combinations of RCS + Each Sign**			**Combinations of RCS + Triple Test**	
	RCS-T	Triple	RCS-T and PHTS	RCS-T and PAS	RCS-T and NAAS	RCS-T and Triple	RCS-T or Triple
CI							
Sensitivity %	85.83	29.66	58.47	29.66	79.66	29.17	86.44
Specificity %	88.19	96.51	96.94	98.69	92.14	98.7	85.59
PPV %	78.63	81.40	90.79	92.11	83.93	92.11	75.56
NPV %	92.48	72.70	81.92	73.14	89.79	72.76	92.45
AD							
Sensitivity %	86.67	42.37	69.49	40.48	86.44	39.49	88.33
Specificity %	90.91	93.75	94.77	98.61	93.03	98.89	85.76
PPV %	65.82	58.14	73.21	85.71	71.83	86.82	56.38
NPV %	97.12	88.82	93.79	88.73	97.09	87.06	97.24
MCI							
Sensitivity %	73.33	15.52	78.79	16.95	61.02	15.25	61.54
Specificity %	88.19	96.51	87.06	98.69	92.14	99.13	87.11
PPV %	61.11	52.94	44.07	76.92	66.67	81.82	45.28
NPV %	92.89	81.85	96.94	82.18	90.17	81.95	92.89

AD, Alzheimer's disease; CI, Cognitive impairment; MCI, Mild cognitive impairment; NAAS, Negative for attended alone sign; NPV, Negative predictive value; PAS, Positive for applause sign; PHTS, Positive for head-turning sign; PPV, Positive predictive value; RCS, Rapid Cognitive Screen test.

4. Discussion

The present study demonstrated that RCS-T and the Triple Test are easy to perform together and are highly specific tools to screen elderly patients with CI, AD or MCI while the combination of RCS-T and negative for AAS is sensitive and specific enough to accurately screen those with CI.

Discrimination between cognitively normal and CI in older adults, especially in early stage, requires long, time-consuming cognitive tests and sophisticated evaluations. For this purpose, many tests are currently available for cognitive screening. Out of them, the sensitivity and specificity of MMSE, Montreal cognitive assessment, Turkish version of SLUMS, and Cognitive state test screening tests are 0.91 and 0.95; 0.81 and 0.78; 0.84 and 0.87; and 0.81 and 0.78, respectively [19,23–25]; however, they tend to be time consuming and may be inappropriate for both bedside clinical evaluation and daily clinical practice, especially in the primary care setting. In a recent study, SLUMS-derived RCS [6,7] has been reported to be a simple, fast and practical tool that is sensitive and specific enough to screen CI in older adults and reflects deterioration in daily living activities [7] which is confirmed once again in the present study.

In addition, it is highly important that physicians consider cognitive screening tools as well as the early clinical signs of specific neurodegenerative diseases, such as HTS, AAS, and AS in order to make a differential diagnosis. The neuropsychological properties of HTS are potentially heterogeneous, including amnesia, impaired comprehension and lack of insight [10]. Previous studies showed that AAS is effective in detecting cognitively robust patients [12,26]. AAS is also thought to give information about instrumental activities of daily living and noncognitive functions in the same domain such as mobility, gait, balance and vision [4,27]. AS is a motor perseveration indicative of frontal lobe dysfunction in different types of dementia [28]. In a recent study, the combination called the Triple Test has been demonstrated to be a simple, quick and efficient screening tool for detecting CI [4].

The present study showed that the combination of RCS-T or the Triple Test positivity has a good sensitivity for discriminating between patients with CI, AD, and MCI (0.86, 0.88 and 0.62, respectively) and also better with higher NPV for all (0.92, 0.97 and 0.93, respectively). It means that the combination can correctly identify older patients without CI among those with memory problems, and that it can be used for older adults with memory complaints in bedside evaluation or primary care setting. Hence, those who are negative for the combination may not need to be referred to the relevant memory centers for detailed cognitive assessment. Additionally, in the present study, RCS-T plus AAS has good sensitivity and high specificity to detect CI in older adults.

When the current results were compared with our previous ones [4], it was found that sensitivity and specificity of the Triple Test were not similar in these studies, which can be explained by gender and educational differences, considering the fact that some cultural and methodological differences should be kept in mind while assessing the results of the studies [29].

Of particular note in this study, the RCS-T test together with HTS showed a remarkable NPV (0.97), which may be a signal or alert to closely monitor individuals with the possibility of MCI or to refer to the memory centers. With this finding, using RCS-T and positive for HTS together can be considered as a daily questionnaire because the RCS-T test is a reliable and valid measure, and indeed doctors inevitably evaluate HTS during routine history taking. Unfortunately, there is no specific applicable measurement to differentiate those with MCI from those that are cognitively robust, but measurements are increasingly being investigated for early detection of AD/MCI. Recently, it has been shown that Addenbrooke's Cognitive Examination III has a sensitivity of 0.77 and specificity 0.92 in capturing individuals with MCI in Japan [30], and a sensitivity of 0.63 and specificity of 0.63 in Malay [31]. Our finding, with a sensitivity of 0.78 and specificity of 0.87, is also compatible with the aforementioned studies.

RCS-T alone is also very valuable due to the fact that it differentiated cognitively robust older adults accurately from those who had MCI or cognitive impairment. In the present study, RCS-T is combined with Triple Test, which is performed by physicians during the physical examination. It is striking that specificity of the combination was high enough to show that individuals with a good test performance are healthy. Furthermore, patients who have poor performance for either RCS-T or Triple Test are more likely to be cognitively impaired, with a sensitivity of 0.86. Therefore, older people with memory problems could be better directed for further neurocognitive analysis if either of them is positive.

The strengths of this study are the large sample size and that all the cases included in the study were over 60 years of age. As far as we are concerned, this is the first study to evaluate the diagnostic value of the combination; however, it has still some limitations. Since it was conducted at a memory center, the generalizability of our findings might be limited. Another limitation is that HTS requires the presence of a person accompanying the patient to the clinic.

5. Conclusions

Our study has demonstrated that the combination of RCS-T and negative for AAS is simple, effective and rapid way to identify possible CI in older adults. The combination of RCS-T and Triple Test has the ability to identify the cognitively robust older adults with subjective memory complaints, while those with poor performance for either of them may require further neurocognitive evaluation for CI. Therefore, the combination of both tests could serve as an indicator of those patients in need of further neurocognitive analysis, especially in daily busy clinical practice.

Author Contributions: Conceptualization, P.S. and A.T.I.; formal analysis, O.D.; investigation, S.K.O. and D.K.; methodology, A.T.I.; writing—review & editing, S.K.O., P.S. and A.T.I.

References

1. Ates Bulut, E.; Soysal, P.; Yavuz, I.; Kocyigit, S.E.; Isik, A.T. Effect of Vitamin D on Cognitive Functions in Older Adults: 24-Week Follow-Up Study. *Am. J. Alzheimers Dis. Other Demen* **2019**, *34*, 112–117. [CrossRef] [PubMed]
2. Reitz, C.; Brayne, C.; Mayeux, R. Epidemiology of Alzheimer disease. *Nat. Rev. Neurol.* **2011**, *7*, 137–152. [CrossRef] [PubMed]
3. Cordell, C.B.; Borson, S.; Boustani, M.; Chodosh, J.; Reuben, D.; Verghese, J.; Thies, W.; Fried, L.B. Alzheimer's Association recommendations for operationalizing the detection of cognitive impairment during the Medicare Annual Wellness Visit in a primary care setting. *Alzheimers Dement.* **2013**, *9*, 141–150. [CrossRef] [PubMed]
4. Isik, A.T.; Soysal, P.; Kaya, D.; Usarel, C. Triple test, a diagnostic observation, can detect cognitive impairment in older adults. *Psychogeriatrics* **2018**, *18*, 98–105. [CrossRef] [PubMed]
5. Annoni, J.; Chouiter, L.; Demonet, J. Age-related cognitive impairment: Conceptual changes and diagnostic strategies. *Rev. Méd. Suisse* **2016**, *12*, 774–779. [PubMed]
6. Malmstrom, T.K.; Voss, V.B.; Cruz-Oliver, D.M.; Cummings-Vaughn, L.A.; Tumosa, N.; Grossberg, G.T.; Morley, J.E. The Rapid Cognitive Screen (RCS): A point-ofcare screening for dementia and mild cognitive impairment. *J. Nutr. Health Aging* **2015**, *19*, 741–744. [CrossRef]
7. Koc Okudur, S.; Dokuzlar, O.; Usarel, C.; Soysal, P.; Isik, A.T. Validity and Reliability of Rapid Cognitive Screening Test for Turkish Older Adults. *J. Nutr. Health Aging* **2019**, *23*, 68–72. [CrossRef]
8. Larner, A.J. 'Who came with you?' A diagnostic observation in patients with memory problems? *J. Neurol. Neurosurg. Psychiatry* **2005**, *76*, 1739. [CrossRef]
9. Fukui, T.; Yamazaki, T.; Kinno, R. Can the 'head-turning sign' be a clinical marker of Alzheimer's disease? *Dement. Geriatr. Cogn. Disord. Extra* **2011**, *1*, 310–317. [CrossRef]
10. Larner, A.J. Head turning sign: Pragmatic utility in clinical diagnosis of cognitive impairment. *J. Neurol. Neurosurg. Psychiatry* **2012**, *83*, 852–853. [CrossRef]
11. Dubois, B.; Slachevsky, A.; Pillon, B.; Beato, R.; Villalponda, J.M.; Liyvan, I. 'Applause sign' helps to discriminate PSP from FTD and PD. *Neurology* **2005**, *64*, 2132–2133. [CrossRef] [PubMed]
12. Soysal, P.; Usarel, C.; Ispirli, G.; Isik, A.T. Attended with and headturning sign can be clinical markers of cognitive impairment in older adults. *Int. Psychogeriatr.* **2017**, *29*, 1–7. [CrossRef] [PubMed]

13. Wu, L.J.; Sitburana, O.; Davidson, A.; Jankovic, J. Applause sign in Parkinsonian disorders and Huntington's disease. *Mov. Disord.* **2008**, *23*, 2307–2311. [CrossRef] [PubMed]
14. Isella, V.; Rucci, F.; Traficante, D.; Mapelli, C.; Ferri, F.; Appollonio, I.M. The applause sign in cortical and cortical-subcortical dementia. *J. Neurol.* **2013**, *260*, 1099–1103. [CrossRef] [PubMed]
15. Larner, A. History and neurological examination. In *Dementia in Clinical Practice: A Neurological Perspective*, 2nd ed.; Larner, A.J., Ed.; Springer: London, UK, 2014; pp. 41–69.
16. American Psychiatric Association. *Diagnostic and Statistical Manual of Mental Disorders*, 5th ed.; American Psychiatric Association: Arlington, VA, USA, 2013.
17. McKhann, G.M.; Knopman, D.S.; Chertkow, H.; Hyman, B.T.; Jack, C.R., Jr.; Kawas, C.H.; Klunk, W.E.; Koroshetz, W.J.; Manly, J.J.; Mayeux, R.; et al. The diagnosis of dementia due to Alzheimer's disease: Recommendations from the National Institute on Aging Alzheimer's Association workgroups on diagnostic guidelines for Alzheimer's disease. *Alzheimers Dement.* **2011**, *7*, 263–269. [CrossRef]
18. Isik, A.T.; Bozoglu, E.; Yay, A.; Soysal, P.; Ateskan, U. Which cholinesterase inhibitor is the safest for heart in elderly patients with Alzheimer's disease? *Am. J. Alzheimers Dis. Other Dement.* **2012**, *27*, 171–174. [CrossRef] [PubMed]
19. Gungen, C.; Ertan, T.; Eker, E.; Yasar, R.; Engin, F. Reliability and validity of the standardized Mini Mental State Examination in the diagnosis of mild dementia in Turkish population. *Turk. Psikiyatr. Dergisi* **2002**, *13*, 273–281.
20. Durmaz, B.; Soysal, P.; Ellidokuz, H.; Isik, A.T. Validity and reliability of geriatric depression scale-15 (short form) in Turkish older adults. *North. Clin. Istanbul* **2018**, *5*, 216–220. [CrossRef]
21. Lawton, M.P.; Brody, E.M. Assessment of older people: Selfmaintaining and instrumental activities of daily living. *Gerontologist* **1969**, *9*, 179–186. [CrossRef]
22. Mahoney, F.I.; Barthel, D. Functional evaluation: The Barthel Index: A simple index of independence useful in scoring improvement in the rehabilitation of the chronically ill. *Md. State Med. J.* **1965**, *14*, 61–65.
23. Selekler, K.; Cangöz, B.; Uluc, S. Montreal bilissel degerlendirme ölceginin hafif bilissel bozukluk ve Alzheimer hastalarini ayırtedebilme gücünün incelenmesi. *Turk. J. Geriatr.* **2010**, *13*, 166–171.
24. Kaya, D.; Isik, A.T.; Usarel, C.; Soysal, P.; Ellidokuz, H.; Grossberg, G.T. The Saint Louis University Mental Status Examination is better than the Mini-Mental State Examination to determine the cognitive impairment in Turkish elderly people. *J. Am. Med. Dir. Assoc.* **2016**, *17*, 370.e11–370.e15. [CrossRef] [PubMed]
25. Babacan-Yildiz, G.; Isik, A.T.; Ur, E.; Aydemir, E.; Ertas, C.; Cebi, M.; Soysal, P.; Gursoy, E.; Kolukisa, M.; Kocaman, G.; et al. COST: Cognitive state test, a brief screening battery for Alzheimer disease in illiterate and literate patients. *Int. Psychogeriatr.* **2013**, *25*, 403–412. [CrossRef] [PubMed]
26. Larner, A.J. Screening utility of the "attended alone" sign for subjective memory impairment. *Alzheimer Dis. Assoc. Disord.* **2014**, *28*, 364–365. [CrossRef] [PubMed]
27. Larner, A.J. 'Attended alone'sign: Validity and reliability for the exclusion of dementia. *Age Ageing* **2009**, *38*, 476–478. [CrossRef] [PubMed]
28. Bonello, M.; Larner, A.J. Applause sign: Screening utility for dementia and cognitive impairment. *Postgrad. Med.* **2016**, *128*, 250–253. [CrossRef]
29. Soysal, P.; Isik, A.T. Factors affecting sensitivity and specificity of head-turning sign in the studies. *Int. Psychogeriatr.* **2018**, *30*, 1571–1572. [CrossRef] [PubMed]
30. Takenoshita, S.; Terada, S.; Yoshida, H.; Yamaguchi, M.; Yabe, M.; Imai, N.; Horiuchi, M.; Miki, T.; Yokota, O.; Yamada, N. Validation of Addenbrooke's cognitive examination III for detecting mild cognitive impairment and dementia in Japan. *BMC Geriatr.* **2019**, *19*, 123. [CrossRef]
31. Kan, K.C.; Subramaniam, P.; Shahrizaila, N.; Kamaruzzaman, S.B.; Razali, R.; Ghazali, S.E. Validation of the Malay Version of Addenbrooke's Cognitive Examination III in Detecting Mild Cognitive Impairment and Dementia. *Dement. Geriatr. Cogn. Disord. Extra* **2019**, *9*, 66–76. [CrossRef]

11

MACE for Diagnosis of Dementia and MCI: Examining Cut-Offs and Predictive Values

Andrew J. Larner

Cognitive Function Clinic, Walton Centre for Neurology and Neurosurgery, Liverpool L9 7LJ, UK; a.larner@thewaltoncentre.nhs.uk or A.J.Larner@thewaltoncentre.nhs.uk

Abstract: The definition of test cut-offs is a critical determinant of many paired and unitary measures of diagnostic or screening test accuracy, such as sensitivity and specificity, positive and negative predictive values, and correct classification accuracy. Revision of test cut-offs from those defined in index studies is frowned upon as a potential source of bias, seemingly accepting any biases present in the index study, for example related to sample bias. Data from a large pragmatic test accuracy study examining the Mini-Addenbrooke's Cognitive Examination (MACE) were interrogated to determine optimal test cut-offs for the diagnosis of dementia and mild cognitive impairment (MCI) using either the maximal Youden index or the maximal correct classification accuracy. Receiver operating characteristic (ROC) and precision recall (PR) curves for dementia and MCI were also plotted, and MACE predictive values across a range of disease prevalences were calculated. Optimal cut-offs were found to be a point lower than those defined in the index study. MACE had good metrics for the area under the ROC curve and for the effect size (Cohen's d) for both dementia and MCI diagnosis, but PR curves suggested the superiority for MCI diagnosis. MACE had high negative predictive value at all prevalences, suggesting that a MACE test score above either cut-off excludes dementia and MCI in any setting.

Keywords: diagnosis; dementia; mild cognitive impairment; Mini-Addenbrooke's Cognitive Examination

---

1. Introduction

The Mini-Addenbrooke's Cognitive Examination (MACE) is a shortened version of the Addenbrooke's Cognitive Examination-Revised (ACE-R) and ACE-III developed by Mokken scaling analysis of these longer instruments [1]. MACE comprises tests of attention, memory (7-item name and address), verbal fluency, clock drawing and memory recall (score range 0–30, impaired to normal), and takes between 5–10 min to administer.

In the index MACE study, two cut-off points were identified in the cohort examined (n = 242; Alzheimer's disease 28, behavioural variant frontotemporal dementia 23, primary progressive aphasia 82, corticobasal syndrome 21, controls 78): ≤25/30 had high sensitivity (0.85) and high specificity (0.87); and ≤21/30 had high specificity (1.00), and hence an abnormal score was almost certain to have come from a dementia patient. MACE was found to be more sensitive than the Mini-Mental State Examination (MMSE) and less likely to have ceiling effects [1].

The general applicability of these MACE cut-offs for the diagnosis of dementia and mild cognitive impairment (MCI) has not been widely examined. A Spanish translation administered to a cohort of mixed dementia patients and controls (n = 175) with relatively low educational experience found that a cut-off between 16/30 and 17/30 had optimal sensitivity (0.867) and specificity (0.870) for dementia diagnosis [2].

MACE was adopted in the author's practice, based in a dedicated Cognitive Function Clinic located at a regional neuroscience centre in the northwest United Kingdom in June 2014 [3], and has been routinely used since then. Access to a large dataset has provided the opportunity to examine a variety of parameters not hitherto examined. The aims of this study were:

- To determine optimal MACE cut-off points for the diagnosis of dementia and MCI, with the anticipation that cut-offs optimising sensitivity would also minimise false negative rate (FNR) and optimise negative predictive value (NPV) whilst cut-offs optimising specificity would minimise false positive rate (FPR) and optimise positive predictive value (PPV);
- To plot receiver operating characteristic (ROC) and precision recall (PR) curves for dementia and MCI, and to calculate areas under the ROC curves and Q* index (a measure of diagnostic value);
- To calculate MACE effect sizes (Cohen's d) for diagnosis of dementia and MCI;
- To calculate MACE predictive values across a range of disease prevalences.

2. Methods

Consecutive new patient referrals administered the MACE were included, seen over the period June 2014–December 2018 (inclusive), including data reported in previous studies [3–5]. Other than those with a pre-existing diagnosis of dementia, there were no exclusion criteria. As previously detailed [3–5], criterion diagnosis of dementia or mild cognitive impairment was by judgement of an experienced clinician using standard diagnostic criteria (DSM-IV; Petersen); in those without evidence of cognitive impairment, a diagnosis of subjective memory complaint (SMC) was made. MACE scores were not used to make criterion diagnoses to avoid review bias. Subjects gave informed consent, and the study protocol was approved by the institute's committee on human research.

MACE scores were plotted against diagnosis, and the Pearson 2 skewness coefficient (Sk2) was used to assess skew, where:

$$\text{Sk2} = 3(\text{mean} - \text{median})/\text{standard deviation},$$

with values lying between –1 and +1 deemed acceptable for the elimination of floor or ceiling effects [6].

Various measures were calculated for all MACE cut-offs within the range deemed clinically sensible. Paired measures were: sensitivity (Sens, or recall) and specificity (Spec); positive and negative predictive values (PPV or precision, and NPV); positive and negative likelihood ratios (LR+ and LR–); and positive and negative clinical utility indexes (CUI+ and CUI–). Unitary or global measures were: correct classification accuracy (Acc); Youden index (Y, where Y = Sens + Spec – 1) [7]; predictive summary index (PSI, where PSI = PPV = NPV – 1) [8]; and identification index (II, where II = 2(Acc – 1) [9].

Two methods to optimise test cut-offs were examined [10,11], namely, maximising either Acc or Youden index.

In addition, various "number needed to" metrics were calculated: number needed to diagnose (NND, where NND = 1/Y); number needed to predict (NNP, where NNP = 1/PSI) [8]; and number needed to misdiagnose (NNM, where NNM = 1/(1 – Acc)) [12]. Also calculated were the "likelihood to be diagnosed or misdiagnosed" ratio (LDM, where LDM = NNM/NND or NNM/NNP) [13,14], and the "summary utility index" (SUI, where SUI = (CUI+ + CUI–)) [15]. The multiplicative inverse of the latter—the "number needed for screening utility" (NNSU = 1/SUI) [15]—was compared to the "number needed to screen" (NNS) metric, the multiplicative inverse of the "identification index" (II) [9], both rounded to the next highest integer value since they represent numbers of patients.

ROC curves were plotted (false positive rate versus sensitivity) and areas under the curve (AUC ROC) were calculated and categorised according to the scale of Metz [16]. The Q* index, a measure of diagnostic value [17], was determined as the point in ROC space where the anti-diagonal intersected the ROC curve (i.e., where Sens = Spec). Precision recall (PR) curves [18] were also plotted, as these have been recommended over ROC curves when analysing highly skewed datasets [19]. The F measure, or F1 score—the harmonic mean of precision and sensitivity—was also calculated as a global measure of accuracy [20].

Effect sizes (Cohen's d) were calculated as the difference of the means of diagnostic groups divided by the weighted pooled standard deviations of the groups [21]. Cohen's d values were categorised according to Sawilowsky's extension of Cohen's rules of thumb [22].

Predictive values across a range of disease prevalence (Prev) were calculated from observed sensitivity and specificity at the maximum Youden index for dementia and MCI, specifically at prevalence rates of 5%, 10%, 20% and 40% using the standard formulae:

$$PPV = Sens \times Prev/(Sens \times Prev) + [(1 - Spec) \times (1 - Prev)],$$

$$NPV = Spec \times (1 - Prev)/[Spec \times (1 - Prev)] + [(1 - Sens) \times Prev].$$

3. Results

A total of 755 patients were assessed with MACE (F:M = 352:403, 47% female; median age 60 years), of whom 114 were diagnosed with dementia (prevalence = 0.15) and 222 with MCI (prevalence = 0.29). The distribution of MACE scores by diagnosis, as seen in Figure 1, showed the anticipated unimodal negative skew (to the right, i.e., higher test scores = better performance). The Pearson 2 skewness coefficient (Sk2) was −0.48, suggesting that the population sampled was not from a normal distribution, although, as the value was between −1 and +1, the presence of floor or ceiling effects was probably excluded.

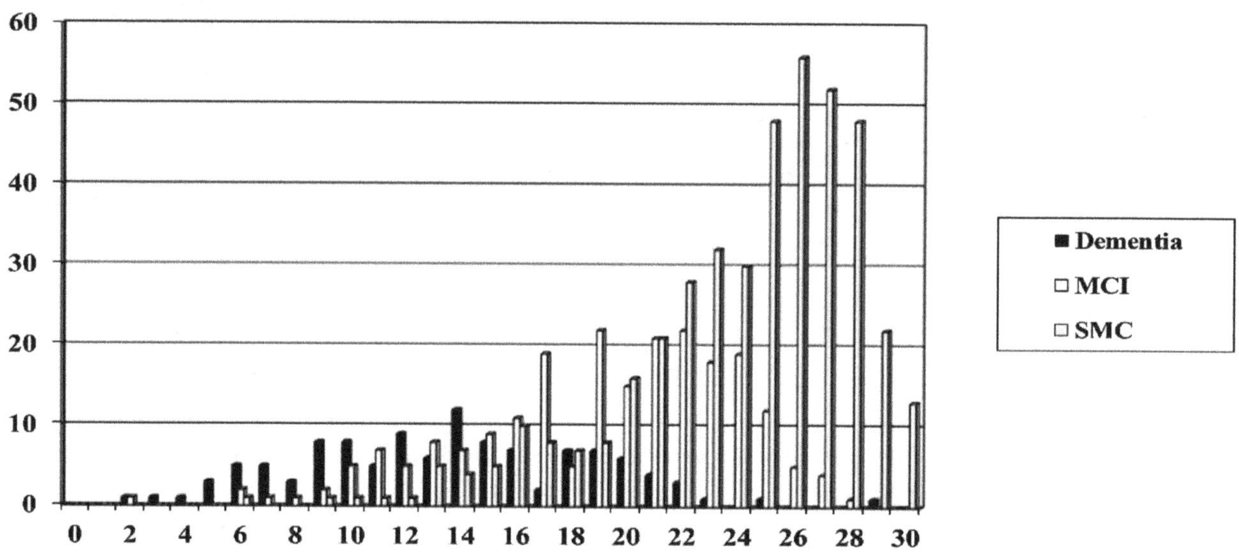

Figure 1. Mini-Addenbrooke's Cognitive Examination (MACE) scores versus patient diagnosis ($n = 755$). MCI: mild cognitive impairment; SMC: subjective memory complaint.

For the diagnosis of dementia (Tables 1 and 2), looking at all MACE cut-off values, the optimal cut-off determined by maximal Youden index was ≤20/30 (sensitivity 0.91, specificity 0.71). By maximal correct classification accuracy the optimal cut-off was ≤14/30 (sensitivity 0.59, specificity 0.92). This latter cut-off also had the maximal values of PSI and LDM (Table 3), the latter also found at ≤15/30, which was also the cut-off for the maximal value of SUI and F measure.

For the diagnosis of MCI (Tables 4 and 5), looking at all MACE cut-off values, the optimal cut-off determined by maximal Youden index was ≤24/30 (sensitivity 0.90, specificity 0.57). By maximal correct classification accuracy the optimal cut-off was ≤19/30 (sensitivity 0.47, specificity 0.88). Both cut-offs coincided with the maximal values of LDM (Table 6), whereas maximum PSI and F measure were at the same cut-off as maximal Youden index (cf. diagnosis of dementia), whilst maximal SUI was at ≤22/30 and ≤21/30.

Table 1. Diagnosis of dementia: paired measures of discrimination at various MACE cut-offs.

Cut-off	Sensitivity (= Recall); Specificity	False Positive Rate (FPR); False Negative Rate (FNR)	PPV (= Precision); NPV	LR+; LR−	CUI+; CUI−
≤29/30	1.00; 0.02	0.98; 0	0.15; 1.00	1.02; 0	0.15; 0.02
≤28/30	0.99; 0.06	0.94; 0.01	0.16; 0.97	1.05; 0.16	0.16; 0.05
≤27/30	0.99; 0.13	0.87; 0.01	0.17; 0.99	1.14; 0.07	0.17; 0.13
≤26/30	0.99; 0.22	0.78; 0.01	0.18; 0.99	1.27; 0.04	0.18; 0.22
≤25/30 *	0.99; 0.32	0.68; 0.01	0.20; 0.99	1.45; 0.03	0.20; 0.32
≤24/30	0.98; 0.41	0.59; 0.02	0.23; 0.99	1.66; 0.04	0.23; 0.41
≤23/30	0.98; 0.49	0.51; 0.02	0.25; 0.99	1.91; 0.04	0.25; 0.49
≤22/30	0.97; 0.56	0.44; 0.03	0.28; 0.99	2.23; 0.05	0.27; 0.55
≤21/30 *	0.95; 0.64	0.36; 0.05	0.32; 0.99	2.64; 0.08	0.30; 0.63
≤20/30	0.91; 0.71	0.29; 0.09	0.36; 0.98	3.11; 0.12	0.33; 0.70
≤19/30	0.86; 0.76	0.24; 0.14	0.38; 0.97	3.51; 0.19	0.33; 0.74
≤18/30	0.80; 0.80	0.20; 0.20	0.42; 0.96	4.03; 0.25	0.34; 0.77
≤17/30	0.74; 0.82	0.18; 0.26	0.42; 0.95	4.11; 0.32	0.31; 0.78
≤16/30	0.72; 0.86	0.14; 0.28	0.48; 0.95	5.24; 0.33	0.35; 0.82
≤15/30	0.66; 0.90	0.10; 0.34	0.53; 0.94	6.29; 0.38	0.35; 0.85
≤14/30	0.59; 0.92	0.08; 0.41	0.56; 0.93	7.11; 0.45	0.33; 0.86
≤13/30	0.48; 0.93	0.07; 0.52	0.57; 0.91	7.36; 0.55	0.27; 0.85

CUI+ and CUI−: positive and negative clinical utility indices; LR+ and LR−: positive and negative likelihood ratios; NPV: negative predictive value; PPV: positive predictive value. * Test cut-off established in index study (Hsieh et al. 2015 [1]).

Table 2. Diagnosis of dementia: unitary measures of discrimination at various MACE cut-offs.

Cut-off	Acc; Inacc	Y (= Sens + Spec − 1)	PSI (= PPV + NPV − 1)	II (= 2(Acc − 1))	DOR (= LR+/LR−)	SUI (= CUI+ + CUI−)	F Measure (F1 Score)
≤29/30	0.17; 0.83	0.02	0.15	−0.66	∞	0.15	0.27
≤28/30	0.20; 0.80	0.05	0.13	−0.61	6.72	0.21	0.27
≤27/30	0.26; 0.74	0.12	0.16	−0.48	17.3	0.30	0.29
≤26/30	0.37; 0.63	0.21	0.17	−0.33	31.9	0.40	0.31
≤25/30 *	0.42; 0.58	0.31	0.19	−0.17	52.0	0.52	0.34
≤24/30	0.49; 0.51	0.39	0.22	−0.01	38.7	0.64	0.37
≤23/30	0.56; 0.44	0.47	0.24	0.12	52.8	0.74	0.40
≤22/30	0.63; 0.37	0.53	0.27	0.25	47.7	0.82	0.44
≤21/30 *	0.69; 0.31	0.59	0.31	0.37	32.2	0.93	0.48
≤20/30	0.74; 0.26	0.619	0.34	0.48	25.1	1.03	0.51
≤19/30	0.77; 0.23	0.614	0.35	0.54	18.9	1.07	0.53
≤18/30	0.80; 0.20	0.60	0.38	0.60	16.0	1.11	0.55
≤17/30	0.81; 0.19	0.56	0.37	0.62	12.8	1.09	0.54
≤16/30	0.84; 0.16	0.58	0.43	0.68	16.1	1.17	0.58
≤15/30	0.859; 0.14	0.56	0.46	0.72	16.5	1.20	0.59
≤14/30	0.867; 0.13	0.51	0.49	0.74	15.8	1.19	0.57
≤13/30	0.866; 0.13	0.41	0.49	0.73	13.3	1.12	0.52

Acc: correct classification accuracy; DOR: diagnostic odds ratio; II: identification index; Inacc: inaccuracy; PSI: predictive summary index; Sens: sensitivity; Spec: specificity; SUI: summary utility index; Y: Youden index. * Test cut-off established in index study (Hsieh et al. 2015 [1]).

Table 3. Diagnosis of dementia: "number needed to" measures (rounded to next highest integer value) and "likelihood to be diagnosed or misdiagnosed" at various MACE cut-offs.

Cut-off	NND (= 1/Y)	NNP (= 1/PSI)	NNM (= 1/Inacc)	NNS (= 1/II)	NNSU (= 1/SUI)	LDM (= NNM/NND; NNM/NNP)
≤29/30	50	7	2	−2	7	0.04; 0.29
≤28/30	20	8	2	−2	5	0.10; 0.25
≤27/30	9	7	2	−3	4	0.22; 0.29
≤26/30	5	6	2	−4	3	0.40; 0.33
≤25/30 *	4	6	2	−7	2	0.50; 0.33
≤24/30	3	5	2	−108	2	0.67; 0.40
≤23/30	3	5	3	9	2	1.00; 0.60
≤22/30	2	4	3	4	2	1.50; 0.75
≤21/30 *	2	4	4	3	2	2.00; 1.00
≤20/30	2	3	4	3	1	2.00; 1.33
≤19/30	2	3	5	2	1	2.50; 1.67
≤18/30	2	3	5	2	1	2.50; 1.67
≤17/30	2	3	6	2	1	3.00; 2.00
≤16/30	2	3	7	2	1	3.50; 2.33
≤15/30	2	3	8	2	1	4.00; 2.67
≤14/30	2	3	8	2	1	4.00; 2.67
≤13/30	3	3	8	2	1	2.67; 2.67

LDM: likelihood to diagnose or misdiagnose; NND: number needed to diagnose; NNM: number needed to misdiagnose; NNP: number needed to predict; NNS: number needed to screen; NNSU: number needed for screening utility. * Test cut-off established in index study (Hsieh et al. 2015 [1]).

Table 4. Diagnosis of MCI: paired measures of discrimination at various MACE cut-offs.

Cut-off	Sensitivity (= Recall); Specificity	False Positive (FPR); False Negative (FNR)	PPV (= Precision); NPV	LR+; LR−	CUI+; CUI−
≤29/30	1.00; 0.03	0.97; 0	0.35; 1.00	1.03; 0	0.35; 0.03
≤28/30	1.00; 0.09	0.91, 0	0.37; 1.00	1.09; 0	0.37; 0.09
≤27/30	0.99; 0.20	0.80; 0.01	0.40; 0.99	1.25; 0.02	0.40; 0.20
≤26/30	0.98; 0.32	0.68; 0.02	0.43; 0.96	1.45; 0.07	0.42; 0.31
≤25/30 *	0.95; 0.46	0.54; 0.05	0.48; 0.95	1.76; 0.10	0.46; 0.44
≤24/30	0.90; 0.57	0.43; 0.10	0.53; 0.92	2.11; 0.17	0.48; 0.52
≤23/30	0.82; 0.64	0.36; 0.18	0.55; 0.87	2.29; 0.29	0.45; 0.56
≤22/30	0.73; 0.72	0.28; 0.27	0.58; 0.84	2.63; 0.37	0.42; 0.60
≤21/30 *	0.64; 0.79	0.21; 0.36	0.61; 0.80	2.99; 0.46	0.39; 0.63
≤20/30	0.54; 0.84	0.16; 0.46	0.63; 0.77	3.33; 0.55	0.34; 0.65
≤19/30	0.47; 0.88	0.12; 0.53	0.67; 0.76	3.81; 0.60	0.31; 0.67
≤18/30	0.37; 0.89	0.11; 0.63	0.65; 0.73	3.56; 0.70	0.24; 0.65

LR+; LR− = positive and negative likelihood ratio; CUI+; CUI− = positive and negative clinical utility index. * = test cut-off established in index study (Hsieh et al. 2015 [1]).

Table 5. Diagnosis of MCI: unitary measures of discrimination at various MACE cut-offs.

Cut-off	Acc; Inacc	Y (= Sens + Spec − 1)	PSI (= PPV + NPV − 1)	II (= 2(Acc − 1))	DOR (= LR+/LR−)	SUI (= CUI+ + CUI−)	F Measure (F1 Score)
≤29/30	0.37; 0.63	0.03	0.35	−0.26	∞	0.38	0.52
≤28/30	0.40; 0.60	0.09	0.37	−0.20	∞	0.46	0.54
≤27/30	0.48; 0.52	0.19	0.39	−0.05	55.4	0.60	0.57
≤26/30	0.55; 0.45	0.30	0.39	0.10	20.9	0.73	0.60
≤25/30 *	0.63; 0.37	0.41	0.43	0.26	17.9	0.90	0.64
≤24/30	0.69; 0.31	0.47	0.45	0.37	12.2	1.00	0.67
≤23/30	0.70; 0.30	0.46	0.42	0.41	8.00	1.01	0.66
≤22/30	0.73; 0.27	0.45	0.42	0.45	7.13	1.02	0.65
≤21/30*	0.73; 0.27	0.43	0.41	0.47	6.45	1.02	0.62
≤20/30	0.73; 0.27	0.38	0.40	0.47	6.07	0.99	0.58
≤19/30	0.74; 0.26	0.35	0.43	0.47	6.33	0.98	0.55
≤18/30	0.71; 0.29	0.26	0.38	0.43	5.09	0.89	0.48

Acc: correct classification accuracy; DOR: diagnostic odds ratio; II: identification index; Inacc: inaccuracy; PSI: predictive summary index; SUI: summary utility index; Y: Youden index. * Test cut-off established in index study (Hsieh et al. 2015 [1]).

Table 6. Diagnosis of MCI: "number needed to" measures (rounded to next highest integer value) and "likelihood to be diagnosed or misdiagnosed" at various MACE cut-offs.

Cut-off	NND (= 1/Y)	NNP (= 1/PSI)	NNM (= 1/Inaccuracy)	NNS (= 1/II)	NNSU (= 1/SUI)	LDM (= NNM/NND; NNM/NNP)
≤29/30	34	3	2	−4	3	0.06; 0.67
≤28/30	12	3	2	−6	3	0.17; 0.67
≤27/30	6	3	2	−21	2	0.33; 0.67
≤26/30	4	3	3	10	2	0.75; 1.00
≤25/30 *	3	3	3	4	2	1.00; 1.00
≤24/30	3	3	4	3	1	1.33; 1.33
≤23/30	3	3	4	3	1	1.33; 1.33
≤22/30	3	3	4	3	1	1.33; 1.33
≤21/30 *	3	3	4	3	1	1.33; 1.33
≤20/30	3	3	4	3	2	1.33; 1.33
≤19/30	3	3	4	3	2	1.33; 1.33
≤18/30	4	3	4	3	2	1.00; 1.33

LDM: likelihood to diagnose or misdiagnose; NND: number needed to diagnose; NNM: number needed to misdiagnose; NNP: number needed to predict; NNS: number needed to screen; NNSU: number needed for screening utility. * Test cut-off established in index study (Hsieh et al. 2015 [1]).

Comparison of the values for NNS and NNSU (Tables 3 and 6) showed negative values of NNS (which are clinically meaningless) when identification index (II) had negative values, but this was not the case with NNSU, since by definition SUI cannot be <0.

A ROC curve was plotted for the diagnosis of dementia and MCI (Figure 2). The AUC ROC was 0.89 (95% confidence interval (CI) 0.86–0.92) for the diagnosis of dementia and 0.81 (95% CI 0.77–0.84) for the diagnosis of MCI, hence the AUC ROC values were categorised as good [16] for the diagnosis of both dementia vs. no dementia and MCI vs. SMC. The Q* index for dementia was 0.8 (comparable to the value of 0.76 found in a previous study examining the first 135 patients in this cohort [3]) and for MCI it was 0.73. PR curves (Figure 3) did not show the desired approximation to the top-right corner of the graph, reflecting the relatively poor PPV of MACE, but did show greater area under the curve for MCI versus dementia.

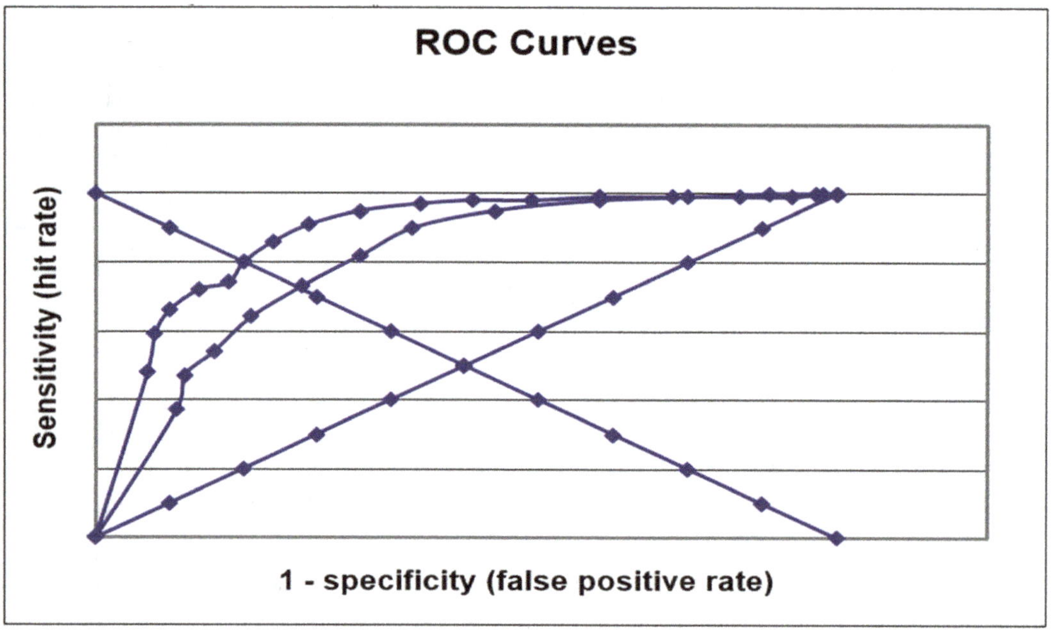

Figure 2. MACE receiver operating characteristic (ROC) plots for the diagnosis of dementia (upper; area under the curve (AUC) = 0.89) and MCI (lower; AUC = 0.81) with chance diagonal ($y = x$) and anti-diagonal ($y = 1 - x$) lines.

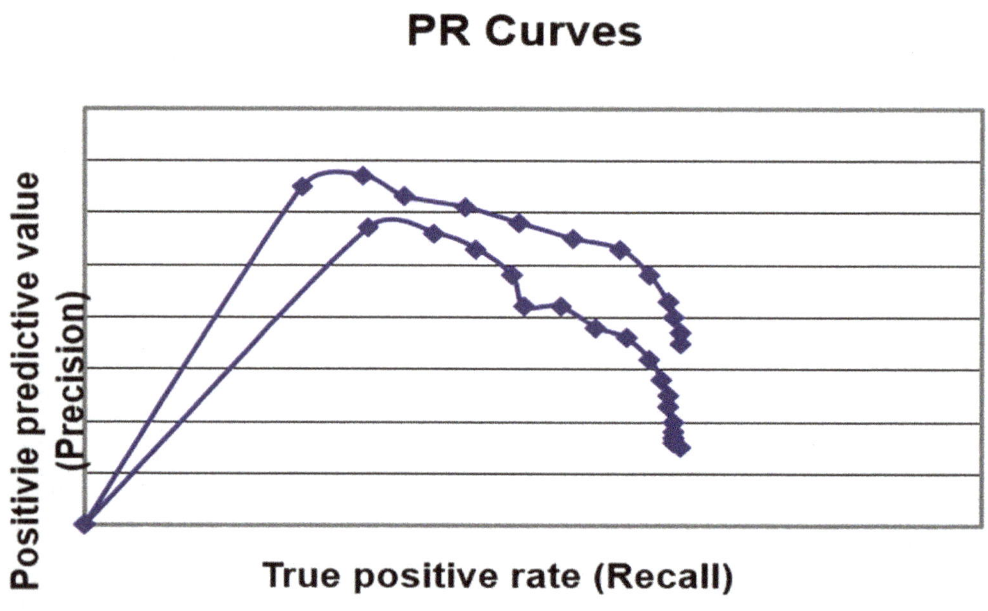

Figure 3. MACE precision recall (PR) curves for the diagnosis of dementia (lower) and MCI (upper); note the reversal of position versus ROC curves.

Effect sizes (Cohen's d) were 1.74 for dementia and 1.13 for MCI, hence very large and large, respectively [22].

PPV and NPV for MACE calculated at prevalence rates of 5%, 10%, 20% and 40% using the sensitivity and specificity figures at the maximum Youden index showed high NPV (≥0.9) at all prevalences examined, but with less-impressive figures for PPV, optimal at higher disease prevalences (Table 7).

Table 7. MACE predictive values at differing disease prevalence of dementia and MCI (0.05–0.4).

	Prevalence					
	0.05	**0.1**	**0.15 (Observed)**	**0.2**	**0.29 (Observed)**	**0.4**
PPV dementia (cut-off ≤20/30)	0.14	0.26	0.36	0.44	-	0.68
NPV dementia (cut-off ≤20/30)	0.99	0.99	0.98	0.97	-	0.92
PPV MCI (cut-off ≤24/30)	0.10	0.19	-	0.34	0.53	0.58
NPV MCI (cut-off ≤24/30)	0.99	0.98	-	0.96	0.92	0.90

4. Discussion

This study of a large cohort of patients examined with the Mini-Addenbrooke's Cognitive Examination suggested that the optimal test cut-offs differ slightly from those suggested in the index study, being a point lower for both high-sensitivity (≤24/30 vs. ≤25/30) and high-specificity (≤20/30 vs. ≤21/30) cut-offs. Even allowing for the objections raised to changing test cut-offs because of risk of bias [23], these findings suggest a possible need for cut-off revision when using MACE in general cognitive clinics, as well as for patient educational level [2].

ROC curves suggested that MACE had adequate accuracy for the diagnosis of dementia and MCI—a finding corroborated by the measure of effect size (Cohen's d). The Q* index for dementia (0.80) was comparable to that found for other cognitive screening instruments [24], but the Q* index for MCI was lower (0.73). However, PR curves suggested better MACE performance (i.e., distinguishable classification performance) for the diagnosis of MCI than for dementia, consistent with findings in previous comparative studies of MACE with the Montreal Cognitive Assessment (MoCA)—a test designed specifically for MCI diagnosis (equivalent MACE performance) [25,26], and Free-Cog (superior MACE performance) [5]. The use of PR curves [18] in diagnostic test accuracy studies is worth emphasizing (to the author's knowledge this is the first such use for dementia test accuracy studies), since these avoid some of the "optimism" of ROC curves (resulting from their combining test accuracy over a range of thresholds which may be both clinically relevant and clinically nonsensical) [27]. PR curves are more informative than ROC curves for skewed datasets [19]. Area under the PR curve may be calculated, although this is not straightforward [28], and visual interpretation may be adequate to denote better classification performance (as for ROC curves).

The comparison of NNS [9] and NNSU [15] in this study was also instructive, demonstrating some of the difficulties in working with reciprocals (multiplicative inverses). By definition, the identification index (II) ranges from -1 to $+1$, and hence NNS ranges from $-\infty$ to $+\infty$ [9]. As II approaches 0, values of NNS are inflated (e.g., Table 3, cut-off ≤24/30; Table 6, cut-off ≤27/30), and when II is negative then NNS also has a negative value. The latter finding is problematic from the clinical standpoint: "number needed to" metrics were originally designed to appeal intuitively at the individual level, so negative values (representing non-individuals?) are meaningless. The construction of SUI is such that by definition its range is from 0 to 2, and hence NNSU ranges from ∞ (no screening value) to 0.5 (perfect screening utility) [15], avoiding the problems encountered with II and NNS.

The high NPV (≥0.9) at all disease prevalences examined (0.05 to 0.4) suggests that a MACE test score above either cut-off excludes dementia and MCI in any setting. PPV was less impressive, but improved with increasing disease prevalence, suggesting a case-finding role for MACE in dedicated cognitive and memory clinics.

In summary, in addition to being quick, easy to use and score and acceptable to patients [1,3,4], when using appropriate cut-offs MACE is a sensitive test for the identification of cognitive impairment and for excluding dementia and MCI with scores below the cut-offs.

Acknowledgments: Nil.

References

1. Hsieh, S.; McGrory, S.; Leslie, F.; Dawson, K.; Ahmed, S.; Butler, C.R.; Rowe, J.B.; · Mioshi, E.; · Hodges, J.R. The Mini-Addenbrooke's Cognitive Examination: A new assessment tool for dementia. *Dement. Geriatr. Cogn. Disord.* **2015**, *39*, 1–11. [CrossRef] [PubMed]
2. Matias-Guiu, J.A.; Fernandez-Bobadilla, R. Validation of the Spanish-language version of Mini-Addenbrooke's Cognitive Examination as a dementia screening tool [in Spanish]. *Neurologia* **2016**, *31*, 646–648. [CrossRef] [PubMed]
3. Larner, A.J. Mini-Addenbrooke's Cognitive Examination: A pragmatic diagnostic accuracy study. *Int. J. Geriatr. Psychiatry* **2015**, *30*, 547–548. [CrossRef] [PubMed]
4. Williamson, J.C.; Larner, A.J. MACE for diagnosis of dementia and MCI: 3-year pragmatic diagnostic test accuracy study. *Dement. Geriatr. Cogn. Disord.* **2018**, *45*, 300–307. [CrossRef] [PubMed]
5. Larner, A.J. Free-Cog: Pragmatic test accuracy study. *Dement. Geriatr. Cogn. Disord.* **2019**, *48*. accepted.
6. Doane, D.P.; Seward, L.E. Measuring skewness: A forgotten statistic? *J. Stat. Educ.* **2011**, *19*, 1–18. [CrossRef]
7. Youden, W.J. Index for rating diagnostic tests. *Cancer* **1950**, *3*, 32–35. [CrossRef]
8. Linn, S.; Grunau, P.D. New patient-oriented summary measure of net total gain in certainty for dichotomous diagnostic tests. *Epidemiol. Perspect. Innov.* **2006**, *3*, 11. [CrossRef] [PubMed]
9. Mitchell, A.J. Index test. In *Encyclopedia of Medical Decision Making*; Kattan, M.W., Ed.; Sage: Los Angeles, CA, USA, 2009; pp. 613–617.
10. Larner, A.J. Optimizing the cutoffs of cognitive screening instruments in pragmatic diagnostic accuracy studies: Maximising accuracy or Youden index? *Dement. Geriatr. Cogn. Disord.* **2015**, *39*, 167–175. [CrossRef] [PubMed]
11. O'Caoimh, R.; Gao, Y.; Svendovski, A.; Gallagher, P.; Eustace, J.; Molloy, D.W. Comparing approaches to optimize cut-off scores for short cognitive screening instruments in mild cognitive impairment and dementia. *J. Alzheimers Dis.* **2017**, *57*, 123–133. [CrossRef] [PubMed]
12. Habibzadeh, F.; Yadollahie, M. Number needed to misdiagnose: A measure of diagnostic test effectiveness. *Epidemiology* **2013**, *24*, 170. [CrossRef] [PubMed]
13. Larner, A.J. Number needed to diagnose, predict, or misdiagnose: Useful metrics for non-canonical signs of cognitive status? *Dement. Geriatr. Cogn. Dis. Extra* **2018**, *8*, 321–327. [CrossRef] [PubMed]
14. Larner, A.J. Evaluating cognitive screening instruments with the "likelihood to be diagnosed or misdiagnosed" measure. *Int. J. Clin. Pract.* **2019**, *73*, e13265. [CrossRef]
15. Larner, A.J. *Manual of Screeners for Dementia: Pragmatic Test Accuracy Studies*; Springer: London, UK, 2019, in press.
16. Metz, C.E. Basic principles of ROC analysis. *Semin. Nucl. Med.* **1978**, *8*, 283–298. [CrossRef]
17. Walter, S.D. Properties of the summary receiver operating characteristic (SROC) curve for diagnostic test data. *Stat. Med.* **2002**, *21*, 1237–1256. [CrossRef]
18. Davis, J.; Goadrich, M. The relationship between Precision-Recall and ROC curves. In *ICML '06: Proceedings of the 23rd International Conference on Machine Learning*; ACM: New York, NY, USA, 2006; pp. 233–240.
19. Saito, T.; Rehmsmeier, M. The precision-recall plot is more informative than the ROC plot when evaluating binary classifiers on imbalanced datasets. *PLoS ONE* **2015**, *10*, e0118432. [CrossRef]
20. Powers, D.M.W. Evaluation: From precision, recall and F-measure to ROC, informedness, markedness and correlation. *J. Mach. Learn. Technol.* **2011**, *2*, 37–63.
21. Cohen, J. *Statistical Power Analysis for the Behavioral Sciences*, 2nd ed.; Lawrence Erlbaum: Hillsdale, NJ, USA, 1988.
22. Sawilowsky, S.S. New effect sizes rules of thumb. *J. Mod. Appl. Stat. Methods* **2009**, *8*, 597–599. [CrossRef]
23. Davis, D.H.; Creavin, S.T.; Noel-Storr, A.; Quinn, T.J.; Smailagic, N.; Hyde, C.; Brayne, C.; McShane, R.; Cullum, S. Neuropsychological tests for the diagnosis of Alzheimer's disease dementia and other dementias: A generic protocol for cross-sectional and delayed-verification studies. *Cochrane Database Syst. Rev.* **2013**, *3*, CD010460. [CrossRef]
24. Larner, A.J. The Q* index: A useful global measure of dementia screening test accuracy? *Dement. Geriatr. Cogn. Dis. Extra* **2015**, *5*, 265–270. [CrossRef]

25. Nasreddine, Z.S.; Phillips, N.A.; Bédirian, V.; Charbonneau, S.; Whitehead, V.; Collin, I.; Cummings, J.L.; Chertkow, H. The Montreal Cognitive Assessment, MoCA: A brief screening tool for mild cognitive impairment. *J. Am. Geriatr. Soc.* **2005**, *53*, 695–699. [CrossRef] [PubMed]
26. Larner, A.J. MACE versus MoCA: equivalence or superiority? Pragmatic diagnostic test accuracy study. *Int. Psychogeriatr.* **2017**, *29*, 931–937. [CrossRef] [PubMed]
27. Ozenne, B.; Subtil, F.; Maucort-Boulch, D. The precision-recall curve overcame the optimism of the receiver operating characteristic curve in rare diseases. *J. Clin. Epidemiol.* **2015**, *68*, 855–859. [CrossRef] [PubMed]
28. Keilwagen, J.; Grosse, I.; Grau, J. Area under precision-recall curves for weighted and unweighted data. *PLoS ONE* **2014**, *9*, e92209. [CrossRef] [PubMed]

12

Test Your Memory (TYM) and Test Your Memory for Mild Cognitive Impairment (TYM-MCI): A Review and Update Including Results of Using the TYM Test in a General Neurology Clinic and Using a Telephone Version of the TYM Test

Jeremy M. Brown [1,*], Julie Wiggins [2], Kate Dawson [2], Timothy Rittman [1,2] and James B. Rowe [1,2]

1 Department of Neurology, Box 83, Addenbrooke's Hospital, Hills Road, Cambridge CB2 2QQ, UK; timothy.rittman@nhs.net (T.R.); james.rowe@mrc-cbu.cam.ac.uk (J.R.B.)

2 Department of Clinical Neurosciences, University of Cambridge, Cambridge CB2 0SZ, UK; jkw41@medschl.cam.ac.uk (J.W.); ced35@cam.ac.uk (K.D.)

* Correspondence: jmb75@medschl.cam.ac.uk

Abstract: This paper summarises the current status of two novel short cognitive tests (SCT), known as Test Your Memory (TYM) and Test Your Memory for Mild Cognitive Impairment (TYM-MCI). The history of and recent research on the TYM and TYM-MCI are summarised in applications for Alzheimer's and non-Alzheimer's dementia and mild cognitive impairment. The TYM test can be used in a general neurology clinic and can help distinguish patients with Alzheimer's disease (AD) from those with no neurological cause for their memory complaints. An adapted tele-TYM test administered by telephone to patients produces scores which correlate strongly with the clinic-administered Addenbrookes Cognitive Examination revised (ACE-R) test and can identify patients with dementia. Patients with AD decline on the TYM test at a rate of 3.6–4.1 points/year.

Keywords: dementia; TYM; TYM-MCI; Alzheimer's

1. Introduction

NICE has recommended the use of the TYM test in non-specialised settings, and this paper is intended to facilitate its use and understanding [1].

1.1. The TYM Test

The original TYM test is a series of 10 cognitive tasks printed on both sides of a thin sheet of card that is filled in by a patient under minimal supervision by a non-specialist healthcare worker [2]. How much help the patient needs is used as an 11th scored "task" of the test. The TYM test can be viewed and downloaded free from the website tymtest.com. The vast majority of patients needs little help completing the TYM test and this allows the supervising health worker to continue to perform other tasks at the same time, e.g., welcoming patients to the clinic, booking patients in and out, or filling in a scan form. Scoring the TYM test takes approximately two minutes. The TYM test therefore takes a minimal amount of medical time to administer. Much of the administration and scoring of the test is intuitive, meaning staff need minimal training to supervise and score the test. JMB (Jeremy M. Brown) has successfully taught many nurses at the Queen Elizabeth Hospital, King's Lynn, and elsewhere to supervise the test at the start of the clinic, even if they have no experience of memory clinics. It is possible to obtain valid results with patients' relatives rather than health professionals supervising the test [3]. A sheet is available from the website tymtest.com to aid scoring and more detailed scoring sheets are available from JMB.

The 11 tasks cover a wide range of cognitive skills similar to those tested by the Addenbrookes Cognitive Examinations (ACE) [4–6] and in all our studies the TYM score is very strongly correlated to the ACE-R (Addenbrookes Cognitive Examination Revised) score (with high Pearson co-efficient). The ACE-R and ACE-III are the gold standard short cognitive tests in use in memory clinics, and are widely used throughout the world. The TYM test is scored out of 50 and the ACE-R and ACE-III are scored out of 100; doubling the TYM score will give a good estimate of the ACE-R or ACE-III score.

1.2. Domains of the TYM Test

1. Orientation to time and person (orientation)—scored out of 10
2. Copying a sentence (copying)—scored out of 2
3. Recall of facts (facts)—scored out of 3
4. Arithmetic (sums)—scored out of 4
5. Animal Fluencies (fluencies)—scored out of 4
6. Similarities—scored out of 4
7. Naming—scored out of 5
8. Spotting the letter W (visuospatial 1)—scored out of 3
9. Completing a clock (visuospatial 2)—scored out of 4
10. Recall of the sentence (recall)—scored out of 6
11. Help needed to complete the test (help)—scored out of 5

2. History

The TYM test was invented and developed by the author from 2007 to 2009 and the original validation paper was published in the BMJ (British Medical Journal) in 2009 [2]. This showed that the TYM test detected the majority of patients with Alzheimer's disease. There was considerable initial publicity and interest and almost immediately a large number of validation projects began throughout the world. Many of these have now been published in peer-reviewed journals. A table giving a review of these papers was included in a chapter in 2015, and since then more validation studies have been published. Table 1 includes a summary of the results of all of these studies, which include over 4000 individuals. The protocols for the different studies vary and the populations studied were very different, so there is limited value in comparing sensitivities and specificities.

All of the studies published are positive, demonstrating that the TYM test is a good short cognitive test for the detection of dementia in a wide range of cultures, in different languages, and using different alphabets. The test was developed in the United Kingdom and does show a cultural bias. This has necessitated some country-specific modifications of the TYM test, which are usually minor, e.g., changing important national dates or the letter for animal fluencies. The sentence about "stout shoes" is very British and the alternative sentence "Great cooks always bake chocolate cakes" has been used in several validations. It is important that the sentence is not a well-known phrase and it needs to be counter-intuitive to avoid a patient guessing the end by remembering the first couple of words. The sentence should not be directly translated, as to do so may undermine its critical features for cognitive assessment. Information on how to adapt the TYM test for different languages is available from JMB.

The tymtest.com website was launched in 2010. Health professionals can view the test and download the TYM test from the site free of charge for healthcare and research purposes. They can also download scoring instructions and advice on how to administer the test. The website continues to be widely used and the TYM test has now been downloaded more than 20,500 times from the website.

The website is currently being upgraded and videos will be added to aid the use and standardisation of the TYM test. The TYM-MCI will also be available from the site.

Table 1. Summary of TYM validation studies.

Country	First Author Reference	Numbers Recruited	Setting and Disease	Cut off Used Sensitivity/Specificity or Other Parameter
Japan	Hanyui [7]	159	Memory Clinic AD	Cut off varied Sensitivity 0.96 Specificity 0.88
Japan	Kotuku [8]	334	Memory Clinic AD	Cut off 42 Sensitivity 0.82 Specificity 0.72
United Kingdom	Hancock [3]	224	2 Memory Clinics Dementia	Cut off 30 Sensitivity 0.73 Specificity 0.88
Poland	Szczesniak [9]	225	Memory Clinic AD	Cut off 39 Sensitivity 0.91 Specificity 0.90
Poland	Derkacz [10]	65	Memory Clinic	Cut off 36 Improvement on MMSE (mini-mental state examination)
France	Postel-Vinay [11]	201	Memory Clinic Dementia	Cut off 39 Sensitivity 0.90 Specificity
Greece	Iatraki [12,13]	373	Community and Neurology Clinic Dementia	Cut off varied Sensitivity 0.82 (0.80) Specificity 0.71 (0.77)
South Africa	Van Schalkwyk [14]	100	Primary Care Dementia	Strong correlation with MMSE
Chile Spanish	Munoz-Neira [15]	74	Memory Clinic Dementia	Cut off 39 Specificity 0.93 Sensitivity 0.82
Netherlands	Koekkoek [16]	86	Memory Clinic	AUC = 0.88 Correlated with neuropsychological tests
Netherlands	Van der Zande [17]		Memory Clinic Dementia	Better than MMSE
Turkey	Mavis [18]	395	Memory Clinic Dementia	Cut off 34 Sensitivity 0.97 Specificity 0.96
Argentina Spanish	Serrani [19]	300	Memory Clinic Dementia	Cut off 40 Sensitivity 0.84 Specificity 0.95
Norway	Breitve [20]	33	Memory Clinic	Cut off 42 Specificity 0.84 Sensitivity 1.00 For dementia
Spain	Ferrero-Arias [21]	1049	Neurology Clinic Dementia	Cut off 36 Sensitivity 0.94 Specificity 0.89 For dementia
Iran	Salami [22]	175	Community AD	Cut off 31 Sensitivity 0.9 Specificity 1.0
EgyptArabic	Abd-Al-Atty [23]	206	Hospital Dementia	Cut off 39/40 in well-educated patients only. Sensitivity 0.80 Specificity 0.97
China Mandarin	Xuemei [24]	237	Neurology Clinic AD	Cut off 39.5 Sensitivity 0.95 Specificity 0.95
Hungary	Kolozsvari [25]	50	Community AD	Cut off 35/36 Sensitivity 0.94 Specificity 0.94
Singapore	Dong [26]	90	Memory Clinic AD	Cut off 38 As good as MOCA (Montreal Cognitive Assessment) Better than MMSE AUC 0.96

2.1. TYM Tests for Non-Alzheimer's Dementia

Further studies on the TYM test by the author have also confirmed the initial findings [27]. Recently the author published a validation study of the TYM test in non-Alzheimer's dementia [28]. These included the behavioural variant of frontotemporal dementia, semantic dementia, vascular dementia, progressive non-fluent aphasia, corticobasal syndrome, progressive supranuclear palsy and atypical focal presentations of Alzheimer's disease (posterior cortical atrophy and logopaenic aphasia).

The TYM test was a useful test in detecting each of these different dementia types. The standard TYM test (cut off 42) detected 80% of non-Alzheimer's or atypical Alzheimer's dementia, whereas the ACE-R (cut off 82) detected 69% of cases and the MMSE (Mini-mental state examination) (cut off 23) detected only 27%. When grouping all of the different diseases together, the TYM test had a positive predictive value of 0.80 and a negative predictive value of 0.84, with an area under the ROC curve of 0.89, similar to its accuracy at detection of typical Alzheimer's disease. The pattern of scoring on the TYM test differed between conditions, and the pattern of deficits can be useful in supporting a clinical diagnosis, particularly for semantic dementia and posterior cortical atrophy.

2.2. *The TYM-MCI*

The TYM test has been shown to be useful in the detection of both Alzheimer's and non-Alzheimer's dementia. Empirically it is unlikely to be as useful in detecting amnestic mild cognitive impairment, an important role in the memory clinic, as it has 9 points for memory, and so a patient with single cognitive domain deficits in memory may need to score just 2/9 in order for them to reach the threshold of 43/50.

The detection of early or mild clinical cases of aMCI (amnestic Mild Cognitive Impairment) or early symptomatic AD is important, particularly as disease modifying treatments are developed. JMB recognised the need for a short cognitive test aimed at better sensitivity to aMCI and this led to the TYM-MCI test. During its development, the TYM-MCI was known first as the Hard TYM (H-TYM) or the Tricky TYM. The current and more formal name TYM-MCI is the most apt name, describing exactly what it does—it detects mild cognitive impairment.

The TYM-MCI is the first short cognitive test to examine both visual and verbal episodic memory. It looks rather similar to the TYM test and will be available shortly on the website tymtest.com. However, the usage of the TYM-MCI is very different from the TYM test—the TYM-MCI is administered by a health professional. The administration takes approximately 7 minutes. The TYM-MCI should only be used for the detection of aMCI or mild AD (unlike the TYM test, which can be used in many clinical scenarios), and the patient should have completed and performed well on a standard SCT (either TYM or other appropriate SCT) prior to attempting the TYM-MCI. It can be run immediately following the standard TYM in a clinic setting. As the diagnostic value rests on the patient's recall of recently learnt visual and verbal information, only the recall tasks on page 2 are scored. The scoring system will be released shortly on the website tymtest.com and is available from JMB. Visual recall and verbal recall are both scored out of 15, giving a maximum total score of 30.

Two validation studies of the TYM-MCI have been reported [29,30] and both showed very striking results. The initial validation compared the TYM-MCI scores in patients with mild AD and normal controls [29]. This kind of validation study, a proof of principle, sets a fairly low bar, which the TYM-MCI nonetheless passed very easily and with very clear results. Patients with mild AD scored 6.7/30 on the TYM-MCI compared to normal controls who scored 20.4/30. The area under the ROC (receiver operating characteristic) curve was 0.99. The results were particularly impressive for recall of visual encoded information with both a modal and median score of 0/15 for patients with mild AD or aMCI compared to a mean of 10/15 for the controls. The greater deficit in visual recall may reflect preferential involvement of recall of visual information in the earliest stages of AD or may reflect that it is a more difficult sub-test of the TYM-MCI than the recall of verbally encoded information. One other H-TYM study confirmed it was a useful test [31].

The second validation study [30] was more clinically relevant, examining the usefulness of the TYM-MCI in the separation of patients with aMCI or mild AD from patients presenting to the same memory clinic with memory complaints that were felt not to have a neurological cause (subjective memory complaints). These patients could be "worried well", depressed, or have conditions such as obstructive sleep apnoea. The study was a thorough assessment of the TYM-MCI, for example including only patients who scored in the normal range on the MMSE.

The TYM-MCI performed very well, with a specificity of 0.79 and a sensitivity of 0.91 in distinguishing the two groups of patients. An important result of this study was that the TYM-MCI was shown to provide additional information to the ACE-R and add information to the overall clinical assessment. Three useful practical conclusions from this paper were:

1. The combination of the TYM-MCI with the ACE-R detects virtually all cases of aMCI or mild AD.

2. The TYM-MCI is a useful test in patients with borderline ACE-R scores. A total of 72% of patients with aMCI or mild AD who had a borderline score on the ACE-R (scoring between the 2 thresholds of 82 and 89) were detected on the TYM-MCI and 79% of patients with subjective memory complaints and a borderline ACE-R score passed the TYM-MCI.
3. Patients initially felt to have subjective memory problems who were later re-diagnosed with organic aMCI scored poorly on their initial TYM-MCI (mean score 9.8/30).

The TYM-MCI is now used routinely in the Addenbrooke's memory clinic for patients whom we suspect have early AD/aMCI as the cause of their memory problems but whom have scored well (>82/100) on the ACE-R.

2.3. TYM Testing in a Non-Specialised Clinical Settings

The TYM was designed for use in non-specialised clinics and NICE (National Institute for Health and Care Excellence) has recommended the use of the TYM test in non-specialised settings [1]. The validation research studies were undertaken in primary, secondary, and tertiary care settings. In this section, we outline the use of TYM testing in a NHS (National Health Service) Trust hospital's general neurology clinic at Queen Elizabeth Hospital, King's Lynn, United Kingdom.

Research validation of the TYM test in general clinics has different endpoints to the memory clinical validation against ACE-R or ACE-III and multidisciplinary team review. In the generalist setting, there is often no definitive "memory" outcome to the consultation. However, feedback on its widespread use suggests that it does provide useful information. One study has reported on the results of TYM testing in a general neurology clinic [21], but again outcomes regarding diagnostic accuracy are difficult to assess. Here we describe our own work on the TYM test in general neurology clinics.

Materials and Methods: Between January 2013 and August 2018, a total of 938 TYM tests were administered in general neurology clinics at Queen Elizabeth Hospital, King's Lynn, United Kingdom. The age of the patients tested ranged from 18 to 93 years of age. The average age was 65.9 years. The majority of TYM tests were performed on patients with memory complaints either as a sole problem or as part of a neurological illness, such as Parkinson's disease, multiple sclerosis or epilepsy. The general clinic nurses supervised the TYM tests with minimal training and in addition to their usual clinic duties. There were no major problems or complaints from supervising staff or patients.

Results: Many of the diagnoses recorded in the letters were not definitive and patients were not necessarily followed-up, so we do not present its diagnostic accuracy against a gold standard of specialist review and extensive investigations. The final diagnosis could not be determined for many patients and these individuals are not included in the analysis. These data are therefore "pragmatic" and embedded in a real-world setting. The diagnoses were clinical and not made according to international criteria, so detailed analysis is not appropriate. The data are summarized in Table 2.

Table 2. Characteristics and TYM test results of patients with various diseases in a general neurology clinic. The diagnoses were clinical.

Diagnosis	No.	Age Range Years	Age: Mean and SD Years	TYM Score Range	TYM: Mean and SD
Clinical Alzheimer's disease	81	48–89	74.7 ± 9.1	0–48	29.6 ± 11.1
Clinical Parkinson's disease	132	46–90	71.2 ± 9.9	21–50	40.2 ± 7.3
Clinical dementia with Lewy bodies	31	68–84	75.9 ± 5.0	20–46	35.2 ± 7.6
Clinical MCI (Mild Cognitive Impairment)	43	52–86	71.7 ± 9.5	24–49	40.2 ± 7.7
Clinical Epilepsy	30	21–73	58.0 ± 18.1	26–49	39.7 ± 7.2
Subjective memory loss	116	23–88	57.6 ± 14.3	24–50	42.3 ± 5.3

Patients with a clinical diagnosis of Alzheimer's disease had significantly lower TYM scores than those with subjective memory loss ($p < 0.001$)

2.4. Rates of Change in Clinical Alzheimer's Disease, Clinical Parkinson's Disease and Patients Felt to Have Subjective Memory Complaints

Seventeen patients with a final diagnosis of clinical Alzheimer's disease completed the TYM test on more than one visit (follow-up 6–50 months). The rate of decline was variable between individuals and there was no clear relationship to disease severity. The mean rate of deterioration was 4.1 points/year, in keeping with a typical rate of decline of 10 points per year on the ACE-R.

Twenty patients with clinical Parkinson's disease had TYM tests on more than one visit (range 5–60 months). Four patients had an improvement in their score, 4 scored the same, and 12/20 (60%) showed a decline. The rate of decline was variable between individuals and there was no clear relationship to disease severity. Overall, the rate of decline in TYM scores in PD was 1.4 points/year.

Twenty-five patients with a final baseline diagnosis of subjective memory problems completed the TYM test on more than one visit (follow-up 4–50 months). Interestingly, 18/25 showed a small improvement in their TYM score, 4 had the same score, and only 3 declined. The mean rate of change in the TYM score was plus 1.2 points/year. It seems most likely that a mild practice effect was responsible for the improvement in TYM scores.

3. Conclusions

The TYM test has been used since 2013 without any complications or complaints. Patients were tested because they had memory complaints or were suspected of having cognitive problems. The major categories of patients were those suspected of having Alzheimer's disease or other dementia, patients with subjective memory problems, Parkinson's disease, epilepsy and mild cognitive impairment. In patients who were followed-up with, the TYM test proved very useful, as patients with AD declined at an average rate of 4.1 points per year, whereas patients with subjective complaints tended to show a small increase in TYM scores with time. Patients with Parkinson's disease had an average score of 40.2/50 on the TYM test—below the threshold for supporting a diagnosis of dementia. PD patients did decline on the TYM test but at a much slower rate than patients with AD (1.4 points/year). The TYM test reveals memory problems in the other groups of patients seen in a General Neurology clinic but the numbers of these patients were too small to make clear conclusions.

3.1. The Telephone TYM or Tele-TYM

While supervised TYM testing in a clinic setting works well, there are situations where a remote assessment would be helpful, such as pre-admission clerking or follow-up. Patients may also be more relaxed and perform better at home, while it could save an outpatient appointment or allow better planning of appointments (e.g., to decide who might benefit from a pre-clinic brain scan). In principle, one could assess cognitive function over the telephone or using an internet-based consultation. Cognitive testing of patients by telephone is not straightforward but could bring advantages to both health care professionals and patients. A telephone TYM test could be used to help assess the response of a patient to a cholinesterase inhibitor and save a journey to outpatients.

As the TYM test is filled in by the patient, it has the potential to be administered by telephone, and we investigated this in a pilot study in 2017.

The protocol was as follows. Patients who were due to be seen in a specialised memory clinic in approximately 6 weeks were contacted by a research nurse and offered the chance to participate in the telephone TYM study. If they consented to the trial, a date about 2 weeks in advance of the clinic was agreed. They were asked to ensure that a relative or friend who was able to help them was available at that time.

They were sent an envelope with details of the trial, including an envelope containing the TYM test, which was marked "not to be opened before nurse phones". There was also a stamped, addressed envelope for the patient to return the completed test to the clinic nurse.

The nurse would phone the patient at the agreed time. She would ask them to sit down in a comfortable chair at a table with their reading glasses, a pen and a helper. They were then asked to open the envelope. The nurse encouraged them to fill in the TYM test themselves as much as possible but remained on the end of the phone and provided assistance or reassurance when required. She recorded how much time and help the patient needed. She reminded them to remember the sentence at the end of page 1 and not to turn the page back. Once they finished, the nurse asked them to place the completed TYM test in the envelope and post it to her.

When the patient came to the clinic they had the usual assessment, which includes seeing an experienced nurse who would administer the ACE-R and MMSE, followed by a neurologist, imaging as required, and multidisciplinary team review. Results of the telephone TYM test were then compared to the ACE-R and MMSE results. A subset of the patients had an additional TYM test in the clinic (often a different version of the TYM test, such as the TYM-B (Test Your Memory version B). Practice effects can be seen in the TYM test if it is administered twice at short intervals. This can be only partially alleviated by using a different version of the TYM test and we normally do not repeat the TYM test at an interval of less than 3 months.

117 patients were recruited. Of these, 16 failed to complete the TYM test or did not attend their clinic appointment. Additionally, 22 patients had diagnoses such as Parkinson's disease, stroke or epilepsy which may or may not be associated with an organic dementia, and so were not included in the analysis. A total of 81 patients were included in the analysis—43 patients were felt to have subjective memory problems with no identified neurological cause for their memory problems after their assessment by a consultant with a special interest in cognition; 38 patients were given organic cognitive diagnoses. The breakdown of the organic cases was: mild cognitive impairment, 18; Alzheimer's disease, 9; unspecified organic dementia, 5; semantic dementia, 2; mixed dementia, 2; dementia with Lewy bodies, 1; progressive supranuclear palsy, 1.

Patients with an organic cause for their memory problems were significantly older than patients with subjective memory complaints. However, in this study there was no correlation between TYM score and age. Patients with organic disease scored lower in all three cognitive tests than those with subjective memory complaints but no underlying neurological disease (Table 3). There was a strong correlation between the telephone TYM score and the clinic ACE-R score in both groups (Pearson r = 0.83 organic, r = 0.60 subjective memory complaints). There were no complications from the study and no complaints from the patients concerning the telephone testing. Very occasionally the nurse suspected some cheating.

Table 3. Telephone TYM scores, clinic ACE-R (Addenbrooke's Cognitive Examination Revised) and clinic MMSE scores in patients with organic dementia or MCI and no organic dementia.

Characteristics	Organic Dementia/MCI	Subjective Memory Complaints
Number in study	38	43
Mean age	69.7	60.5
Telephone TYM score	36.9	43.8
Clinic ACE-R score	71.4	87.6
Clinic MMSE	24.5	27.7

This study shows that it is possible to administer the TYM test over the telephone. The telephone TYM test shows very good correlation with an ACE-R test administered by an experienced ACE tester in clinic. Used alone as a cognitive test the tele-TYM shows a sensitivity of 78% and specificity of 69%, with a cut-off set at ≥43. Comparing the patients with organic and subjective memory diagnoses, the tele-TYM score was significantly lower in the organic group ($p < 0.001$, Wilcoxon rank sum test, corrected for multiple comparisons). The results are summarised in Table 4 below.

Table 4. Results of the Telephone TYM study.

Score	Organics Mean	Subjective Memory Complaints Mean	*p* Value Corrected
Tele-TYM overall score	36.9	43.8	<0.001
Orientation	8.9	9.7	0.011
Copy	1.5	1.8	ns
Facts	1.5	2.2	ns
Sums	3.3	3.6	ns
Fluencies	2.2	3.2	0.008
Similarities	3.1	3.5	ns
Naming	4.5	4.6	ns
Visuospatial 1	1.8	2.4	ns
Visuospatial 2	2.9	3.7	0.006
Recall	2.4	4.0	ns
Help	4.7	5.0	0.01

Note: ns = non-significant.

3.2. Longitudinal TYM Studies

Thirty-four patients with Alzheimer's disease had more than 1 TYM test administered in the Cambridge memory clinic with an interval of between 2 months and 52 months (mean 15 months). There was an average decline in the TYM test of 3.6 points per year.

3.3. TYM Passers with a Diagnosis of Amnestic Mild Cognitive Impairment

One of the drawbacks of the TYM test is that it does not reliably detect patients with amnestic mild cognitive impairment or very mild Alzheimer's disease on total score. To examine this further we selected the 46 patients with a diagnosis of aMCI or mild AD who passed the TYM test and compared them to 157 normal controls. Their results are shown in Table 5.

Table 5. Comparison of TYM and TYM subtest scores in patients with aMCI (amnestic mild cognitive impairment) who passed the TYM test compared to controls.

Characteristic	aMCI	Percentage	Controls	Percentage	*p* = corrected
n =	46		157		
Age	68.3		67.5		ns
TYM total/50	45.0	90	46	92	ns
Orientation/10	9.9	99	9.8	98	ns
Copying/2	2.0	98	1.8	90	ns
Facts/3	2.4	81	2.6	87	ns
Sums/4	3.2	81	3.7	93	ns
Fluencies/4	3.4	84	3.4	85	ns
Similarities/4	3.8	94	3.3	83	ns
Naming/5	4.9	99	4.9	98	ns
Visuospatial 1/3	2.8	92	2.8	92	ns
Visuospatial 2/4	3.1	78	3.7	93	ns
Recall/6	3.5	58	5.0	83	<0.001
Help/5	4.7	95	5.0	100	<0.001

4. Discussion

We looked retrospectively to see whether the pattern of TYM scoring can help distinguish patients with mild amnestic AD who pass the TYM test from controls. The only significant differences between the 2 groups were in recall and help given. Patients with aMCI tended to score comparatively poorly on the second page of the TYM test. One other study [32] has examined the value of the TYM test in the diagnosis of aMCI in a community-based cohort of patients and showed that the TYM test had a specificity of 0.87 and sensitivity of 0.63 in the diagnosis of aMCI.

5. Conclusions

1. The TYM test is a useful short cognitive test in the support of a diagnosis of AD.
2. The TYM test detects a majority of patients with non-Alzheimer's dementia and unusual presentations of AD.
3. The usefulness of the TYM test has been shown in over 20 published studies in peer-reviewed journals covering different languages, cultures and alphabets.
4. Patients with AD show a decline on the TYM test of 3.6 and 4.1 points/year in two different studies.
5. The TYM test can be used in a general neurology clinic. Patients with AD score significantly lower on the TYM test than patients with no identified neurological cause for their subjective memory problems. Follow-up TYM testing shows that patients with AD decline at an average rate of 4.1 points per year, whilst the patients with subjective memory complaints show a small improvement on average.
6. The TYM test can be used over the telephone with results that correlate with clinic-administered tests, and show a significant difference between patients with organic disease and those with no neurological cause for their subjective memory problems.
7. Patients with amnestic MCI score more poorly than controls on recall and help given on subtests of the TYM.
8. The TYM-MCI is a short cognitive test that can support a clinical diagnosis of mild AD and amnestic MCI.

Author Contributions: Formal analysis, T.R.; investigation, J.M.B., J.W., and K.D.; project administration, J.B.R.; writing—original draft, J.M.B.

References

1. National Institute for Health and Care Excellence, London. *Dementia: Assessment, Management and Support for People Living with Dementia and Their Carers*; National Institute for Health and Care Excellence (UK): London, UK, 2018.
2. Brown, J.M.; Pengas, G.; Dawson, K.; Brown, L.A.; Clatworthy, P. Self-administered cognitive screening test (TYM) for detection of Alzheimer's disease: Cross sectional study. *BMJ* **2009**, *338*, b2030. [CrossRef]
3. Hancock, P.; Larner, A.J. Test Your Memory: Diagnostic utility in a memory clinic population. *Int. J. Geriatr Psychiatry* **2011**, *26*, 976–980. [CrossRef] [PubMed]
4. Mathuranath, P.S.; Nestor, P.J.; Berrios, G.E.; Rakowicz, W.; Hodges, J. A brief cognitive test battery to differentiate Alzheimer's disease and frontotemporal dementia. *Neurology* **2000**, *55*, 1613–1620. [CrossRef] [PubMed]
5. Mioshi, E.; Dawson, K.; Mitchell, J.; Arnold, R.; Hodges, J. The Addenbrooke's cognitive examination revised (ACE-R). A brief cognitive test battery for dementia screening. *Int. J. Geriatr. Psychiatry* **2006**, *21*, 1078–1085. [CrossRef] [PubMed]
6. Hodges, J.R.; Larner, A.J. Addenbrooke's Cognitive Examinations: ACE, ACE-R, ACE-111, ACE app and M-ACE. In *Cognitive Screening Instruments a Practical Approach.*, 2nd ed.; Larner, A.J., Ed.; Springer: London, UK, 2017; pp. 109–137.
7. Hanyu, H.; Maezone, M.; Sakurai, H.; Kume, K.; Kanetaka, H.; Iwamoto, T. Japanese version of the Test Your Memory as a screening test in a Japanese memory clinic. *Psychiatry Res.* **2011**, *190*, 145–148. [CrossRef] [PubMed]
8. Kutoku, Y.; Oshsawa, Y.; Kushida, R.; Fuki, Y.; Izawa, N.; Rikimaru, M.; Miyazaki, Y.; Kurokawa, K.; Murakami, T.; Sunada, Y. Diagnostic utility of the Japanese version of Test Your Memory (TYM-J) for Alzheimer's disease. *Kawasaki Med. J.* **2011**, *37*, 177–184.
9. Szczesniak, D.; Wojtynska, R.; Rymaszewska, J. Test Your Memory (TYM) as a screening instrument in clinical practice—the Polish validation study. *Aging Ment. Health* **2013**, *17*, 863–868. [CrossRef]

10. Derkacz, M.; Chmiel-Perzynska, I.; Kowal, A.; Pawlos, J.; Michalojic-Derkacz, M.; Olajossy, M.; Marczewski, K. Tym Test—Novel diagnostic tool to assess cognitive functions—study on inhabitants of social welfare house. *Curr. Probl. Psychiatry* **2011**, *12*, 152–159.
11. Postel-Vinay, N.; Hanon, O.; Clerson, P.; Brown, J.; Menard, J.; Paillaud, E.; Alonso, E.; Pasquier, F.; Pariel, S.; Belliard, S.; et al. Validation of the Test Your Memory (F-TYM Test) in a French memory clinic population. *Clin. Neuropsychol.* **2014**, *28*, 994–1007. [CrossRef]
12. Iatraki, E.; Simos, P.; Lionis, C.; Zaganas, I.; Symvoulakis, E.; Papastefanakis, E.; Panagiotakis, S.; Pantelidakis, H.; Papadopoulos, K.; Tziraki, C. Cultural adaption, standardization and clinical validity of the Test Your Memory dementia screening instrument in Greek. *Dement. Geriatr. Cogn. Disord.* **2014**, *37*, 163–180. [CrossRef]
13. Iatraki, E.; Simos, P.; Bertias, A.; Duijker, G.; Zagamas, I.; Tziraki, C.; Vgontzas, A.; Lionis, C.; Thalis Primary Health Care Research Team/Network. Cognitive screening tools for primary care settings: Examining the "Test Your Memory" and "General Practice Assessment of Cognition" tools in a rural aging population in Greece. *Eur. J. Gen. Pract.* **2017**, *23*, 172–179. [CrossRef] [PubMed]
14. Van Schalkwyk, G.; Botha, H.; Seedat, S. Comparison of 2 dementia screeners, the Test Your Memory Test and the Mini-Mental State Examination, in a Primary Care Setting. *J. Geriatr. Psychiatry Neurol.* **2012**, *25*, 85–88. [CrossRef] [PubMed]
15. Munoz-Neira, C.; Chaparro, F.; Delgado, C.; Brown, J.; Slachevsky, A. Test Your Memory—Spanish version (TYM-S): A validation study of a self-administered cognitive screening test. *Int. J. Geriatr. Psychiatry* **2014**, *29*, 730–740. [CrossRef] [PubMed]
16. Koekkoek, P.; Rutten, G.; van der Berg, E.; van Sonsbeek, S.; Gorter, K.; Kappelle, L.; Biessels, G. The "Test Your Memory" test performs better than the MMSE in a population without known cognitive dysfunction. *J. Neurol. Sci.* **2013**, *328*, 92–97. [CrossRef] [PubMed]
17. Van de Zande, E.; Van de Nes, J.; Jansen, I.; van den Berg, M.; Zwart, A.; Bimmel, D.; Rijkers, G.; Andringa, G. The Test Your Memory (TYM) Test Outperforms the MMSE in the Detection of MCI and Dementia. *Curr. Alz. Res.* **2017**, *14*, 598–607. [CrossRef] [PubMed]
18. Mavis, I.; Ozbabalik Adapinar, B.; Yenilmez, C.; Aydin, A.; OLgun, E.; Bal, C. Test your memory—Turkish version. *Turk. J. Med. Sci.* **2015**, *45*, 1178–1185. [PubMed]
19. Serrani, D. Spanish validation of the TYM Test for dementia screening in the Argentine population. *Univ. Psychol.* **2014**, *13*, 265–284.
20. Breitve, M.; Chwiszuk, L.; Hynninen, M. A Norwegian pilot study of the TYM test. An alternative to the Norwegian MMSE. *Tidsskr. Nor. Psykologforening* **2015**, *52*, 49–53.
21. Ferrero-Arias, J.; Turrion-Rojo, M. Validation of a Spanish version of the Test Your Memory. *Neurologia* **2016**, *31*, 33–42. [CrossRef]
22. Salami, M.; Alinaghipour, A.; Daneshvar, R.; Hamidi, G.; Agahi, A.; Soheili, M.; Akbari, H.; Taba, S. Adapted MMSE and TYM cognitive tests: How much powerful in screening for Alzheimer's disease in Iranian people. *Aging Ment. Health* **2019**. [CrossRef]
23. Abd-Al-Atty, M.; Abou-Hashem, R.; Abd El Gawad, W.; Elgazzar, Y. Test Your Memory, Arabic Version. Is it practical in a different culture? *J. Am. Geriatr. Soc.* **2012**, *60*, 596–597. [CrossRef] [PubMed]
24. Xuemei, L.; Zhang, J.; Zhu, J.; Zhang, Y.; Zhang, W.; Tin, D. Construct validity and reliability of the Test Your Memory Chinese version in older neurology outpatient attendees. *Int. J. Ment. Health Sys.* **2018**, *12*, 64.
25. Kolozsvari, L.; Kovacs, Z.; Szollosi, G.; Frecska, E.; Egerhazi, A. Validation of the Hungarian version of the Test Your Memory. *Ideggyogy* **2017**, *70*, 267–272. [CrossRef]
26. Dong, Y.; Ling, T.; Ng, K.; Wang, A.; Wan, E.; Merchant, R.; Venketasubramanian, N.; Chen, C.; Amahendran, R.; Collinson, S. The Clinical Utility of the TYM and RBANS in a One-Stop Memory Clinic in Singapore: A Pilot Study. *J. Geriatr. Psychiatry Neurol.* **2019**, *32*, 68–73. [CrossRef] [PubMed]
27. Brown, J.M. TYM (Test Your Memory) Testing. In *Cognitive Screening Instruments. A Practical Approach*, 2nd ed.; Larner, A.J., Ed.; Springer: London, UK, 2017; pp. 209–229.
28. Brown, J.; Wiggins, J.; Lansdall, C.J.; Dawson, K.; Rittman, T.; Rowe, J. Test Your Memory: Diagnostic evaluation of patients with non-Alzheimer dementias. *J. Neurol.* **2019**. [CrossRef] [PubMed]
29. Brown, J.; Wiggins, J.; Dong, H.; Harvey, R.; Richardson, F.; Hunter, K.; Dawson, K.; Parker, R. The hard Test Your Memory. Evaluation of a short cognitive test to detect mild Alzheimer's disease and amnestic mild cognitive impairment. *Int. J. Geriatr. Psychaitry* **2014**, *29*, 272–280. [CrossRef]

30. Brown, J.; Lansdall, C.J.; Wiggins, J.; Dawson, K.; Hunter, K.; Rowe, J.; Parker, R. The Test Your Memory for Mild Cognitive Impairment (TYM-MCI). *J. Neurol. Neurosurg. Psychiatry* **2017**, *88*, 1045–1051. [CrossRef]
31. Larner, A.J. Hard TYM: A pragmatic study. *Int. J. Geriatr. Psychiatry* **2015**, *30*, 330–331. [CrossRef]
32. Ozer, S.; Noonan, K.; Burke, M.; Young, J.; Barber, S.; Forster, A.; Jones, R. The validity of the Memory Alteration Test and the Test Your Memory test for community-based identification of amnestic mild cognitive impairment. *Alzheimers Dement.* **2016**, *12*, 987–995. [CrossRef]

13

Causes and Mechanisms of Hematopoietic Stem Cell Aging

Jungwoon Lee [1,†], Suk Ran Yoon [2,3,†], Inpyo Choi [2,3,*] and Haiyoung Jung [2,*]

1 Environmental Disease Research Center, Korea Research Institute of Bioscience and Biotechnology (KRIBB), 125 Gwahak-ro, Yuseong-gu, Daejeon 34141, Korea; jwlee821@kribb.re.kr
2 Immunotherapy Research Center, Korea Research Institute of Bioscience and Biotechnology (KRIBB), 125 Gwahak-ro, Yuseong-gu, Daejeon 34141, Korea; sryoon@kribb.re.kr
3 Department of Functional Genomics, University of Science and Technology (UST), 113 Gwahak-ro, Yuseong-gu, Daejeon 34113, Korea
* Correspondence: ipchoi@kribb.re.kr (I.C.); haiyoung@kribb.re.kr (H.J.)
† These authors contributed equally to this work.

Abstract: Many elderly people suffer from hematological diseases known to be highly age-dependent. Hematopoietic stem cells (HSCs) maintain the immune system by producing all blood cells throughout the lifetime of an organism. Recent reports have suggested that HSCs are susceptible to age-related stress and gradually lose their self-renewal and regeneration capacity with aging. HSC aging is driven by cell-intrinsic and -extrinsic factors that result in the disruption of the immune system. Thus, the study of HSC aging is important to our understanding of age-related immune diseases and can also provide potential strategies to improve quality of life in the elderly. In this review, we delineate our understanding of the phenotypes, causes, and molecular mechanisms involved in HSC aging.

Keywords: hematopoietic stem cell aging; rejuvenation; self-renewal; differentiation

1. Introduction

In the hematopoietic system, hematopoietic stem cells (HSCs) continuously replenish the blood cells including B and T lymphocytes, erythrocytes, myeloid cells, platelets, natural killer (NK) cells, mast cells, and dendritic cells (DCs), throughout the lifetime of an organism [1–3]. HSCs were the first stem cells to be identified and isolated and remain the most-studied tissue-specific stem cells. HSCs constitute the pool of long-term HSCs (LT-HSCs), short-term HSCs (ST-HSCs), and multipotent progenitors (MPPs). They can be identified with specific cell-surface markers using fluorescence-activated cell sorting (FACS) technology. All murine HSCs are lineage (Lin^-), stem cell antigen-1 $(Sca\text{-}1)^+$, and $cKit^+$ (LSKs) that can be characterized as more or less primitive with CD150 (Slamf1), CD48 (Slamf2), CD34, and Flt3 [4,5]. Human HSCs can also be isolated and identified by the expression of cell surface markers such as Lin^-, $CD34^+$, $CD38^-$, $Thy1.1^+$, and $CD45RA^-$ [6–8] (Figure 1).

HSCs have the ability to self-renew and differentiate into immune cells; however, similar to other adult stem cells, HSCs are vulnerable to age-related stress [7,8]. With aging, HSCs gradually lose their self-renewal capacity and reconstitution potential and are therefore different from pluripotent embryonic stem cells (ESCs) and induced pluripotent stem cells (iPSCs) [9]. HSC aging is driven by both cell-intrinsic and -extrinsic factors. Although the functional change of HSCs with aging is mostly regulated by cell-intrinsic factors, including DNA damage, reactive oxygen species (ROS), epigenetic changes and polarity changes, it is also known that the hematopoietic niche or microenvironment-derived cell-extrinsic factors are essential for the maintenance of HSCs [7,10]. Hematopoietic aging alters the immune system, inducing many types of immune diseases including both myeloid and lymphoid leukemias, anemia, declining adaptive immunity, autoimmunity, increased susceptibility to infectious diseases, and vaccine failure [11,12]. Thus, the study of HSC aging is important to our understanding of age-related immune diseases and can also provide potential strategies to improve quality of life in the elderly. In this review, we summarized the hallmarks, causes and mechanisms, and rejuvenation of HSC aging, and also introduced recent emerging technologies for HSC study.

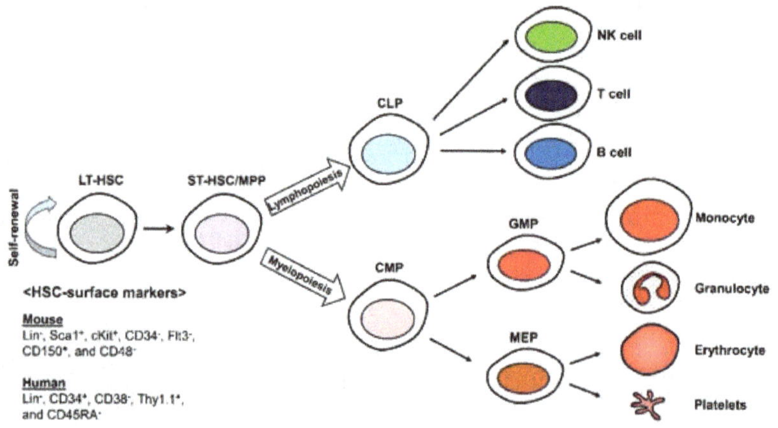

Figure 1. Differentiation of hematopoietic stem cells (HSCs). Long-term HSCs (LT-HSCs) are able to self-renew and are responsible for generating blood cells. CLP; the common lymphoid progenitor, CMP; the common myeloid progenitor, GMP; the granulocyte macrophage progenitor, and MEP; the megakaryocytic and erythroid progenitor.

2. Hallmarks of HSC Aging

2.1. Defect in Repopulating Capacity

Though we know that the number of HSCs in bone marrow (BM) increases 2- to 10-fold with aging in both mice and humans [12–14], the mechanisms by which such increases in HSC numbers occur in aged organisms remain elusive. One hypothesis proposes that the increase in the number of aged HSCs is a compensatory mechanism to overcome their loss of function in normal hematopoiesis [12]. Another study suggested that an increase in the frequency of self-renewing symmetric cell divisions might contribute to the increased numbers and impaired function of aged HSCs [15]. Recent reports show that aged HSCs are less quiescent, with larger fractions undergoing cell division than young HSCs [8,16], having accumulated more oxidative DNA damage [17]. These reports go on to suggest that the function of aged HSCs may be limited by these factors. To determine the functional differences between young and aged HSCs, a competitive transplantation assay was developed as a gold standard test to assess the long-term self-renewal and multi-lineage potential of HSCs. In this method, HSCs are mixed with young BM cells that are able to restore immunity in the recipient animal post-irradiation [3,5,11,12]. We and other research groups have reported that aged HSCs exhibited a functional decline in repopulation capacity [13,18,19]. These results imply that the increased number of aged HSCs does not compensate for their loss of function, thereby resulting in immune cell homeostasis defects in aged organisms [12,15].

2.2. Defect in Homing and Increase in Mobilization

HSCs reside in the marrow cavity of long bones during adult life, co-existing in close association with many other cell types in BM in a highly organized structure supported by stromal cells referred to as the niche [20–22]. The engraftment of HSCs into nonmyeloablative hosts resulted in spatial localization of stem cell "niches," while other transplanted BM cells were detected as flattened bone lining cells on the periosteal bone surface [23]. Osteoblastic cells constitute an important cellular component of the HSC niche [24,25]. Other groups assessed that different hematopoietic cell subsets are localized to distinct areas according to their stage of differentiation using live-imaging techniques [20,26,27]. Interestingly, transplanted HSCs tended to home to the endosteum in irradiated recipients but were randomly distributed and unstable in nonirradiated mice [27]. The homing ability of HSCs, involving the trafficking of a transplanted donor HSC to the BM of a recipient, is critical in BM transplantation procedures for the successful treatment of many blood disorders and malignancies including leukemia, lymphoma, and myeloma [28]. Liang and colleagues found that the BM homing efficiency of aged mouse HSCs was approximately three-fold lower than that of young HSCs; we also reported a reduction in the homing ability of aged HSCs in BM [1,19,29].

Systemic administration of cytokines and chemokines or cytotoxic agents mobilizes hematopoietic stem and progenitor cells (HSPCs) from the BM into peripheral blood, where they are collected in clinically useful quantities for stem cell therapies [22]. Granulocyte colony-stimulating factor (G-CSF) mobilizes hematopoietic cells from the marrow into circulation, with increased progenitor cells of all lineages detected in the spleens of G-CSF-treated mice [30,31]. In a G-CSF-receptor (G-CSFR)-deficient mice study, they found that expression of the G-CSFR on BM cells is required for mobilization of hematopoietic progenitor cells (HPCs), but this is not dependent on the expression of the G-CSFR on hematopoietic progenitor cells (HPCs). From these results, they suggested that the indirect effect of G-CSF on hematopoietic cells is essential for HSC mobilization [30,32]. G-CSF causes transient upregulation of stromal cell-derived factor-1 (SDF-1) and subsequently activates CXC chemokine receptor-4 (CXCR4) signaling for the production of hepatocyte growth factor (HGF). HGF binds to c-Met and thus activates c-Met signaling to regulate the mTOR/FOXO3a signaling pathway. Finally, G-CSF signaling causes ROS production and promotes the egress of HSCs out of the BM [31,33]. Xing and colleagues revealed that the mobilization of HSPCs from BM to peripheral blood in response to G-CSF requires the de-adhesion of HSPCs from the niche. This ability to mobilize HSCs is approximately five-fold greater in aged mice [22].

2.3. Lineage Skewing

Under normal conditions, HSCs differentiate into balanced myeloid and lymphoid lineages. However, aged adults show a higher prevalence of anemia and compromised adaptive immunity, due to reduced HSC number and function, caused by thymic involution and aged lymphoid progenitors [34,35]. Aging forces the differentiation of HSCs to myeloid bias, characterized by a higher percentage of myeloid cells in peripheral blood, both upon transplantation and at steady state [1,8,29,36]. Sudo and colleagues showed that although aged HSCs exhibit abnormal differentiation, they were able to regenerate blood cells over long periods of time and could self-renew. These aged HSCs exhibited myeloid biased differentiation [3,15]. This characteristic is also reflected in the relative expansion of myeloid progenitor numbers in aged compared to young mice—a feature of aged HSCs known to be a cell autonomous function [37]. The lineage skewing associated with HSC aging has been linked to an upregulation of myeloid-specific genes and a downregulation of lymphoid-specific genes [38,39].

3. Causes and Mechanisms of HSC Aging

3.1. DNA Damage

The DNA damage response (DDR) in cells is involved in cell cycle regulation, cell death and senescence, transcriptional regulation, as well as chromatin remodeling [40]. HSCs are also exposed to DDR stress due to their continuous self-renewal process as well as their microenvironment during aging. It has been proposed that DNA damage may be a principal mechanism regulating age-dependent stem cell decline; furthermore, the accumulation of genomic instability has been implicated in hematopoietic malignancy, possibly derived from transformed HSCs [40,41]. Researchers have reported that HSCs experience genomic instability during physiological aging. Rossi and colleagues tested these hypotheses in mice deficient in several genomic maintenance pathways including nucleotide excision repair, telomere maintenance, and non-homologous end-joining. DDR-deficient HSCs exhibited an accumulation of high levels of DNA double strand breaks (DSBs), reduced repopulation ability and self-renewal, as well as stem cell exhaustion, such as occurs in aged HSCs [1,40,42]. Similar to mouse HSCs, human CD34$^+$ HSCs and hematopoietic progenitors showed a significant accumulation of DSBs during the normal aging process [43]. These reports strongly suggest that the appropriate DDR is important for the maintenance of HSCs and may prevent the functional decline of HSCs from aging.

3.2. ROS (Reactive Oxygen Species)

HSCs reside in hypoxic niches in the BM—an environment that presumably ensures HSCs are protected from oxidative stress and can maintain their self-renewal ability [31]. HSCs are quiescent, have a low metabolic rate, and therefore, generate low levels of reactive oxygen species (ROS). However, with aging, ROS levels accumulate and can result in ROS-induced oxidative stress in HSCs [1,44,45]. Aging increases ROS levels, which contribute to increased proliferation, senescence, or apoptosis. HSCs exposed to low ROS levels maintained a higher self-renewal potential in serial transplantation. However, HSCs exposed to high ROS levels failed to self-renew and showed higher levels of expression of activated p38 mitogen-activated protein kinase (p38) and mammalian target of rapamycin (mTOR) [46]. Porto and colleagues found that aged HSCs showed increased oxidative stress compared to young HSCs; mitochondria and NADPHox were the major sources of ROS production, whereas CYP450 contributed in middle and aged HSCs and xanthine oxidase only in aged HSCs [47]. Thus, oxidative stress might be considered an important cause of HSC dysfunction during the aging process [48]. We have reported the regulatory mechanisms of ROS in aged HSCs using specific gene knockout mice. We found that thioredoxin-interacting protein (TXNIP) regulated ROS levels in HSCs by regulating p53 activity via interference with p53-mouse double minute 2 (MDM2) interactions [5]. More recently, we revealed that TXNIP regulated p38 activity—a critical inducer of ROS in aged HSCs [19]. Recent reports have also demonstrated that ROS acted as critical regulators of HSC aging and go on to determine regulatory mechanisms. The Forkhead O (FOXO) subfamily of transcription factors—including Foxo1, Foxo3a, and Foxo4—regulated pools of HSCs and progenitors as well as ROS in HSCs [49,50]. Hypoxia-inducible factor-1α (HIF-1α) was highly expressed in HSCs. HIF-1α changed cellular metabolism of HSCs from mitochondrial respiration to glycolysis and thereby reduced ROS production. Deletion of HIF-1α in HSCs induced ROS levels and reduced long-term repopulation capacity [31,51]. Altogether, the importance of ROS as an inducer of aging in HSCs was determined by cellular regulatory mechanism studies.

3.3. Epigenetic Changes

Epigenetics refers to changes in gene expression that do not involve changes to the underlying DNA sequence, that is a change in phenotype without a change in genotype [52]. Analysis of gene transcriptional profiles indicated that myeloid differentiation-linked and inflammation- and stress response-related genes were upregulated, but lymphopoiesis, DNA repair, and chromatin silencing genes were downregulated in aged HSCs [13,53]. Aged HSCs exhibited broader H3K4me3 peaks across HSC identity and self-renewal genes, exhibiting increased DNA methylation at transcription factor binding sites associated with differentiation-promoting genes. There is a strong correlation between altered H3K4me3 levels and transcriptional activity, involving genes that undergo increased expression levels, most significantly with age [53]. These gene expression changes are in accordance with age-induced myeloid skewing, at the level of gene transcription. It also implies that HSC aging is related to epigenetic changes that impact transcriptional regulation. The function of DNA methylation includes the induction of physiological processes such as stem cell differentiation [52]. Genetic inactivation of DNA methyltransferase 1 (DNMT1), induced nearly immediate and complete loss of HSCs in vivo [54]. Reduced DNMT1 activity in HSCs restricted myeloerythroid differentiation due to both impaired silencing of key lineage determinant genes and an inability to prime master lymphoid regulators [55]. DNMT3a also regulates HSC fate decisions, as evidenced by the conditional inactivation of DNMT3a, which skews HSC divisions toward self-renewal at the expense of differentiation [56]. The expression of genes encoding DNA methyltransferase enzymes decreases in aged HSCs compared to young; moreover, aged HSCs are characterized by a gradual increase in global DNA methylation levels [53]. Corresponding with the DNA hypermethylation of aged HSCs, there is a concomitant reduction in 5-hmC in aged HSCs compared to young, with all three TET enzymes decreasing in abundance, with age [52,53]. Florian and colleagues demonstrated that young HSCs expressed higher levels of AcH4K16 and aged HSCs presented decreased levels of AcH4K16 [57]. However, these mechanisms are inadequate to explain the exact correlation between epigenetic changes and HSC aging; therefore, the functional consequences of epigenetic changes in HSCs remain to be determined.

3.4. Polarity Changes

The small RhoGTPase Cdc42 (Cdc42) cycles between an active (GTP-bound) and an inactive (GDP-bound) state and is known to regulate actin and tubulin organization, cell-cell and cell-extracellular matrix adhesion, and cell polarity in distinct cell types [57–59]. Florian and colleagues reported Cdc42 as a new aging marker for HSCs. They found that elevated Cdc42 activity in aged HSCs was causally linked to HSC aging and correlated with a loss of polarity in aged HSCs. Constitutively activated Cdc42 resulted in premature aging of HSCs and induced depolarization of Cdc42 and tubulin in aged HSCs. Pharmacological reduction of Cdc42 activity reversed the polarity of Cdc42 and tubulin and restored cellular function of aged HSCs [57]. We also demonstrated that aged HSCs showed depolarization of Cdc42 allowing us to use it as an aging marker for HSCs in our study [19].

4. Rejuvenation of Aged HSCs

4.1. Reduction of Nutrient Supply

Mutations in growth signaling pathways extend the life span while protecting against age-dependent DNA damage in yeast [60]. Prolonged fasting (PF) reduces progrowth signaling and activates pathways that enhance cellular resistance to toxins in mice and humans [60–62]. One group has suggested that caloric restriction by PF can rejuvenate aged HSCs. They reported that PF reduced circulating IGF-1 levels and PKA activity in various cell populations and rejuvenated the aging-associated phenotypes of aged HSCs including myeloid bias. PF also protected mice from chemotherapy-induced immunosuppression and mortality [63].

Reversible acetylation of metabolic enzymes regulates metabolic pathways in response to nutrient availability [64]. The sirtuin family are key regulators of the nutrient-sensitive metabolic regulatory circuit. Calorie restriction reduced ROS by inducing the activation of SIRT3-mediated superoxide dismutase 2 (SOD2) [65]. Brown and colleagues demonstrated that SIRT3 regulated the global acetylation of mitochondrial proteins, which are enriched in HSCs. The expression of SIRT3 decreased with aging; moreover, SIRT3 was dispensable for young HSCs but was essential under stress or for aged HSCs. Finally, the authors suggested that the plasticity of mitochondrial homeostasis controls HSC aging and showed that aged HSCs can be rejuvenated by SIRT3 expression [66]. Mohrin and colleagues have reported on the interaction between SIRT7 and nuclear respiratory factor 1 (NRF1). SIRT7-deficient HSCs showed a reduction in repopulating capacity and myeloid-biased differentiation in transplantation assays. The upregulation of SIRT7 improved the regenerative capacity of aged HSCs [67].

4.2. ROS Scavenging

HSCs exhibit low metabolic rates and produce less ROS. The ataxia telangiectasia mutated (ATM) gene is essential for HSC self-renewal and quiescence; ATM regulates ROS levels in HSCs. ATM-deficient mice showed a defect in HSC function and elevated ROS levels in HSCs. Treatment with the ROS scavenging agent, N-acetyl-L-cysteine (NAC), rescued the repopulating capacity of

ATM-deficient HSCs [68]. p38 limits the lifespan of HSCs in vivo by inducing ROS; the inhibition of p38 by treatment with SB203580, a p38 inhibitor, rescued ROS-induced defects in HSC repopulating capacity and HSC quiescence maintenance [69]. Recently, we developed a new p38 inhibitor—TN13—which is a cell-penetrating peptide-(CPP-), a conjugated peptide derived from the TXNIP-p38 interaction motif in TXNIP. TN13 inhibited p38 activity and rejuvenated aged HSCs by reducing ROS levels [19]. G protein-coupled receptor kinases (GRKs) regulate cytokine receptors in mature leukocytes. GRK6$^{-/-}$ mice exhibited HSC loss and impaired HSC self-renewal. GRK6 also regulates ROS response, and ROS scavenger α-lipoic acid treatment rescued HSC loss in GRK6$^{-/-}$ mice [70].

4.3. Epigenetic Modulation

Elevated Cdc42 activity is associated with HSC aging and induces decreased levels of H4K16Ac in aged HSCs. Treatment with a specific inhibitor of Cdc42 activity (CASIN) can restore aged HSC phenotypes by regulating both Cdc42 activity and epigenetic reprograming by elevating H4K16Ac levels to those of young cells [1,57]. Special AT-rich sequence binding 1 (Satb1), a nuclear architectural protein, regulates chromatin structure by epigenetic regulation and plays an important role in lymphoid lineage specification. The expression of Satb1 increased with early lymphoid differentiation and Satb1-deficient HSCs showed a reduction in lymphopoiesis, while induced Satb1 expression enhanced lymphocyte production. Exogenous Satb1 expression primed the lymphoid potential of aged HSCs [71].

4.4. Clearance of Senescent Cells

Aging and genotoxic stress induce cellular senescence of HSCs [72,73]. Senescent cells (SCs) accumulate in various tissues and organs with aging, thereby disrupting tissue structure and function by secreting cellular components. Clearance of SCs in a mouse model using a transgenic approach revealed delays in several age-associated disorders [74]. Chang and colleagues developed a potent senolytic drug ABT263—a specific inhibitor of BCL-2 and BCL-xL, that selectively kills SCs. Oral administration of ABT263 effectively depleted SCs—including senescent HSCs in both sub-lethally irradiated and normally aged mice. Depletion of SCs mitigated irradiation-induced premature aging of the hematopoietic system and rejuvenated aged HSCs in normally aged mice [75]. Given these results, Chang et al. determined that ABT263 may represent a new class of radiation mitigators and anti-aging agents.

5. Emerging Technologies for HSC Study

5.1. Single-Cell RNA-Sequencing (scRNA-Seq)

HSCs are heterogeneous and HSC fate decisions are performed at the individual cell level. Thus, single-cell profiling may be an essential tool for characterizing the heterogeneity of HSCs. Most recently, single-cell RNA-sequencing (scRNA-Seq) was developed to profile single cells and was applied in the studies of HSCs [76]. Kowalczyk and colleagues used scRNA-Seq to dissect variability in HSCs and HPCs from young and old mice. They found that transcriptional changes in HSCs during aging are inversely related to those upon HSC differentiation, and old ST-HSCs exist in a less differentiated state than young ST-HSCs [77]. One group have revealed that the megakaryocyte lineage is developed independently of other hematopoietic fates using scRNA-Seq. They have also found a functional hierarchy of unilineage- and oligolineage-producing clones within the MPPs [78]. Grover and colleagues identified an unrecognized class of HSCs that exclusively produce platelets with age. They suggested that increased platelet bias may contribute to the age-associated decrease in lymphopoiesis [79]. More recently, Baron and colleagues reported the genes and transcription factor networks activated during the endothelial-to-haematopoietic switch using scRNA-Seq. From this study, they provide an unprecedented complete resource to study in depth HSC generation in vivo [80].

5.2. Single-Cell Transplantation

HSC transplantation assays evaluate the capacity of HSCs to repopulate the hematopoietic system. HSC heterogeneity was initially identified by tracking of myeloid and lymphoid lineage output from transplanted single HSCs [81–83]. Single-cell transplantation has shown considerable heterogeneity of HSCs and different propensities of myeloid-, lymphoid- and platelet-biased HSCs in fate decision [84]. Carrelha and colleagues applied single-cell transplantation assays to investigate lineage-restricted fates of long-term self-renewing HSCs. They found that a distinct class of HSCs adopts a fate towards megakaryocyte/platelet-lineage tree, but not of other blood cell lineages. Finally, they suggested that a limited repertoire of distinct HSC subsets adopt a fate towards replenishment of a restricted set of blood lineages, before loss of self-renewal and multipotency [84]. Yamamoto and colleagues investigated the age-related functional changes in HSCs using single-cell transplantation assays. They found that myeloid-restricted repopulating progenitor (MyRPs) frequency increased dramatically with age. Interestingly, they identified new subsets, latent-HSCs, that were myeloid restricted in primary recipients but displayed multipotent (five blood-lineage) output in secondary recipients. From these results, they have raised a question about the traditional dogma of HSC aging and our current approaches to assay [85].

6. Conclusions

Here, we introduced the hallmarks of HSC aging including defects in repopulation capacity, homing, and an increase in mobilization and myeloid-biased skewing. HSC aging is driven by multiple cell-intrinsic factors such as DNA damage, ROS, epigenetic changes and polarity changes, and cell-extrinsic factors including cytokines and chemokines derived from the HSC niche. We also mentioned recent emerging technologies for single-HSC profiling such as scRNA-Seq and single-cell transplantation. These methods have proven highly valuable in the unravelling of HSC heterogeneity, as described above. Surprisingly, aged HSCs could be rejuvenated by reduction of the nutrient supply, ROS scavenging, epigenetic modulation or the clearance of senescent cells (Figure 2). Although we have described the defined mechanisms and the physiological or biological changes involved in HSC aging, this does not explain all the aspects of aging, many of which remain elusive. However, our accumulated knowledge may be helpful for understanding HSC aging and designing HSC aging studies. Fortunately, many HSC aging studies have suggested that the dysregulated functions of aged HSCs can be reversed or rescued by rejuvenating agents or the overexpression of specific genes. In the future, these approaches may shine a light on treating age-related immune diseases and can also provide a promising tool to improve quality of life for the elderly.

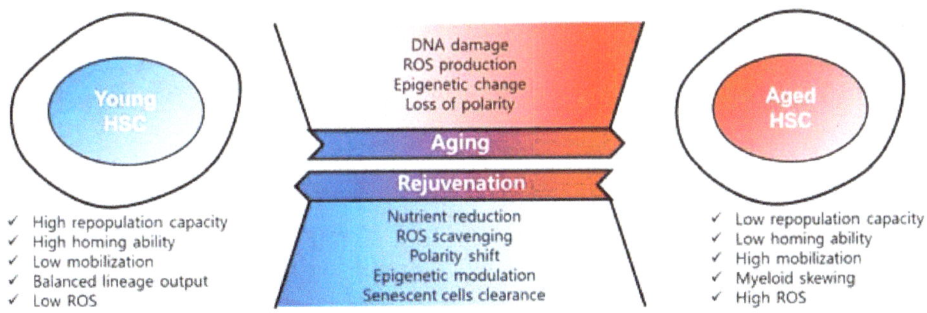

Figure 2. Regulation of HSC aging and rejuvenation. Aged HSCs have the hallmarks of low repopulation capacity, low homing ability, high mobility, myeloid skewing, and high ROS, among others. HSC aging is driven by DNA damage, ROS, epigenetic change, and loss of polarity. Aged HSCs can be rejuvenated by nutrient reduction, ROS scavenging, polarity shift, epigenetic modulation, and senescent cells clearance.

Author Contributions: J.L. and S.R.Y. wrote the manuscript. I.C. and H.J. wrote and supervised the manuscript.

References

1. Akunuru, S.; Geiger, H. Aging, Clonality, and Rejuvenation of Hematopoietic Stem Cells. *Trends Mol. Med.* **2016**, *22*, 701–712. [CrossRef]
2. Moehrle, B.M.; Geiger, H. Aging of hematopoietic stem cells: DNA damage and mutations? *Exp. Hematol.* **2016**, *44*, 895–901. [CrossRef] [PubMed]
3. Ergen, A.V.; Goodell, M.A. Mechanisms of hematopoietic stem cell aging. *Exp. Gerontol.* **2010**, *45*, 286–290. [CrossRef]
4. Kiel, M.J.; Yilmaz, O.H.; Iwashita, T.; Yilmaz, O.H.; Terhorst, C.; Morrison, S.J. SLAM family receptors distinguish hematopoietic stem and progenitor cells and reveal endothelial niches for stem cells. *Cell* **2005**, *121*, 1109–1121. [CrossRef]
5. Jung, H.; Kim, M.J.; Kim, D.O.; Kim, W.S.; Yoon, S.J.; Park, Y.J.; Yoon, S.R.; Kim, T.D.; Suh, H.W.; Yun, S.; et al. TXNIP maintains the hematopoietic cell pool by switching the function of p53 under oxidative stress. *Cell Metab.* **2013**, *18*, 75–85. [CrossRef]
6. Notta, F.; Doulatov, S.; Laurenti, E.; Poeppl, A.; Jurisica, I.; Dick, J.E. Isolation of single human hematopoietic stem cells capable of long-term multilineage engraftment. *Science* **2011**, *333*, 218–221. [CrossRef]
7. Latchney, S.E.; Calvi, L.M. The aging hematopoietic stem cell niche: Phenotypic and functional changes and mechanisms that contribute to hematopoietic aging. *Semin. Hematol.* **2017**, *54*, 25–32. [CrossRef] [PubMed]
8. Pang, W.W.; Schrier, S.L.; Weissman, I.L. Age-associated changes in human hematopoietic stem cells. *Semin. Hematol.* **2017**, *54*, 39–42. [CrossRef]
9. De Haan, G.; Lazare, S.S. Aging of hematopoietic stem cells. *Blood* **2018**, *131*, 479–487. [CrossRef] [PubMed]
10. Morrison, S.J.; Scadden, D.T. The bone marrow niche for haematopoietic stem cells. *Nature* **2014**, *505*, 327–334. [CrossRef]
11. Warren, L.A.; Rossi, D.J. Stem Cells and aging in the hematopoietic system. *Mech. Ageing Dev.* **2009**, *130*, 46–53. [CrossRef]
12. Geiger, H.; de Haan, G.; Florian, M.C. The ageing haematopoietic stem cell compartment. *Nat. Rev. Immunol.* **2013**, *13*, 376–389. [CrossRef]
13. Rossi, D.J.; Bryder, D.; Zahn, J.M.; Ahlenius, H.; Sonu, R.; Wagers, A.J.; Weissman, I.L. Cell intrinsic alterations underlie hematopoietic stem cell aging. *Proc. Natl. Acad. Sci. USA* **2005**, *102*, 9194–9199. [CrossRef] [PubMed]
14. De Haan, G.; Nijhof, W.; Van Zant, G. Mouse strain-dependent changes in frequency and proliferation of hematopoietic stem cells during aging: Correlation between lifespan and cycling activity. *Blood* **1997**, *89*, 1543–1550. [PubMed]
15. Sudo, K.; Ema, H.; Morita, Y.; Nakauchi, H. Age-associated characteristics of murine hematopoietic stem cells. *J. Exp. Med.* **2000**, *192*, 1273–1280. [CrossRef]
16. Pang, W.W.; Price, E.A.; Sahoo, D.; Beerman, I.; Maloney, W.J.; Rossi, D.J.; Schrier, S.L.; Weissman, I.L. Human bone marrow hematopoietic stem cells are increased in frequency and myeloid-biased with age. *Proc. Natl. Acad. Sci. USA* **2011**, *108*, 20012–20017. [CrossRef] [PubMed]
17. Yahata, T.; Takanashi, T.; Muguruma, Y.; Ibrahim, A.A.; Matsuzawa, H.; Uno, T.; Sheng, Y.; Onizuka, M.; Ito, M.; Kato, S.; et al. Accumulation of oxidative DNA damage restricts the self-renewal capacity of human hematopoietic stem cells. *Blood* **2011**, *118*, 2941–2950. [CrossRef] [PubMed]
18. Kim, M.; Moon, H.B.; Spangrude, G.J. Major age-related changes of mouse hematopoietic stem/progenitor cells. *Ann. N. Y. Acad. Sci.* **2003**, *996*, 195–208. [CrossRef]
19. Jung, H.; Kim, D.O.; Byun, J.E.; Kim, W.S.; Kim, M.J.; Song, H.Y.; Kim, Y.K.; Kang, D.K.; Park, Y.J.; Kim, T.D.; et al. Thioredoxin-interacting protein regulates haematopoietic stem cell ageing and rejuvenation by inhibiting p38 kinase activity. *Nat. Commun.* **2016**, *7*, 13674. [CrossRef]
20. Chen, J. Hematopoietic stem cell development, aging and functional failure. *Int. J. Hematol.* **2011**, *94*, 3–10. [CrossRef]
21. Spangrude, G.J.; Heimfeld, S.; Weissman, I.L. Purification and characterization of mouse hematopoietic stem cells. *Science* **1988**, *241*, 58–62. [CrossRef]
22. Xing, Z.; Ryan, M.A.; Daria, D.; Nattamai, K.J.; Van Zant, G.; Wang, L.; Zheng, Y.; Geiger, H. Increased hematopoietic stem cell mobilization in aged mice. *Blood* **2006**, *108*, 2190–2197. [CrossRef]

23. Nilsson, S.K.; Dooner, M.S.; Weier, H.U.; Frenkel, B.; Lian, J.B.; Stein, G.S.; Quesenberry, P.J. Cells capable of bone production engraft from whole bone marrow transplants in nonablated mice. *J. Exp. Med.* **1999**, *189*, 729–734. [CrossRef]
24. Calvi, L.M.; Adams, G.B.; Weibrecht, K.W.; Weber, J.M.; Olson, D.P.; Knight, M.C.; Martin, R.P.; Schipani, E.; Divieti, P.; Bringhurst, F.R.; et al. Osteoblastic cells regulate the haematopoietic stem cell niche. *Nature* **2003**, *425*, 841–846. [CrossRef]
25. Zhang, J.; Niu, C.; Ye, L.; Huang, H.; He, X.; Tong, W.G.; Ross, J.; Haug, J.; Johnson, T.; Feng, J.Q.; et al. Identification of the haematopoietic stem cell niche and control of the niche size. *Nature* **2003**, *425*, 836–841. [CrossRef] [PubMed]
26. Lo Celso, C.; Fleming, H.E.; Wu, J.W.; Zhao, C.X.; Miake-Lye, S.; Fujisaki, J.; Cote, D.; Rowe, D.W.; Lin, C.P.; Scadden, D.T. Live-animal tracking of individual haematopoietic stem/progenitor cells in their niche. *Nature* **2009**, *457*, 92–96. [CrossRef]
27. Xie, Y.; Yin, T.; Wiegraebe, W.; He, X.C.; Miller, D.; Stark, D.; Perko, K.; Alexander, R.; Schwartz, J.; Grindley, J.C.; et al. Detection of functional haematopoietic stem cell niche using real-time imaging. *Nature* **2009**, *457*, 97–101. [CrossRef]
28. Domingues, M.J.; Nilsson, S.K.; Cao, B. New agents in HSC mobilization. *Int. J. Hematol.* **2017**, *105*, 141–152. [CrossRef]
29. Liang, Y.; Van Zant, G.; Szilvassy, S.J. Effects of aging on the homing and engraftment of murine hematopoietic stem and progenitor cells. *Blood* **2005**, *106*, 1479–1487. [CrossRef]
30. Bendall, L.J.; Bradstock, K.F. G-CSF: From granulopoietic stimulant to bone marrow stem cell mobilizing agent. *Cytokine Growth Factor Rev.* **2014**, *25*, 355–367. [CrossRef]
31. Lee, J.; Cho, Y.S.; Jung, H.; Choi, I. Pharmacological Regulation of Oxidative Stress in Stem Cells. *Oxid. Med. Cell. Longev.* **2018**, *2018*, 4081890. [CrossRef]
32. Liu, F.; Poursine-Laurent, J.; Link, D.C. Expression of the G-CSF receptor on hematopoietic progenitor cells is not required for their mobilization by G-CSF. *Blood* **2000**, *95*, 3025–3031.
33. Tesio, M.; Golan, K.; Corso, S.; Giordano, S.; Schajnovitz, A.; Vagima, Y.; Shivtiel, S.; Kalinkovich, A.; Caione, L.; Gammaitoni, L.; et al. Enhanced c-Met activity promotes G-CSF-induced mobilization of hematopoietic progenitor cells via ROS signaling. *Blood* **2011**, *117*, 419–428. [CrossRef]
34. Dorshkind, K.; Montecino-Rodriguez, E.; Signer, R.A. The ageing immune system: Is it ever too old to become young again? *Nat. Rev. Immunol.* **2009**, *9*, 57–62. [CrossRef]
35. Geiger, H.; Rudolph, K.L. Aging in the lympho-hematopoietic stem cell compartment. *Trends Immunol.* **2009**, *30*, 360–365. [CrossRef]
36. Wahlestedt, M.; Erlandsson, E.; Kristiansen, T.; Lu, R.; Brakebusch, C.; Weissman, I.L.; Yuan, J.; Martin-Gonzalez, J.; Bryder, D. Clonal reversal of ageing-associated stem cell lineage bias via a pluripotent intermediate. *Nat. Commun.* **2017**, *8*, 14533. [CrossRef]
37. Beerman, I.; Bhattacharya, D.; Zandi, S.; Sigvardsson, M.; Weissman, I.L.; Bryder, D.; Rossi, D.J. Functionally distinct hematopoietic stem cells modulate hematopoietic lineage potential during aging by a mechanism of clonal expansion. *Proc. Natl. Acad. Sci. USA* **2010**, *107*, 5465–5470. [CrossRef]
38. Cho, R.H.; Sieburg, H.B.; Muller-Sieburg, C.E. A new mechanism for the aging of hematopoietic stem cells: Aging changes the clonal composition of the stem cell compartment but not individual stem cells. *Blood* **2008**, *111*, 5553–5561. [CrossRef]
39. Rundberg Nilsson, A.; Soneji, S.; Adolfsson, S.; Bryder, D.; Pronk, C.J. Human and Murine Hematopoietic Stem Cell Aging Is Associated with Functional Impairments and Intrinsic Megakaryocytic/Erythroid Bias. *PLoS ONE* **2016**, *11*, e0158369. [CrossRef]
40. Li, T.; Zhou, Z.W.; Ju, Z.; Wang, Z.Q. DNA Damage Response in Hematopoietic Stem Cell Ageing. *Genom. Proteom. Bioinform.* **2016**, *14*, 147–154. [CrossRef]
41. Park, Y.; Gerson, S.L. DNA repair defects in stem cell function and aging. *Annu. Rev. Med.* **2005**, *56*, 495–508. [CrossRef]
42. Rossi, D.J.; Bryder, D.; Seita, J.; Nussenzweig, A.; Hoeijmakers, J.; Weissman, I.L. Deficiencies in DNA damage repair limit the function of haematopoietic stem cells with age. *Nature* **2007**, *447*, 725–729. [CrossRef]
43. Rube, C.E.; Fricke, A.; Widmann, T.A.; Furst, T.; Madry, H.; Pfreundschuh, M.; Rube, C. Accumulation of DNA damage in hematopoietic stem and progenitor cells during human aging. *PLoS ONE* **2011**, *6*, e17487. [CrossRef]

44. Hamilton, M.L.; Van Remmen, H.; Drake, J.A.; Yang, H.; Guo, Z.M.; Kewitt, K.; Walter, C.A.; Richardson, A. Does oxidative damage to DNA increase with age? *Proc. Natl. Acad. Sci. USA* **2001**, *98*, 10469–10474. [CrossRef]
45. Simsek, T.; Kocabas, F.; Zheng, J.; Deberardinis, R.J.; Mahmoud, A.I.; Olson, E.N.; Schneider, J.W.; Zhang, C.C.; Sadek, H.A. The distinct metabolic profile of hematopoietic stem cells reflects their location in a hypoxic niche. *Cell Stem Cell* **2010**, *7*, 380–390. [CrossRef]
46. Jang, Y.Y.; Sharkis, S.J. A low level of reactive oxygen species selects for primitive hematopoietic stem cells that may reside in the low-oxygenic niche. *Blood* **2007**, *110*, 3056–3063. [CrossRef]
47. Porto, M.L.; Rodrigues, B.P.; Menezes, T.N.; Ceschim, S.L.; Casarini, D.E.; Gava, A.L.; Pereira, T.M.; Vasquez, E.C.; Campagnaro, B.P.; Meyrelles, S.S. Reactive oxygen species contribute to dysfunction of bone marrow hematopoietic stem cells in aged C57BL/6 J mice. *J. Biomed. Sci.* **2015**, *22*, 97. [CrossRef]
48. Urao, N.; Ushio-Fukai, M. Redox regulation of stem/progenitor cells and bone marrow niche. *Free Rad. Biol. Med.* **2013**, *54*, 26–39. [CrossRef]
49. Tothova, Z.; Kollipara, R.; Huntly, B.J.; Lee, B.H.; Castrillon, D.H.; Cullen, D.E.; McDowell, E.P.; Lazo-Kallanian, S.; Williams, I.R.; Sears, C.; et al. FoxOs are critical mediators of hematopoietic stem cell resistance to physiologic oxidative stress. *Cell* **2007**, *128*, 325–339. [CrossRef]
50. Miyamoto, K.; Araki, K.Y.; Naka, K.; Arai, F.; Takubo, K.; Yamazaki, S.; Matsuoka, S.; Miyamoto, T.; Ito, K.; Ohmura, M.; et al. Foxo3a is essential for maintenance of the hematopoietic stem cell pool. *Cell Stem Cell* **2007**, *1*, 101–112. [CrossRef]
51. Wheaton, W.W.; Chandel, N.S. Hypoxia. 2. Hypoxia regulates cellular metabolism. *Am. J. Physiol. Cell Physiol.* **2011**, *300*, C385–C393. [CrossRef]
52. Kramer, A.; Challen, G.A. The epigenetic basis of hematopoietic stem cell aging. *Semin. Hematol.* **2017**, *54*, 19–24. [CrossRef]
53. Sun, D.; Luo, M.; Jeong, M.; Rodriguez, B.; Xia, Z.; Hannah, R.; Wang, H.; Le, T.; Faull, K.F.; Chen, R.; et al. Epigenomic profiling of young and aged HSCs reveals concerted changes during aging that reinforce self-renewal. *Cell Stem Cell* **2014**, *14*, 673–688. [CrossRef]
54. Trowbridge, J.J.; Snow, J.W.; Kim, J.; Orkin, S.H. DNA methyltransferase 1 is essential for and uniquely regulates hematopoietic stem and progenitor cells. *Cell Stem Cell* **2009**, *5*, 442–449. [CrossRef]
55. Broske, A.M.; Vockentanz, L.; Kharazi, S.; Huska, M.R.; Mancini, E.; Scheller, M.; Kuhl, C.; Enns, A.; Prinz, M.; Jaenisch, R.; et al. DNA methylation protects hematopoietic stem cell multipotency from myeloerythroid restriction. *Nat. Genet.* **2009**, *41*, 1207–1215. [CrossRef]
56. Challen, G.A.; Sun, D.; Jeong, M.; Luo, M.; Jelinek, J.; Berg, J.S.; Bock, C.; Vasanthakumar, A.; Gu, H.; Xi, Y.; et al. Dnmt3a is essential for hematopoietic stem cell differentiation. *Nat. Genet.* **2011**, *44*, 23–31. [CrossRef]
57. Florian, M.C.; Dorr, K.; Niebel, A.; Daria, D.; Schrezenmeier, H.; Rojewski, M.; Filippi, M.D.; Hasenberg, A.; Gunzer, M.; Scharffetter-Kochanek, K.; et al. Cdc42 activity regulates hematopoietic stem cell aging and rejuvenation. *Cell Stem Cell* **2012**, *10*, 520–530. [CrossRef]
58. Cau, J.; Hall, A. Cdc42 controls the polarity of the actin and microtubule cytoskeletons through two distinct signal transduction pathways. *J. Cell Sci.* **2005**, *118*, 2579–2587. [CrossRef]
59. Florian, M.C.; Geiger, H. Concise review: Polarity in stem cells, disease, and aging. *Stem Cells* **2010**, *28*, 1623–1629. [CrossRef]
60. Guevara-Aguirre, J.; Balasubramanian, P.; Guevara-Aguirre, M.; Wei, M.; Madia, F.; Cheng, C.W.; Hwang, D.; Martin-Montalvo, A.; Saavedra, J.; Ingles, S.; et al. Growth hormone receptor deficiency is associated with a major reduction in pro-aging signaling, cancer, and diabetes in humans. *Sci. Transl. Med.* **2011**, *3*, 70ra13. [CrossRef]
61. Fontana, L.; Partridge, L.; Longo, V.D. Extending healthy life span–from yeast to humans. *Science* **2010**, *328*, 321–326. [CrossRef]
62. Holzenberger, M.; Dupont, J.; Ducos, B.; Leneuve, P.; Geloen, A.; Even, P.C.; Cervera, P.; Le Bouc, Y. IGF-1 receptor regulates lifespan and resistance to oxidative stress in mice. *Nature* **2003**, *421*, 182–187. [CrossRef]
63. Cheng, C.W.; Adams, G.B.; Perin, L.; Wei, M.; Zhou, X.; Lam, B.S.; Da Sacco, S.; Mirisola, M.; Quinn, D.I.; Dorff, T.B.; et al. Prolonged fasting reduces IGF-1/PKA to promote hematopoietic-stem-cell-based regeneration and reverse immunosuppression. *Cell Stem Cell* **2014**, *14*, 810–823. [CrossRef]
64. Shin, J.; Zhang, D.; Chen, D. Reversible acetylation of metabolic enzymes celebration: SIRT2 and p300 join the party. *Mol. Cell* **2011**, *43*, 3–5. [CrossRef]

65. Qiu, X.; Brown, K.; Hirschey, M.D.; Verdin, E.; Chen, D. Calorie restriction reduces oxidative stress by SIRT3-mediated SOD2 activation. *Cell Metab.* **2010**, *12*, 662–667. [CrossRef]
66. Brown, K.; Xie, S.; Qiu, X.; Mohrin, M.; Shin, J.; Liu, Y.; Zhang, D.; Scadden, D.T.; Chen, D. SIRT3 reverses aging-associated degeneration. *Cell Rep.* **2013**, *3*, 319–327. [CrossRef]
67. Mohrin, M.; Shin, J.; Liu, Y.; Brown, K.; Luo, H.; Xi, Y.; Haynes, C.M.; Chen, D. Stem cell aging. A mitochondrial UPR-mediated metabolic checkpoint regulates hematopoietic stem cell aging. *Science* **2015**, *347*, 1374–1377. [CrossRef]
68. Ito, K.; Hirao, A.; Arai, F.; Matsuoka, S.; Takubo, K.; Hamaguchi, I.; Nomiyama, K.; Hosokawa, K.; Sakurada, K.; Nakagata, N.; et al. Regulation of oxidative stress by ATM is required for self-renewal of haematopoietic stem cells. *Nature* **2004**, *431*, 997–1002. [CrossRef]
69. Ito, K.; Hirao, A.; Arai, F.; Takubo, K.; Matsuoka, S.; Miyamoto, K.; Ohmura, M.; Naka, K.; Hosokawa, K.; Ikeda, Y.; et al. Reactive oxygen species act through p38 MAPK to limit the lifespan of hematopoietic stem cells. *Nat. Med.* **2006**, *12*, 446–451. [CrossRef]
70. Le, Q.; Yao, W.; Chen, Y.; Yan, B.; Liu, C.; Yuan, M.; Zhou, Y.; Ma, L. GRK6 regulates ROS response and maintains hematopoietic stem cell self-renewal. *Cell Death Dis.* **2016**, *7*, e2478. [CrossRef]
71. Satoh, Y.; Yokota, T.; Sudo, T.; Kondo, M.; Lai, A.; Kincade, P.W.; Kouro, T.; Iida, R.; Kokame, K.; Miyata, T.; et al. The Satb1 protein directs hematopoietic stem cell differentiation toward lymphoid lineages. *Immunity* **2013**, *38*, 1105–1115. [CrossRef] [PubMed]
72. Shao, L.; Feng, W.; Li, H.; Gardner, D.; Luo, Y.; Wang, Y.; Liu, L.; Meng, A.; Sharpless, N.E.; Zhou, D. Total body irradiation causes long-term mouse BM injury via induction of HSC premature senescence in an Ink4a- and Arf-independent manner. *Blood* **2014**, *123*, 3105–3115. [CrossRef] [PubMed]
73. Le, O.N.; Rodier, F.; Fontaine, F.; Coppe, J.P.; Campisi, J.; DeGregori, J.; Laverdiere, C.; Kokta, V.; Haddad, E.; Beausejour, C.M. Ionizing radiation-induced long-term expression of senescence markers in mice is independent of p53 and immune status. *Aging Cell* **2010**, *9*, 398–409. [CrossRef]
74. Baker, D.J.; Wijshake, T.; Tchkonia, T.; LeBrasseur, N.K.; Childs, B.G.; van de Sluis, B.; Kirkland, J.L.; van Deursen, J.M. Clearance of p16Ink4a-positive senescent cells delays ageing-associated disorders. *Nature* **2011**, *479*, 232–236. [CrossRef]
75. Chang, J.; Wang, Y.; Shao, L.; Laberge, R.M.; Demaria, M.; Campisi, J.; Janakiraman, K.; Sharpless, N.E.; Ding, S.; Feng, W.; et al. Clearance of senescent cells by ABT263 rejuvenates aged hematopoietic stem cells in mice. *Nat. Med.* **2016**, *22*, 78–83. [CrossRef] [PubMed]
76. Papalexi, E.; Satija, R. Single-cell RNA sequencing to explore immune cell heterogeneity. *Nat. Rev. Immunol.* **2018**, *18*, 35–45. [CrossRef] [PubMed]
77. Kowalczyk, M.S.; Tirosh, I.; Heckl, D.; Rao, T.N.; Dixit, A.; Haas, B.J.; Schneider, R.K.; Wagers, A.J.; Ebert, B.L.; Regev, A. Single-cell RNA-seq reveals changes in cell cycle and differentiation programs upon aging of hematopoietic stem cells. *Genome Res.* **2015**, *25*, 1860–1872. [CrossRef]
78. Rodriguez-Fraticelli, A.E.; Wolock, S.L.; Weinreb, C.S.; Panero, R.; Patel, S.H.; Jankovic, M.; Sun, J.; Calogero, R.A.; Klein, A.M.; Camargo, F.D. Clonal analysis of lineage fate in native haematopoiesis. *Nature* **2018**, *553*, 212–216. [CrossRef] [PubMed]
79. Grover, A.; Sanjuan-Pla, A.; Thongjuea, S.; Carrelha, J.; Giustacchini, A.; Gambardella, A.; Macaulay, I.; Mancini, E.; Luis, T.C.; Mead, A.; et al. Single-cell RNA sequencing reveals molecular and functional platelet bias of aged haematopoietic stem cells. *Nat. Commun.* **2016**, *7*, 11075. [CrossRef] [PubMed]
80. Baron, C.S.; Kester, L.; Klaus, A.; Boisset, J.C.; Thambyrajah, R.; Yvernogeau, L.; Kouskoff, V.; Lacaud, G.; van Oudenaarden, A.; Robin, C. Single-cell transcriptomics reveal the dynamic of haematopoietic stem cell production in the aorta. *Nat. Commun.* **2018**, *9*, 2517. [CrossRef]
81. Muller-Sieburg, C.E.; Cho, R.H.; Thoman, M.; Adkins, B.; Sieburg, H.B. Deterministic regulation of hematopoietic stem cell self-renewal and differentiation. *Blood* **2002**, *100*, 1302–1309. [PubMed]
82. Dykstra, B.; Kent, D.; Bowie, M.; McCaffrey, L.; Hamilton, M.; Lyons, K.; Lee, S.J.; Brinkman, R.; Eaves, C. Long-term propagation of distinct hematopoietic differentiation programs in vivo. *Cell Stem Cell* **2007**, *1*, 218–229. [CrossRef] [PubMed]
83. Jacobsen, S.E.W.; Nerlov, C. Haematopoiesis in the era of advanced single-cell technologies. *Nat. Cell Biol.* **2019**, *21*, 2–8. [CrossRef] [PubMed]

84. Carrelha, J.; Meng, Y.; Kettyle, L.M.; Luis, T.C.; Norfo, R.; Alcolea, V.; Boukarabila, H.; Grasso, F.; Gambardella, A.; Grover, A.; et al. Hierarchically related lineage-restricted fates of multipotent haematopoietic stem cells. *Nature* **2018**, *554*, 106–111. [CrossRef] [PubMed]
85. Yamamoto, R.; Wilkinson, A.C.; Ooehara, J.; Lan, X.; Lai, C.Y.; Nakauchi, Y.; Pritchard, J.K.; Nakauchi, H. Large-Scale Clonal Analysis Resolves Aging of the Mouse Hematopoietic Stem Cell Compartment. *Cell Stem Cell* **2018**, *22*, 600–607e604. [CrossRef]

14

Expression of Longevity Genes Induced by a Low-Dose Fluvastatin and Valsartan Combination with the Potential to Prevent/Treat "Aging-Related Disorders"

Miodrag Janić [1], Mojca Lunder [2], Srdjan Novaković [3], Petra Škerl [3] and Mišo Šabovič [1,*]

[1] Department of Vascular Diseases, Ljubljana University Medical Centre, Zaloška cesta 7, SI-1000 Ljubljana, Slovenia; miodrag.janic@kclj.si

[2] Department of Endocrinology, Diabetes and Metabolic Diseases, Ljubljana University Medical Centre, Zaloška cesta 7, SI-1000 Ljubljana, Slovenia; mojca.lunder@kclj.si

[3] Department of Molecular Diagnostics, Institute of Oncology Ljubljana, SI-1000 Ljubljana, Slovenia; snovakovic@onko-i.si (S.N.); pskerl@onko-i.si (P.Š.)

* Correspondence: miso.sabovic@kclj.si

Abstract: The incidence of aging-related disorders may be decreased through strategies influencing the expression of longevity genes. Although numerous approaches have been suggested, no effective, safe, and easily applicable approach is yet available. Efficacy of low-dose fluvastatin and valsartan, separately or in combination, on the expression of the longevity genes in middle-aged males, was assessed. Stored blood samples from 130 apparently healthy middle-aged males treated with fluvastatin (10 mg daily), valsartan (20 mg daily), fluvastatin-valsartan combination (10 and 20 mg, respectively), and placebo (control) were analyzed. They were taken before and after 30 days of treatment and, additionally, five months after treatment discontinuation. The expression of the following longevity genes was assessed: *SIRT1*, *PRKAA*, *KLOTHO*, *NFE2L2*, *mTOR*, and *NF-κB*. Treatment with fluvastatin and valsartan in combination significantly increased the expression of *SIRT1* (1.8-fold; $p < 0.0001$), *PRKAA* (1.5-fold; $p = 0.262$) and *KLOTHO* (1.7-fold; $p < 0.0001$), but not *NFE2L2*, *mTOR* and *NF-κB*. Both fluvastatin and valsartan alone significantly, but to a lesser extent, increased the expression of *SIRT1*, and did not influence the expression of other genes. Five months after treatment discontinuation, genes expression decreased to the basal levels. In addition, analysis with previously obtained results revealed significant correlation between *SIRT1* and both increased telomerase activity and improved arterial wall characteristics. We showed that low-dose fluvastatin and valsartan, separately and in combination, substantially increase expression of *SIRT1*, *PRKAA*, and *KLOTHO* genes, which may be attributed to their so far unreported pleiotropic beneficial effects. This approach could be used for prevention of ageing (and longevity genes)–related disorders.

Keywords: aging-related disorders; longevity genes; arterial aging; low-dose fluvastatin and valsartan combination

---

1. Introduction

An aging population, along with increased life expectancy and the prevalence of associated chronic diseases, has become an important medical and economic issue. Consequently, the burden of so-called "aging-related disorders," such as associated cardiovascular diseases, degenerative diseases of the central nervous system, and malignant diseases, is also increasing [1,2]. These diseases represent one of the leading problems of the healthcare systems in developed countries around the globe. Effective strategies for their prevention are therefore needed. Aging-related disorders have been found to be causally associated with the altered expression of aging-related or so-called longevity genes [3]. In addition, telomere length per se [4], as well as telomerase expression [5], are also associated with aging-related disorders. In a narrower context, it seems logical that these genes represent mechanistic intracellular targets that could be altered to change the intracellular pro-aging milieu. It is expected that with the induction of expression of protective and suppression of expression of harmful genes, a new rejuvenated cellular phenotype could be reached that could influence the occurrence and course of aging-related disorders. In summary, so-called rejuvenating strategies, focused on modifying such genes' expression, could possibly importantly impact the prevalence of aging-related disorders [3].

In our prior studies, we explored the functional and structural characteristics of the arterial wall, some of which are also characteristic for arterial aging, and were particularly interested in the improvement of altered characteristics of the arterial wall by low doses of fluvastatin and valsartan [6]. We found significant improvement of arterial wall characteristics after 30 days of treatment in middle-aged males, with the beneficial effect slowly declining within nine months of treatment discontinuation [7–9]. Importantly, for age-related changes, the improvement of arterial wall characteristics was associated with increased telomerase expression and reduced inflammation as well as oxidative stress parameters [10,11]. Both decreased telomerase expression along with decreased telomeres' length and increased activation of inflammation and oxidative stress are characteristic of aging, arterial aging, and aging-related disorders. Therefore, we hypothesized that "anti-aging" or "rejuvenation" effects could be achieved through treatment impacting the longevity genes. This impact should have the capacity to influence "aging-related" disorders. Considering our previous results, this approach could be particularly effective for decreasing aging-related changes of the arterial system.

In the present study, we explored the efficacy of an approach consisting of (short-term) treatment with low-dose fluvastatin and valsartan alone or in combination on the expression of longevity genes in middle-aged males who had already (sub-clinically) impaired functional and structural arterial wall characteristics which could at least partially be attributed to the initial processes of aging.

2. Results

2.1. *Expression of Longevity Genes*

We analyzed the expression of longevity genes in the treatment and control groups. At the beginning of the study, there was no difference in longevity genes expression in the four different groups (low-dose fluvastatin, low-dose valsartan, low-dose fluvastatin and valsartan combination, and the control group). Differences between the groups were only observed after 30 days of treatment. Five months after treatment discontinuation, the expression of longevity genes in all treatment groups decreased almost to initial values. In the control group, the expression of longevity genes did not change during the study (Figure 1A–F).

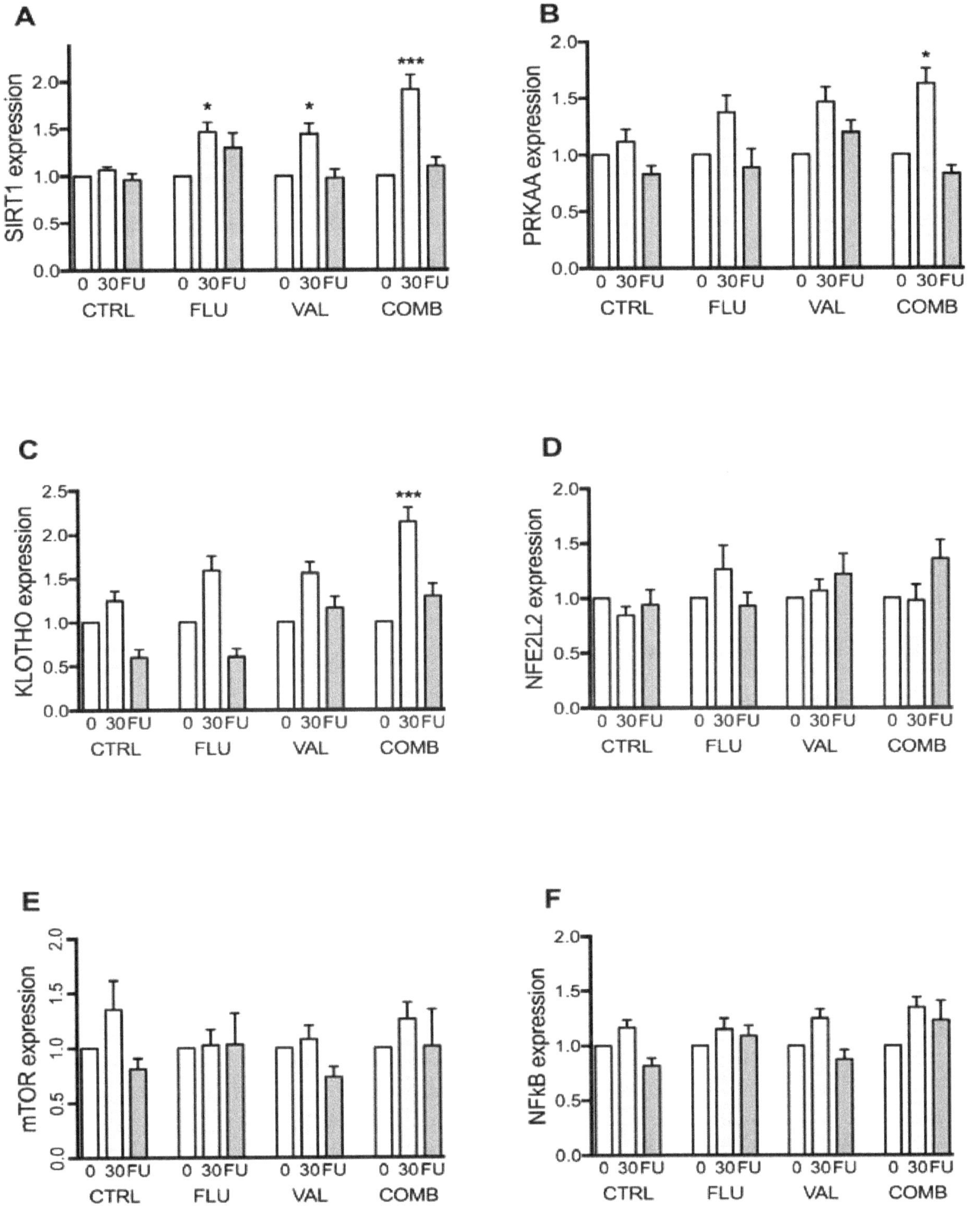

Figure 1. The expression of longevity genes: (**A**) *SIRT1*, (**B**) *PRKAA*, (**C**) *KLOTHO*, (**D**) *NFE2L2*, (**E**) *mTOR*, and (**F**) *NF-κB* in placebo (CTRL), low-dose fluvastatin (FLU), low-dose valsartan (VAL), or low-dose fluvastatin and valsartan combination (COMB). "0" represents the time before treatment, "30" represents the end of treatment, i.e., after 30 days (30) and "FU" represents five months after treatment discontinuation. Values are presented as means ± SEM. Presented p values are after Benjamini-Hochberg false discovery rate (FDR) correction, significance threshold set at $p < 0.05$. * signifies $p < 0.05$ and *** $p < 0.001$, vs. control group. *SIRT1*—sirtuin 1 gene; *PRKAA*—5′-AMP-activated protein kinase catalytic subunit α-2 gene; *NFE2L2*—nuclear factor (erythroid-derived 2)-like 2 gene; *mTOR*—mechanistic target of rapamycin (mTOR) gene; *NF-κB1*—nuclear factor κB gene.

2.1.1. Sirtuin 1 (*SIRT1*) Gene Expression

Both low-dose fluvastatin and valsartan separately increased the expression of the *SIRT1* gene after 30 days of treatment up to 1.4-fold ($p = 0.0165$ and $p = 0.0229$, respectively), while their low-dose combination increased its expression up to 1.8-fold ($p < 0.0001$) compared to the control group. Five months after treatment discontinuation, no significant effects of the treatment on the *SIRT1* gene expression were observed (Figure 1A).

2.1.2. 5′-AMP-Activated Protein Kinase Catalytic Subunit α-2 (*PRKAA*) Gene Expression

After 30 days of treatment, only the low-dose fluvastatin and valsartan combination significantly increased the expression of the *PRKAA* gene, up to 1.5-fold ($p = 0.0262$) compared to the control group. Separate drugs had no influence on the *PRKAA* gene expression (Figure 1B).

2.1.3. *KLOTHO* Gene Expression

After 30 days of treatment, only the low-dose fluvastatin and valsartan combination significantly increased the expression of the *KLOTHO* gene, up to 1.7-fold ($p < 0.0001$) compared to the control group. Separate drugs had no influence on the *KLOTHO* gene expression (Figure 1C).

2.1.4. Nuclear Factor (Erythroid-Derived 2)-Like 2 Gene Expression (*NFE2L2*)

No significant changes of the *NFE2L2* gene expression were observed in any of the study groups (Figure 1D).

2.1.5. Mechanistic Target of Rapamycin (*mTOR*) Gene Expression

No significant changes were observed in the *mTOR* gene expression in any of the study groups (Figure 1E).

2.1.6. Nuclear Factor κB (*NF-κB*) Gene Expression

No statistically significant changes in the expression of the *NF-κB* gene were observed either (Figure 1F).

2.2. Correlations between the Expression of Longevity Genes, Telomerase Activity and Arterial Wall Properties

The correlations between longevity genes expression and previously described telomerase activity and arterial wall properties [7–10], all measured after 30 days of treatment, were calculated. In the separate, low-dose fluvastatin and valsartan groups, the expression of the *SIRT1* gene positively correlated with telomerase activity ($r = 0.42$; $p = 0.04$ and $r = 0.39$; $p = 0.03$, respectively). Importantly, in the low-dose combination group, the expression of the *SIRT1* gene positively correlated with telomerase activity ($r = 0.62$; $p = 0.01$) and with brachial artery flow-mediated dilation (FMD) ($r = 0.52$; $p = 0.05$) while negatively correlated with carotid artery beta stiffness ($r = -0.45$; $p = 0.02$) and pulse wave velocity (PWV) ($r = -0.56$; $p = 0.05$).

3. Discussion

In the present study, we showed that low-dose fluvastatin and valsartan in combination significantly increased the expression of several important longevity genes (*SIRT1, PRKAA, KLOTHO*). Moreover, these changes correlated with an improvement of functional and structural arterial wall characteristics as well as with telomerase activity, both assessed previously [7–10]. Overall, the results revealed increased expression of several longevity genes that seems to be causally associated with increased telomerase activity and improvement of arterial wall (initial aging-related) characteristics. The results are very promising and indicate that our relatively simple but innovative approach could have potential efficacy as a "rejuvenating agent," particularly in the efforts to decrease the occurrence of aging-related disorders.

The present study was designed as a two-part study: The first part comprised the measurement of longevity genes in relation to treatment with low-dose fluvastatin and valsartan, and the second part comprised of a correlation analysis with previously measured relevant parameters (telomerase activity and functional/structural arterial wall characteristics). The studied population was a group of middle-aged males with already present aging-related changes. Since we found that a low-dose combination of fluvastatin and valsartan improved arterial wall characteristics, we aimed to further explore the mechanism behind these beneficial effects. Thus, from the previously obtained samples, we assessed the expression of longevity genes to explore the potential rejuvenating effect of our approach. We found that the low-dose fluvastatin and valsartan combination increased the expression of the *SIRT1* (1.8-fold; $p < 0.0001$), *PRKAA* (1.5-fold; $p = 0.0262$) and *KLOTHO* (1.7-fold; $p < 0.0001$) genes after 30 days, whereas no differences in the expression of the *NFE2L2*, *mTOR*, and *NF-κB* genes were observed. Fluvastatin or valsartan alone were less effective, increasing only the expression of the *SIRT1* gene to a lesser extent. Moreover, the expression of the *SIRT1* gene in the combination group positively correlated with telomerase activity and improvement of the arterial wall characteristics.

Importantly, the FDA recently approved the first interventional "anti-aging" study (MILES—Metformin in Longevity Study). Metformin, which, for this purpose, was repositioned from a solely antidiabetic drug to an "anti-aging" drug, is the interventional drug. This is based on a wealth of data indicating that metformin could influence the aging process, or more importantly, aging-related disorders. Interestingly, one of the most prominent of the several hypotheses underlying the "anti-aging" effects of metformin is the activation of longevity genes with consequent effects on energy metabolism, inflammation and oxidative stress. Several other currently ongoing studies with metformin are focusing on its "anti-aging" effects, such as VA-IMPACT, TAME and ePREDICE. In any event, a new period in which specific treatments of "aging-related disorders" are being studied, has already begun.

Sirtuins are a family of nicotinamide adenine dinucleotide (NAD)-dependent deacetylases, and according to some studies, are one of the key molecules involved in the regulation of aging and aging-related disorders [12]. *SIRT1* regulates DNA transcription and repair as well as cell survival, thus also inducing longevity. It was shown to have an important role in aging-related disorders of the cardiovascular [5] and nervous systems [13]. Some statins in therapeutic doses were shown to induce *SIRT1* expression, for example, simvastatin in endothelial progenitor cells [14]. On the other hand, atorvastatin and rosuvastatin reduced its expression in patients with coronary artery disease [15]. Until now, the effect of fluvastatin in therapeutic or low doses on *SIRT1* expression has not been assessed. To the best of our knowledge and according to the literature, no studies have assessed the effect of valsartan on the *SIRT1* gene in humans, either. A few studies were performed on rats or mice, in which valsartan and other sartans increased the expression of the *SIRT1* gene [16–18]. The *PRKAA* gene encodes the catalytic subunit of the AMPK. AMPK is the primary regulator of cellular responses and acts as a sensor to maintain energy balance within the cell [19]. In animal and cell culture studies, several statins were shown to induce the AMPK and eNOS pathway, acting in a vasoprotective manner [20–22]. Valsartan was also shown to act protectively through activation of the AMPK pathway in diabetic rats [23]; similar effects have been shown for telmisartan in human coronary artery cells [24]. The consequences of AMPK activations were divergent: In acute activation, it caused cell protection, whereas in chronic activation, it might have activated the pro-aging pathways and progressive degeneration during cellular senescence. There are various interactions between sirtuin and AMPK pathways [19]. The expression of *KLOTHO* decreased in aging-related disorders [25]. Valsartan in therapeutic doses increased the amount of plasma-soluble *KLOTHO* and consequently induced cardiorenal beneficial effects in patients with diabetes mellitus and diabetic kidney disease [26]. The effects of valsartan in low doses have not yet been studied in such a setting. The potential beneficial effects of statins on *KLOTHO* expression was only shown in animal studies [27]. The *NFE2L2* gene encodes a transcription factor, which regulates the proteins involved in responding to injury and inflammation. According to some studies, enhancing *NFE2L2* activity may be beneficial in diabetic cardiomyopathy, mitochondrial dysfunction, and as an anti-aging agent, but further studies are needed [28]. Fluvastatin was shown to induce *NFE2L2* in the vascular smooth muscle cells [29,30]. Mammalian target of Rapamycin (mTOR) was shown to have an important role in cardiovascular diseases, oxidative stress and longevity [31]. In animal or cell studies, statins influenced the *mTOR*, which was proven for fluvastatin in rats [32] and for lovastatin in vascular smooth muscle cells [33]. In one study on rats, valsartan induced cardio protection against ischemic-reperfusion injury through the mTOR [34]. *NF-κB* gene expression mediated vascular and myocardial inflammation and was additionally associated with impaired endothelial function [35]. There is evidence that both statins and sartans could reduce the *NF-κB* gene activation in various animal and cell line models [36,37].

To the best of our knowledge, no study like the present one, has been published. In our review of the literature, we found several different studies that assessed the effects of statins or sartans on longevity genes, but most of those studies were performed either on cell lines or animals. Therefore, the present study is the first to show that our new preventive cardiovascular approach, which was proven to induce the improvement of arterial wall functional and structural characteristics, and consequently decrease arterial age, additionally acted through the expression of several longevity genes. This could be one of the mechanisms lying behind the beneficial effects observed in our previous clinical studies [7–9]. Nevertheless, one of the limitations of the present study is that we used only qPCR, but validation by Western blotting would be of added value.

The results of the present study indicate that our innovative approach using short-term low-dose fluvastatin and valsartan has a potential in inducing the expression of certain longevity genes. These effects could be anti-aging or rejuvenating as well as act as a potential specific prevention/treatment for "aging-related" disorders. It can be speculated that using cycling, intermittent treatment with low-dose combination (every 6–12 years) starting at middle-age could postpone the occurrence of aging-related disorders. On the other hand, this approach could be used in the same population and with the same aim as metformin in the MILES trial. One of the major advantages of this approach is its cyclic, intermittent character, which, as previously described, could potentially activate the beneficial longevity genes for a time short enough not activate their contra regulatory mechanisms as well. With intermittently repeating cycles, this could lead to repetitive beneficial activations of the protective longevity genes. Thus, it could be speculated that the cumulative effect of these repeating cycles of treatment might eventually lead to successful specific prevention/treatment of "aging-related" disorders, most likely cardiovascular "aging-related" disorders.

4. Materials and Methods

4.1. Participants and Study Design

The stored blood samples from our three prior studies were used together for the present longevity gene expression study. Overall, 130 middle-aged, apparently healthy male participants were recruited and treated for one month (30 days): 25 persons with fluvastatin 10 mg daily, 20 persons with valsartan 20 mg daily, and 20 persons with a low-dose combination of fluvastatin (10 mg daily) and valsartan (20 mg daily). Accordingly, 65 participants received placebo. All the participants were blindly randomized into the relevant group, as in our previous studies, which are described in more detail elsewhere [7–9]. Blood samples were collected and ultrasound measurements of the arterial wall properties (endothelial function, arterial stiffness) were performed at the beginning and at the end of the treatment period (day 0 and day 30). The measurements were also repeated five months after treatment discontinuation.

The National Medical Ethics Committee of Slovenia approved the studies (Approval date 3 July 2009, Approval No.: 21k/05/09) and informed consent was obtained from all participants. Inclusion criteria were: age between 30 and 50 years, non-smoking status, normal blood pressure values, body mass index values below 30 kg/m^2, no clinical cardiovascular disease, no history of any other chronic disease, and no regular medication therapy. The characteristics of the subjects were already extensively described in our previous publications [7–9].

4.2. Blood Sampling

Three samples of whole peripheral blood were collected from each participant: before treatment (day 0), after treatment conclusion (day 30), and five months after treatment discontinuation (follow-up). The whole blood samples were collected in 10 mL EDTA tubes and stored at −80 °C. Prior to RNA extraction, samples were centrifuged at 4000 rpm for 25 min to obtain the pellet of cells and cell debris. The pellets were then used for RNA extraction.

4.3. RNA Isolation

Total RNA was isolated using a miRNeasy Mini kit (Qiagen, Hilden, Germany) according to the manufacturer's instructions. RNA was quantified using the NanoDrop, and cDNA was synthesized from 300 ng of the total RNA using the High-Capacity cDNA Reverse Transcription Kit with RNase Inhibitor (Applied Biosystems, Foster City, CA, USA) according to the manufacturer's protocol.

4.4. Quantitative Real-Time PCR (qPCR) for Human Telomerase Reverse Transcriptase (hTERT) Expression

The expression of target genes in the tested samples was performed using TaqMan Gene Expression Assays (Applied Biosystems) according to the manufacturer's instructions: Assay Hs00183100_m1 for the *KLOTHO* gene; assay Hs01009006_m1 for the Sirtuin 1 (*SIRT1*) gene; assay Hs01562315_m1 for the 5′AMP-activated protein kinase (*AMPK*) gene; assay Hs00765730_m1 for the Nuclear factor κB (*NF-κB1*) gene; assay Hs00234522_m1 for the Mechanistic target of rapamycin (*mTOR*) gene and assay Hs00975961_g1 for the Nuclear factor (erythroid-derived 2)-like 2 (*NFE2L2*) gene. The housekeeping gene glyceraldehyde 3-phoshate dehydrogenase (*GAPDH*) was used as an endogenous control. Described briefly, qPCR was performed using the ABI 7900 instrument (Applied Biosystems). Individual qPCR reactions were carried out in 10 μL reaction mix with 2xTaqMan Universal PCR Master Mix (Applied Biosystems), 1× TaqMan Gene Expression Assay (Applied Biosystems) and 200 ng cDNA. Each sample was analyzed in triplicate. RNA isolated from healthy volunteers ($n = 5$) was used as a positive control for target genes expression. In each run, the dilutions of control RNA (pool of RNA from healthy volunteers) was included. The data were analyzed by the SDS2.4 software and Ct values were extracted. Fold-differences in *hTERT* expression were calculated using the comparative Ct method as described previously [38], where data were normalized to day 0 for each participant.

4.5. Data Analysis

All values were expressed as means ± SEM. Differences between values were assessed by one-way analysis of variance (ANOVA). When significant interaction was present, the Bonferroni post-test was performed. Benjamini-Hochberg's correction method was used to control false discovery rate (FDR), with significance threshold set at $p < 0.05$. Correlations between arterial wall properties and telomerase activity that were described previously [7–9,11] and longevity genes expression assessed in the present study were calculated after 30 days treatment period using Pearson correlation coefficients. A $p < 0.05$ was considered significant. All statistical analyses were performed using the Graph Pad Prism 5.0 software.

5. Conclusions

In conclusion, the present study has shown that low-dose fluvastatin and valsartan treatment increased the expression of beneficial longevity genes (*SIRT1*, *PRKAA*, and *KLOTHO*) and could therefore represent a promising new treatment approach for "aging-related" disorders. Additional, population-based research is needed to additionally prove the proposed concept.

Author Contributions: Conceptualization, M.Š.; Data curation, M.J., M.L. and M.Š.; Formal analysis, M.J., M.L. and M.Š.; Investigation, M.J., M.L., S.N. and P.Š.; Methodology, S.N. and P. Š.; Supervision, M.Š.; Writing—original draft, M.J., M.L. and M.Š.; Writing—review & editing, M.J., M.L. and M.Š.

Abbreviations

AMPK	AMP-activated protein kinase
ANOVA	Analysis of variance
COMB	Combination group
CTRL	Placebo group
FDA	Food and Drug Administration
FLU	Fluvastatin group
FMD	Flow mediated dilation
hTERT	human telomerase reverse transcriptase
MILES	Metformin in Longevity Study
mTOR	Mechanistic target of rapamycin
NAD	Nicotinamide adenine dinucleotide
NF-κB1	Nuclear factor κB
NFE2L2	Nuclear factor (erythroid-derived 2)-like 2 gene
PRKAA	5′-AMP-activated protein kinase catalytic subunit α-2 gene
PWV	Pulse wave velocity
qPCR	Quantitative real-time polymerase chain reaction
SIRT1	Sirtuin 1 gene
VAL	Valsartan group

References

1. Stevens, W.; Peneva, D.; Li, J.Z.; Liu, L.Z.; Liu, G.; Gao, R.; Lakdawalla, D.N. Estimating the future burden of cardiovascular disease and the value of lipid and blood pressure control therapies in China. *BMC Health Serv. Res.* **2016**, *16*, 175. [CrossRef] [PubMed]
2. Global Burden of Cardiovascular Diseases Collaboration; Roth, G.A.; Johnson, C.O.; Abate, K.H.; Abd-Allah, F.; Ahmed, M.; Alam, K.; Alam, T.; Alvis-Guzman, N.; Ansari, H.; et al. The Burden of Cardiovascular Diseases Among US States, 1990–2016. *JAMA Cardiol.* **2018**. [CrossRef] [PubMed]
3. Van Raamsdonk, J.M. Mechanisms underlying longevity: A genetic switch model of aging. *Exp. Gerontol.* **2017**. [CrossRef]
4. Rizvi, S.; Raza, S.T.; Mahdi, F. Telomere length variations in aging and age-related diseases. *Curr. Aging Sci.* **2014**, *7*, 161–167. [CrossRef]
5. Yeh, J.K.; Wang, C.Y. Telomeres and Telomerase in Cardiovascular Diseases. *Genes* **2016**, *7*, 58. [CrossRef] [PubMed]
6. Janic, M.; Lunder, M.; Sabovic, M. A new anti-ageing strategy focused on prevention of arterial ageing in the middle-aged population. *Med. Hypotheses* **2013**, *80*, 837–840. [CrossRef] [PubMed]
7. Lunder, M.; Janic, M.; Habjan, S.; Sabovic, M. Subtherapeutic, low-dose fluvastatin improves functional and morphological arterial wall properties in apparently healthy, middle-aged males—A pilot study. *Atherosclerosis* **2011**, *215*, 446–451. [CrossRef] [PubMed]
8. Lunder, M.; Janic, M.; Sabovic, M. Reduction of age-associated arterial wall changes by low-dose valsartan. *Eur. J. Prev. Cardiol.* **2012**, *19*, 1243–1249. [CrossRef]
9. Lunder, M.; Janic, M.; Jug, B.; Sabovic, M. The effects of low-dose fluvastatin and valsartan combination on arterial function: A randomized clinical trial. *Eur. J. Int. Med.* **2012**, *23*, 261–266. [CrossRef]
10. Janic, M.; Lunder, M.; Cerkovnik, P.; Prosenc Zmrzljak, U.; Novakovic, S.; Sabovic, M. Low-Dose Fluvastatin and Valsartan Rejuvenate the Arterial Wall Through Telomerase Activity Increase in Middle-Aged Men. *Rejuvenation Res.* **2016**, *19*, 115–119. [CrossRef] [PubMed]

11. Janic, M.; Lunder, M.; Prezelj, M.; Sabovic, M. A combination of low-dose fluvastatin and valsartan decreases inflammation and oxidative stress in apparently healthy middle-aged males. *J. Cardiopulm. Rehabil. Prev.* **2014**, *34*, 208–212. [CrossRef] [PubMed]
12. Park, S.; Mori, R.; Shimokawa, I. Do sirtuins promote mammalian longevity? A critical review on its relevance to the longevity effect induced by calorie restriction. *Mol. Cells* **2013**, *35*, 474–480. [CrossRef] [PubMed]
13. Braidy, N.; Jayasena, T.; Poljak, A.; Sachdev, P.S. Sirtuins in cognitive ageing and Alzheimer's disease. *Curr. Opin. Psychiatry* **2012**, *25*, 226–230. [CrossRef] [PubMed]
14. Du, G.; Song, Y.; Zhang, T.; Ma, L.; Bian, N.; Chen, X.; Feng, J.; Chang, Q.; Li, Z. Simvastatin attenuates TNFα-induced apoptosis in endothelial progenitor cells via the upregulation of *SIRT1*. *Int. J. Mol. Med.* **2014**, *34*, 177–182. [CrossRef] [PubMed]
15. Kilic, U.; Gok, O.; Elibol-Can, B.; Uysal, O.; Bacaksiz, A. Efficacy of statins on sirtuin 1 and endothelial nitric oxide synthase expression: The role of sirtuin 1 gene variants in human coronary atherosclerosis. *Clin. Exp. Pharmacol. Physiol.* **2015**, *42*, 321–330. [CrossRef] [PubMed]
16. Ye, Y.; Qian, J.; Castillo, A.C.; Perez-Polo, J.R.; Birnbaum, Y. Aliskiren and Valsartan reduce myocardial AT1 receptor expression and limit myocardial infarct size in diabetic mice. *Cardiovasc. Drugs Ther.* **2011**, *25*, 505–515. [CrossRef]
17. Shiota, A.; Shimabukuro, M.; Fukuda, D.; Soeki, T.; Sato, H.; Uematsu, E.; Hirata, Y.; Kurobe, H.; Maeda, N.; Sakaue, H.; et al. Telmisartan ameliorates insulin sensitivity by activating the *AMPK/SIRT1* pathway in skeletal muscle of obese db/db mice. *Cardiovasc. Diabetol.* **2012**, *11*, 139. [CrossRef] [PubMed]
18. Pantazi, E.; Bejaoui, M.; Zaouali, M.A.; Folch-Puy, E.; Pinto Rolo, A.; Panisello, A.; Palmeira, C.M.; Rosello-Catafau, J. Losartan activates sirtuin 1 in rat reduced-size orthotopic liver transplantation. *World J. Gastroenterol.* **2015**, *21*, 8021–8031. [CrossRef]
19. Wang, Y.; Liang, Y.; Vanhoutte, P.M. *SIRT1* and *AMPK* in regulating mammalian senescence: A critical review and a working model. *FEBS Lett.* **2011**, *585*, 986–994. [CrossRef] [PubMed]
20. Jia, F.; Wu, C.; Chen, Z.; Lu, G. Atorvastatin inhibits homocysteine-induced endoplasmic reticulum stress through activation of AMP-activated protein kinase. *Cardiovasc. Ther.* **2012**, *30*, 317–325. [CrossRef]
21. Sun, W.; Lee, T.S.; Zhu, M.; Gu, C.; Wang, Y.; Zhu, Y.; Shyy, J.Y. Statins activate AMP-activated protein kinase in vitro and in vivo. *Circulation* **2006**, *114*, 2655–2662. [CrossRef] [PubMed]
22. Hermida, N.; Markl, A.; Hamelet, J.; Van Assche, T.; Vanderper, A.; Herijgers, P.; van Bilsen, M.; Hilfiker-Kleiner, D.; Noppe, G.; Beauloye, C.; et al. HMGCoA reductase inhibition reverses myocardial fibrosis and diastolic dysfunction through AMP-activated protein kinase activation in a mouse model of metabolic syndrome. *Cardiovasc. Res.* **2013**, *99*, 44–54. [CrossRef] [PubMed]
23. Ha, Y.M.; Park, E.J.; Kang, Y.J.; Park, S.W.; Kim, H.J.; Chang, K.C. Valsartan independent of AT(1) receptor inhibits tissue factor, TLR-2 and -4 expression by regulation of Egr-1 through activation of AMPK in diabetic conditions. *J. Cell. Mol. Med.* **2014**, *18*, 2031–2043. [CrossRef]
24. Kurokawa, H.; Sugiyama, S.; Nozaki, T.; Sugamura, K.; Toyama, K.; Matsubara, J.; Fujisue, K.; Ohba, K.; Maeda, H.; Konishi, M.; et al. Telmisartan enhances mitochondrial activity and alters cellular functions in human coronary artery endothelial cells via AMP-activated protein kinase pathway. *Atherosclerosis* **2015**, *239*, 375–385. [CrossRef] [PubMed]
25. Donate-Correa, J.; Martin-Nunez, E.; Mora-Fernandez, C.; Muros-de-Fuentes, M.; Perez-Delgado, N.; Navarro-Gonzalez, J.F. Klotho in cardiovascular disease: Current and future perspectives. *World J. Biol. Chem.* **2015**, *6*, 351–357. [CrossRef] [PubMed]
26. Karalliedde, J.; Maltese, G.; Hill, B.; Viberti, G.; Gnudi, L. Effect of renin-angiotensin system blockade on soluble Klotho in patients with type 2 diabetes, systolic hypertension, and albuminuria. *Clin. J. Am. Soc. Nephrol.* **2013**, *8*, 1899–1905. [CrossRef] [PubMed]
27. Yoon, H.E.; Lim, S.W.; Piao, S.G.; Song, J.H.; Kim, J.; Yang, C.W. Statin upregulates the expression of *KLOTHO*, an anti-aging gene, in experimental cyclosporine nephropathy. *Nephron. Exp. Nephrol.* **2012**, *120*, e123–e133. [CrossRef] [PubMed]
28. Satta, S.; Mahmoud, A.M.; Wilkinson, F.L.; Yvonne Alexander, M.; White, S.J. The Role of Nrf2 in Cardiovascular Function and Disease. *Oxid. Med. Cell. Longev.* **2017**, *2017*, 9237263. [CrossRef]
29. Hwang, A.R.; Han, J.H.; Lim, J.H.; Kang, Y.J.; Woo, C.H. Fluvastatin inhibits AGE-induced cell proliferation and migration via an ERK5-dependent Nrf2 pathway in vascular smooth muscle cells. *PLoS ONE* **2017**, *12*, e0178278. [CrossRef]

30. Makabe, S.; Takahashi, Y.; Watanabe, H.; Murakami, M.; Ohba, T.; Ito, H. Fluvastatin protects vascular smooth muscle cells against oxidative stress through the Nrf2-dependent antioxidant pathway. *Atherosclerosis* **2010**, *213*, 377–384. [CrossRef]
31. Sciarretta, S.; Volpe, M.; Sadoshima, J. Mammalian target of rapamycin signaling in cardiac physiology and disease. *Circ. Res.* **2014**, *114*, 549–564. [CrossRef] [PubMed]
32. Cui, X.; Long, C.; Zhu, J.; Tian, J. Protective Effects of Fluvastatin on Reproductive Function in Obese Male Rats Induced by High-Fat Diet through Enhanced Signaling of mTOR. *Cell. Physiol. Biochem.* **2017**, *41*, 598–608. [CrossRef]
33. Wagner, R.J.; Martin, K.A.; Powell, R.J.; Rzucidlo, E.M. Lovastatin induces VSMC differentiation through inhibition of Rheb and mTOR. *Am. J. Physiol. Cell Physiol.* **2010**, *299*, C119–C127. [CrossRef] [PubMed]
34. Wu, X.; He, L.; Cai, Y.; Zhang, G.; He, Y.; Zhang, Z.; He, X.; He, Y.; Zhang, G.; Luo, J. Induction of autophagy contributes to the myocardial protection of valsartan against ischemiareperfusion injury. *Mol. Med. Rep.* **2013**, *8*, 1824–1830. [CrossRef] [PubMed]
35. Costantino, S.; Paneni, F.; Cosentino, F. Ageing, metabolism and cardiovascular disease. *J. Physiol.* **2016**, *594*, 2061–2073. [CrossRef] [PubMed]
36. Lenglet, S.; Quercioli, A.; Fabre, M.; Galan, K.; Pelli, G.; Nencioni, A.; Bauer, I.; Pende, A.; Python, M.; Bertolotto, M.; et al. Statin treatment is associated with reduction in serum levels of receptor activator of NF-κB ligand and neutrophil activation in patients with severe carotid stenosis. *Mediators Inflamm.* **2014**, *2014*, 720987. [CrossRef]
37. Wu, B.; Lin, R.; Dai, R.; Chen, C.; Wu, H.; Hong, M. Valsartan attenuates oxidative stress and NF-κB activation and reduces myocardial apoptosis after ischemia and reperfusion. *Eur. J. Pharmacol.* **2013**, *705*, 140–147. [CrossRef]
38. Livak, K.J.; Schmittgen, T.D. Analysis of relative gene expression data using real-time quantitative PCR and the $2^{-\Delta\Delta Ct}$ Method. *Methods* **2001**, *25*, 402–408. [CrossRef]

Permissions

All chapters in this book were first published by MDPI; hereby published with permission under the Creative Commons Attribution License or equivalent. Every chapter published in this book has been scrutinized by our experts. Their significance has been extensively debated. The topics covered herein carry significant findings which will fuel the growth of the discipline. They may even be implemented as practical applications or may be referred to as a beginning point for another development.

The contributors of this book come from diverse backgrounds, making this book a truly international effort. This book will bring forth new frontiers with its revolutionizing research information and detailed analysis of the nascent developments around the world.

We would like to thank all the contributing authors for lending their expertise to make the book truly unique. They have played a crucial role in the development of this book. Without their invaluable contributions this book wouldn't have been possible. They have made vital efforts to compile up to date information on the varied aspects of this subject to make this book a valuable addition to the collection of many professionals and students.

This book was conceptualized with the vision of imparting up-to-date information and advanced data in this field. To ensure the same, a matchless editorial board was set up. Every individual on the board went through rigorous rounds of assessment to prove their worth. After which they invested a large part of their time researching and compiling the most relevant data for our readers.

The editorial board has been involved in producing this book since its inception. They have spent rigorous hours researching and exploring the diverse topics which have resulted in the successful publishing of this book. They have passed on their knowledge of decades through this book. To expedite this challenging task, the publisher supported the team at every step. A small team of assistant editors was also appointed to further simplify the editing procedure and attain best results for the readers.

Apart from the editorial board, the designing team has also invested a significant amount of their time in understanding the subject and creating the most relevant covers. They scrutinized every image to scout for the most suitable representation of the subject and create an appropriate cover for the book.

The publishing team has been an ardent support to the editorial, designing and production team. Their endless efforts to recruit the best for this project, has resulted in the accomplishment of this book. They are a veteran in the field of academics and their pool of knowledge is as vast as their experience in printing. Their expertise and guidance has proved useful at every step. Their uncompromising quality standards have made this book an exceptional effort. Their encouragement from time to time has been an inspiration for everyone.

The publisher and the editorial board hope that this book will prove to be a valuable piece of knowledge for researchers, students, practitioners and scholars across the globe.

List of Contributors

Ping-Jen Chen
Centre for Dementia Palliative Care Research, Marie Curie Palliative Care Research Department, Division of Psychiatry, University College London, London W1T 7NF, UK
Department of Family Medicine and Division of Geriatrics and Gerontology, Kaohsiung Medical University Hospital, Kaohsiung Medical University, Kaohsiung 807, Taiwan
School of Medicine, Kaohsiung Medical University, Kaohsiung 807, Taiwan

Chung-Han Ho
Department of Medical Research, Chi-Mei Medical Center, Tainan 710, Taiwan
Department of Hospital and Health Care Administration, Chia Nan University of Pharmacy and Science, Tainan 717, Taiwan

Chao A. Hsiung and Jung-Yu Liao
Institute of Population Health Sciences, National Health Research Institutes, Miaoli 350, Taiwan

Lisanne Smits
Centre for Dementia Palliative Care Research, Marie Curie Palliative Care Research Department, Division of Psychiatry, University College London, London W1T 7NF, UK
Faculty of Medicine, University of Amsterdam, 1105 AZ Amsterdam, The Netherlands

Sang-Ju Yu
Home Clinic Dulan, Taitung 959, Taiwan

Kai-Ping Zhang
Home Clinic Dulan, Taipei 106, Taiwan

Elizabeth L. Sampson
Centre for Dementia Palliative Care Research, Marie Curie Palliative Care Research Department, Division of Psychiatry, University College London, London W1T 7NF, UK
Barnet Enfield and Haringey Mental Health Trust Liaison Psychiatry Team, North Middlesex University Hospital, London N18 1QX, UK

Irene Petersen
UCL Department of Primary Care and Population Sciences, University College London, London NW3 2PF, UK

Roberta Balansin Rigon, Christopher Wolff, Christian Hausmann, Nan Zhang, Monika Schäfer-Korting and Christian Zoschke
Institute of Pharmacy (Pharmacology & Toxicology), Freie Universität Berlin, Königin-Luise-Str. 2+4, 14195 Berlin, Germany

Sabine Kaessmeyer
Institute of Veterinary Anatomy, Department of Veterinary Medicine, Freie Universität Berlin, Koserstr. 20, 14195 Berlin, Germany

Michaela Sochorová, Andrej Kováčik and Kateřina Vávrová
Faculty of Pharmacy, Charles University, Akademika Heyrovského 1203, 50005 Hradec Králové, Czech Republic

Rainer Haag
Institute of Chemistry and Biochemistry, Freie Universität Berlin, Takustr. 3, 14195 Berlin, Germany
Department of Neurology, Addenbrooke's Hospital, Hills Road, Cambridge CB2 2QQ, UK
Department of Neurology, Addenbrooke's Hospital, Hills Road, Cambridge CB2 2QQ, UK

Martina Ulrich
Collegium Medicum Berlin, Luisenstr. 54, 10117 Berlin, Germany

Madhulika Achal and Ruth E. Mauntz
Donald P. Shiley BioScience Center, San Diego State University, San Diego, CA 92182, USA

Sharon Zhang
Donald P. Shiley BioScience Center, San Diego State University, San Diego, CA 92182, USA
Biological and Medical Informatics Research Center, San Diego State University, San Diego, CA 92182, USA
Department of Biology, San Diego State University, San Diego, CA 92182, USA

Eric P. Ratliff, Brandon Molina, Nadja El-Mecharrafie, Jessica Mastroianni, Roxanne W. Kotzebue, Arysa Gonzalez, Ayeh Barekat, Andrew M. Macias and Kim D. Finley
Donald P. Shiley BioScience Center, San Diego State University, San Diego, CA 92182, USA
Department of Biology, San Diego State University, San Diego, CA 92182, USA

William A. Bray
Donald P. Shiley BioScience Center, San Diego State University, San Diego, CA 92182, USA
Department of Biology, San Diego State University, San Diego, CA 92182, USA
Sanford Consortium for Regenerative Medicine, 2880 Torrey Pines Scenic Dr., La Jolla, CA 92037, USA

Daniel Daugherty
The Salk Institute for Biological Studies, Cellular Neurobiology, 10010 North Torrey Pines Road, La Jolla, CA 92037, USA

Greg L. Harris
Department of Biology, San Diego State University, San Diego, CA 92182, USA

Robert A. Edwards
Biological and Medical Informatics Research Center, San Diego State University, San Diego, CA 92182, USA
Department of Biology, San Diego State University, San Diego, CA 92182, USA

Karamat Mohammad, Paméla Dakik, Younes Medkour, Mélissa McAuley, Darya Mitrofanova and Vladimir I. Titorenko
Department of Biology, Concordia University, 7141 Sherbrooke Street, West, SP Building, Room 501-13, Montreal, QC H4B 1R6, Canada

Besa Ziso and Andrew J. Larner
Cognitive Function Clinic, Walton Centre for Neurology and Neurosurgery, Liverpool L9 7LJ, UK

Subapriya Suppiah
Centre for Diagnostic Nuclear Imaging, University Putra Malaysia, Serdang 43400, Selangor, Malaysia
Department of Imaging, Faculty of Medicine and Health Sciences, University Putra Malaysia, Serdang 43400, Selangor, Malaysia

Sobhan Vinjamuri
The Royal Liverpool and Broadgreen University Hospitals NHS Trusts, Prescot St, Liverpool L7 8XP, UK

Mellanie-Anne Didier
The Royal Liverpool and Broadgreen University Hospitals NHS Trusts, Prescot St, Liverpool L7 8XP, UK
Section of Nuclear Medicine, Department of Surgery, Radiology, Anaesthesia & Intensive Care, The University Hospital of The West Indies, The University of TheWest Indies, Mona Campus, Kingston 7, Jamaica

Rüdiger Hardeland
Johann Friedrich Blumenbach Institute of Zoology and Anthropology, University of Göttingen, 37073 Göttingen, Germany

Maialen Palomino-Alonso
Clinical Neuroproteomics Group, Navarrabiomed, Departamento de Salud, Universidad Pública de Navarra, 31008 Pamplona, Spain

Mercedes Lachén-Montes, Andrea González-Morales, Joaquín Fernández-Irigoyen and Enrique Santamaría
Clinical Neuroproteomics Group, Navarrabiomed, Departamento de Salud, Universidad Pública de Navarra, 31008 Pamplona, Spain
Proteored-ISCIII, Proteomics Unit, Navarrabiomed, Departamento de Salud, Universidad Pública de Navarra, 31008 Pamplona, Spain
Instituto de Investigación Sanitaria de Navarra (IdiSNA), Navarra Institute for Health Research, 31008 Pamplona, Spain

Karina Ausín
Proteored-ISCIII, Proteomics Unit, Navarrabiomed, Departamento de Salud, Universidad Pública de Navarra, 31008 Pamplona, Spain

Alberto Pérez-Mediavilla
Instituto de Investigación Sanitaria de Navarra (IdiSNA), Navarra Institute for Health Research, 31008 Pamplona, Spain
Neurobiology of Alzheimer's Disease, Neurosciences Division, Center for Applied Medical Research (CIMA), Department of Biochemistry, University of Navarra, 31008 Pamplona, Spain

Saadet Koc Okudur
Department of Geriatric Medicine, Manisa State Hospital, Manisa 45040, Turkey

Ozge Dokuzlar, Derya Kaya and Ahmet Turan Isik
Unit for Brain Aging and Dementia, Department of Geriatric Medicine, Faculty of Medicine, Dokuz Eylul University, Izmir 35340, Turkey

Pinar Soysal
Department of Geriatric Medicine, Faculty of Medicine, Bezmialem Vakif University, Istanbul 34093, Turkey

Jeremy M. Brown
Department of Neurology, Addenbrooke's Hospital, Hills Road, Cambridge CB2 2QQ, UK

Julie Wiggins and Kate Dawson
Department of Clinical Neurosciences, University of Cambridge, Cambridge CB2 0SZ, UK

Timothy Rittman and James B. Rowe
Department of Neurology, Addenbrooke's Hospital, Hills Road, Cambridge CB2 2QQ, UK Department of Clinical Neurosciences, University of Cambridge, Cambridge CB2 0SZ, UK

Jungwoon Lee
Environmental Disease Research Center, Korea Research Institute of Bioscience and Biotechnology (KRIBB), 125 Gwahak-ro, Yuseong-gu, Daejeon 34141, Korea

Haiyoung Jung
Immunotherapy Research Center, Korea Research Institute of Bioscience and Biotechnology (KRIBB), 125 Gwahak-ro, Yuseong-gu, Daejeon 34141, Korea

Suk Ran Yoon and Inpyo Choi
Immunotherapy Research Center, Korea Research Institute of Bioscience and Biotechnology (KRIBB), 125 Gwahak-ro, Yuseong-gu, Daejeon 34141, Korea
Department of Functional Genomics, University of Science and Technology (UST), 113 Gwahak-ro, Yuseong-gu, Daejeon 34113, Korea

Miodrag Janić and Mišo Šabovič
Department of Vascular Diseases, Ljubljana University Medical Centre, Zaloška cesta 7, SI-1000 Ljubljana, Slovenia

Mojca Lunder
Department of Endocrinology, Diabetes and Metabolic Diseases, Ljubljana University Medical Centre, Zaloška cesta 7, SI-1000 Ljubljana, Slovenia

Srdjan Novaković and Petra Škerl
Department of Molecular Diagnostics, Institute of Oncology Ljubljana, SI-1000 Ljubljana, Slovenia

Index

www.ingramcontent.com/pod-product-compliance
Lightning Source LLC
LaVergne TN
LVHW081015210926
848485LV00004B/867